X線画像解剖ポケットアトラス

第3版

監訳　町田 徹　NTT東日本関東病院放射線科部長
訳　　小林有香　東京共済病院放射線科部長
　　　小塚拓洋　癌研有明病院放射線治療科副部長

Torsten B. Moeller, M.D.
Department of Radiology
Caritas Hospital
Dillingen, Germany

Emil Reif, M.D.
Department of Radiology
Caritas Hospital
Dillingen, Germany

Pocket Atlas of Radiographic Anatomy
3rd edition

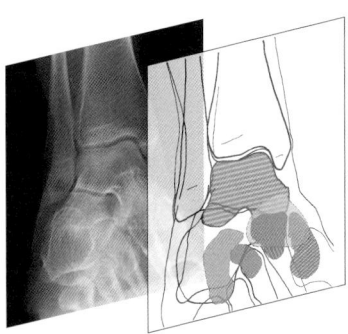

メディカル・サイエンス・インターナショナル

私の米国の親類達に捧ぐ——BernieとArlene, Bryan, Nancy, Rick
とBill, Shirley, Mike, Michael, AustinとAmanda, Audrey, Mike,
KristinとKatelyn, Claudia, Dale, BryanとJamie, そしてMeghan
とJasonへ

Authorized translation of the original edition,
"Pocket Atlas of Radiographic Anatomy", Third Edition
by Torsten B. Moeller, M.D. and Emil Reif, M.D.

Copyright © 2010 by Georg Thieme Verlag, Rüdigerstrasse 14,
70469 Stuttgart, Germany
Thieme New York, 333 Seventh Avenue, New York, NY 10001, USA
All rights reserved.

©Third Japanese Edition 2011 by Medical Sciences International, Ltd.,
Tokyo

Printed and Bound in Japan

監訳者序文

　本書はX線写真の読影に必要な正常X線解剖を詳細に記している．前回の第2版出版時には一般化していなかったデジタルラジオグラフィも今では当たり前の装置として汎用されている．しかし，著者が序文で述べているように従来のX線写真とデジタル化されたX線写真においてなんら変わるところはなく，正常解剖の知識が読影に最も重要である．

　見開きページにX線画像とシェーマを並べた体裁は以前とまったく同様であり，読者にとって分かりやすい配置となっている．今回の改訂でさらに画像とシェーマの追加があり，本書も結構分厚い本となってしまい，姉妹版の「CT/MRI画像解剖ポケットアトラス 第3版」（I，II，III巻）と一緒に白衣のポケットに入れて持ち歩きいつでも参照する，というわけにはいかなくなってしまった．しかし，モニターの横においていつでも簡便に参照することができる良書であることに変わりはない．本書は各科臨床医，コ・メディカル，学生に重用され，有益な書となることを願ってやまない．

2011年1月

町田　徹

序　文

　デジタルラジオグラフィが使用されて十年以上経つにもかかわらず，X線画像を撮り診断する過程はほとんど変化していない．また，従来のX線写真で知られている画像解剖の詳細を知っておくことの重要性はいささかも揺らぐものではない．本書がその好例である．本書の前版が広く読者に受け入れられたことは著者らの大いなる喜びであり，新たな資料を加え手直しをする動機のひとつとなった．

　第3版は Normal Findings in Radiology と Pocket Atlas of Radiographic Positioning と同じ構成とし，それぞれの章での無用な重複を避け，かつ簡潔・明瞭にX線撮影画像を提示することを目指した．同時に，異なる方向からの観察が有効な場合があるので，読者が同じ対象物を違う角度から同様の画質をもって観察できるようにした．本書は一貫したスタイルをとり，同一のX線画像を使って構成してあるので，読者は容易に本書を読み，学びそして参照することができるであろう．

Torsten B. Moeller
Emil Reif

目 次

骨格像 ··· 1
頭 部 ··· 2
- 頭蓋骨 正面（後前） ··· 2
- 頭蓋骨 側面 ··· 4
- 後頭蓋 Towne法 ··· 6
- 副鼻腔 Waters法 ··· 8
- 副鼻腔 正面（後前） ··· 10
- 眼窩 正面（後前） ··· 12
- 眼窩 Rhese法 ··· 14
- 上顎骨 ··· 16
- 下顎枝 ··· 18
- 下顎骨 Clementschitsh法 ··· 20
- 顎・顔面骨 パントモ撮影 ··· 22
- 鼻骨 側面 ··· 24
- 頬骨弓 ··· 26
- 頭蓋底 ··· 28
- 側頭骨（錐体） Altschul法 ··· 30
- 側頭骨（錐体） Schüller法 ··· 32
- 側頭骨（錐体） Stenvers法 ··· 34
- 側頭骨（錐体） Mayer法 ··· 36
- トルコ鞍 側面 ··· 38
- トルコ鞍 正面（前後） ··· 40

脊 椎 ··· 42
- 全脊椎 正面（前後） ··· 42
- 頸椎 正面（前後） ··· 44
- 頸椎 側面 ··· 46
- 頸椎 斜位 ··· 48
- 胸椎 正面（前後） ··· 50
- 胸椎 側面 ··· 52
- 腰椎 正面（前後） ··· 54
- 腰椎 側面 ··· 56
- 腰椎 斜位 ··· 58
- 骨盤 正面（前後） ··· 60

小児骨盤　正面（前後）	62
骨盤　入口撮影（インレット）	64
骨盤　Guthmann法	66
骨盤　腸骨翼斜位	68
骨盤　閉鎖孔斜位	70
仙腸関節　30°前斜位	72
仙骨　正面（前後）	74
仙骨　側面	76
尾骨　正面（前後）	78
尾骨　側面	80

上　肢 …… 82

胸郭	82
胸骨　正面（前後）	84
胸骨　側面	86
肩関節　ストレス撮影	88
鎖骨　正面（前後）	90
鎖骨　斜位	92
肩鎖関節	94
肩甲骨　正面（前後）	96
肩甲骨　側面	98
肩関節　スカプラY法	100
肩関節　正面（前後）	102
肩関節　外転位（挙上位）正面（前後）	104
肩関節　軸位	106
肩関節　接線	108
肩関節　経胸郭撮影	110
上腕骨　正面（前後）	112
上腕骨　側面	114
肘関節　正面（前後）	116
肘関節　側面	118
肘関節　軸位	120
橈骨　斜位	122
前腕骨　正面（前後）	124
前腕骨　側面	126
手　正面（前後）	128
手　斜位	130
手関節　正面（前後）	132

手関節 側面……………………………………………………………134
　手根管撮影………………………………………………………………136
　舟状骨撮影………………………………………………………………138
　豆状骨 特殊撮影………………………………………………………140
　中手骨 斜位……………………………………………………………142
　手指 2方向………………………………………………………………144
下　肢………………………………………………………………………146
　全下肢荷重撮影 正面（前後）…………………………………………146
　股関節 正面（前後）……………………………………………………148
　股関節 Lauenstein法…………………………………………………150
　股関節 接線（SchneiderⅠ法）………………………………………152
　股関節 接線（SchneiderⅡ法）………………………………………154
　股関節 軸位……………………………………………………………156
　大腿骨 正面（前後）……………………………………………………158
　大腿骨 側面……………………………………………………………160
　膝関節 正面（前後）……………………………………………………162
　膝関節 側面……………………………………………………………164
　膝関節 顆間窩撮影（Frik法）…………………………………………166
　膝関節 45°内旋位……………………………………………………168
　膝関節 45°外旋位……………………………………………………170
　膝蓋骨 軸位（30°,60°,90°屈曲位）………………………………172
　下腿骨 正面（前後）……………………………………………………174
　下腿骨 側面……………………………………………………………176
　足関節 正面（前後）……………………………………………………178
　足関節 側面……………………………………………………………180
　足関節 斜位1…………………………………………………………182
　足関節 斜位2…………………………………………………………184
　足 正面（前後）…………………………………………………………186
　足 側面…………………………………………………………………188
　踵骨 側面………………………………………………………………190
　踵骨 接線………………………………………………………………192
　足 立位負荷正面（前後）………………………………………………194
　中足部 正面（前後）……………………………………………………196
　中足部 斜位……………………………………………………………198
　前足部 正面（前後）……………………………………………………200
　前足部 斜位……………………………………………………………202
　母趾 正面（前後）および側面…………………………………………204

いろいろな単純写真解剖 ...207
単純 X 線写真 ...208
- 胸部 正面(後前) ...208
- 胸部 正面(後前)(心臓・脈管) ...210
- 胸部 側面 ...212
- 肺区域解剖 ...214
- 胸部 右前斜位 ...216
- 胸部 左前斜位 ...218
- 腹部 立位正面 ...220
- 腹部 背臥位正面 ...222

スポット像 ...224
- マンモグラフィー CC(頭尾方向) ...224
- マンモグラフィー ML(内外側方向) ...226
- 気管 正面(前後) ...228
- 気管 側面 ...230

断層撮影 ...232
- 肺門部 前後断層 ...232
- 右肺門部 側面断層 ...234
- 仙腸関節 ...236

造影検査 ...239
消化管 ...240
- 下咽頭 正面(前後) ...240
- 下咽頭 側面 ...242
- 食道 ...244
- 胃(食道) ...246
- 胃 ...248
- 胃(十二指腸) ...250
- 胃・小腸 ...252
- 小腸 ...254
- 回盲部 圧迫スポット像 ...256
- 結腸 ...258
- 直腸 ...260
- 排便造影 ...262

経静脈造影検査 ...264
- 排泄性尿路造影 ...264
- 静脈性胆囊胆管造影 ...266

関節造影 ……268
- 手関節造影　正面（前後）……268
- 手関節造影　側面……270
- 肩関節造影　正面（前後）……272
- 肩関節造影　斜位……274
- 膝関節造影……276
- 足関節造影……278

動脈造影 ……280
- 内頸動脈造影　正面（前後）動脈相……280
- 内頸動脈造影　側面　動脈相……282
- 内頸動脈造影　正面（前後）静脈相……284
- 内頸動脈造影　側面　静脈相……286
- 椎骨動脈造影　正面（前後）動脈相……288
- 椎骨動脈造影　側面　動脈相……290
- 椎骨動脈造影　正面（前後）静脈相……292
- 椎骨動脈造影　側面　静脈相……294
- 頸部動脈造影　正面（前後）……296
- 大動脈造影　正面（前後）……298
- 肺動脈造影　動脈相……300
- 肺動脈造影　正面（前後）静脈相……302
- 腹腔動脈幹造影　動脈相……304
- 腹腔動脈幹造影　静脈相……306
- 上陽間膜動脈造影　動脈相……308
- 上陽間膜動脈造影　静脈相……310
- 腎動脈造影　動脈相……312
- 腎動脈造影　静脈相……314
- 骨盤・下肢動脈造影　骨盤部……316
- 骨盤・下肢動脈造影　大腿部……318
- 骨盤・下肢動脈造影　膝部……320
- 骨盤・下肢動脈造影　下腿部……322
- 骨盤・下肢動脈造影　足部……324

静脈造影 ……326
- 上大静脈　正面（前後）……326
- 下大静脈　正面（前後）……328
- 下大静脈　側面……330
- 上腕静脈造影……332
- 前腕静脈造影……334

下肢静脈造影……………………………………………………336

特殊な造影検査……………………………………………………339
胸部ミエログラフィー　正面(前後)……………………………340
胸部ミエログラフィー　側面……………………………………342
腰部ミエログラフィー　正面(前後)……………………………344
腰部ミエログラフィー　側面……………………………………346
腰部ミエログラフィー　斜位……………………………………348
両足リンパ管造影　正面(前後) 注入相…………………………350
両足リンパ管造影　斜位 注入相…………………………………352
両足リンパ管造影　正面(前後) 貯留相…………………………354
左気管支造影　正面(前後)………………………………………356
左気管支造影　側面………………………………………………358
耳下腺造影　側面…………………………………………………360
耳下腺造影　正面(前後)…………………………………………362
子宮卵管造影………………………………………………………364
乳管造影……………………………………………………………366
ERCP(内視鏡的膵胆管造影法)…………………………………368

索　引
和文…………………………………………………………………371
欧文…………………………………………………………………381

注 意

　本書に記載した情報に関しては，正確を期し，一般臨床で広く受け入れられている方法を記載するよう注意を払った．しかしながら，著者(監訳者，訳者)ならびに出版社は，本書の情報を用いた結果生じたいかなる不都合に対しても責任を負うものではない．本書の内容の特定な状況への適用に関しての責任は，医師各自のうちにある．

　著者(監訳者，訳者)ならびに出版社は，本書に記載した薬物の選択，用量については，出版時の最新の推奨，および臨床状況に基づいていることを確認するよう努力を払っている．しかし，医学は日進月歩で進んでおり，政府の規制は変わり，薬物療法や薬物反応に関する情報は常に変化している．読者は，薬物の使用にあたっては個々の薬物の添付文書を参照し，適応，用量，付加された注意・警告に関する変化を常に確認することを怠ってはならない．これは，推奨された薬物が新しいものであったり，汎用されるものではない場合に，特に重要である．

凡　例

本書に使用した和名用語は原則として日本解剖学会により制定された用語に従った．また臨床で一般に使用されている用語も適宜使用した．

骨格像：頭部

脊椎

上肢

下肢

いろいろな単純写真

造影検査

特殊な造影検査

骨 格 像

頭部　2
脊椎　42
上肢　82
下肢　146

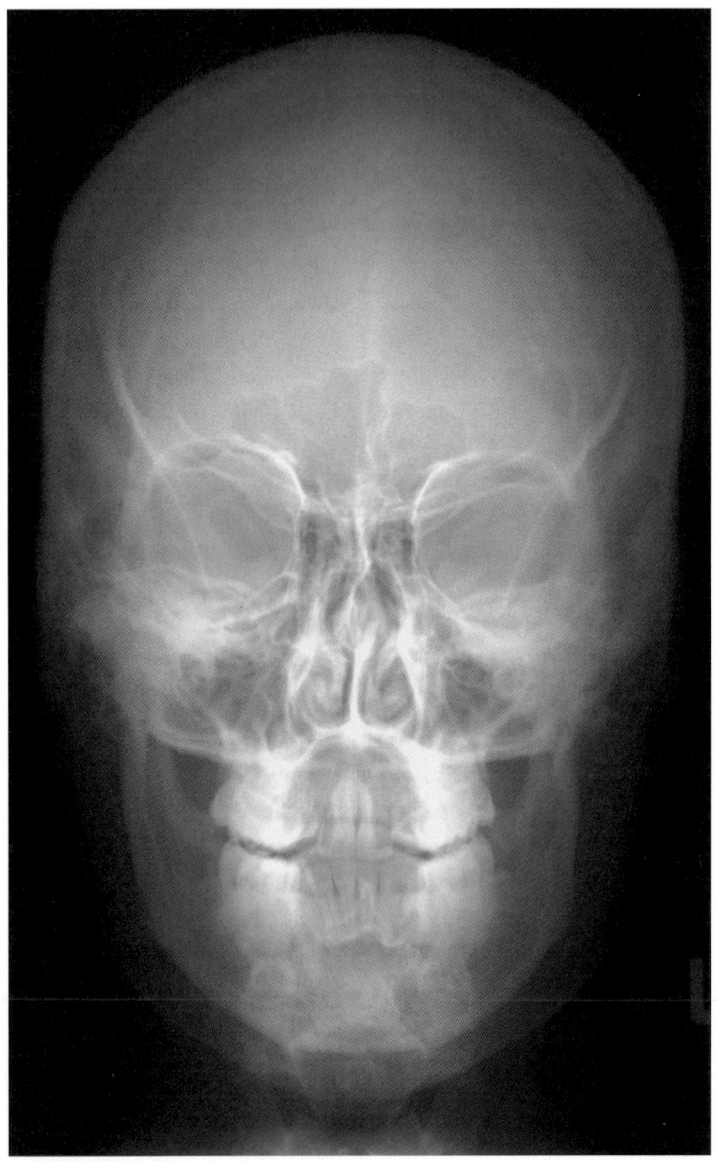

頭蓋骨　正面（後前）

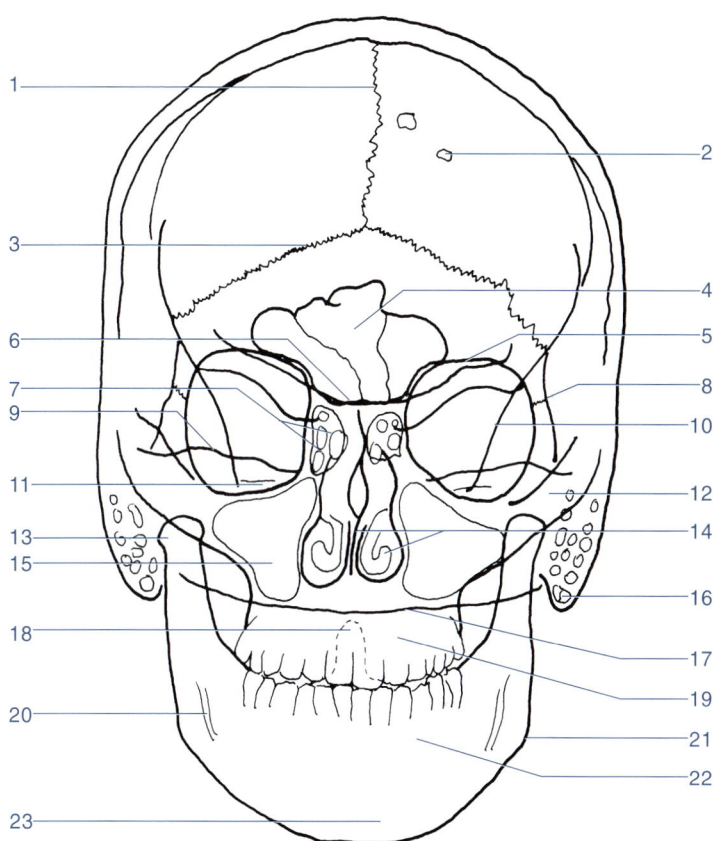

1　矢状縫合 Sagittal suture	13　下顎骨関節突起 Condyle of the mandible
2　クモ膜顆粒（パキオニ顆粒） Pacchionian granulations	14　鼻中隔 Nasal septum
3　ラムダ縫合 Lambdoid suture	下鼻甲介 Inferior nasal turbinate
4　前頭洞 Frontal sinus	15　上顎洞 Maxillary sinus
5　眼窩上壁 Roof of the orbit	16　乳様突起 Mastoid process
6　蝶形骨 Sphenoid	17　後頭部 Occiput
7　篩骨洞 Ethmoid sinus	18　軸椎歯突起 Dens of the axis
8　前頭頬骨縫合 Frontozygomatic suture	19　上顎骨 Maxilla
9　錐体稜 Petrous ridge	20　下顎管 Mandibular canal
10　無名線 Innominate line	21　下顎角 Angle of the mandible
11　内耳道 Internal auditory canal	22　下顎骨 Mandible
12　頬骨弓 Zygomatic arch	23　オトガイ隆起 Mental protuberance

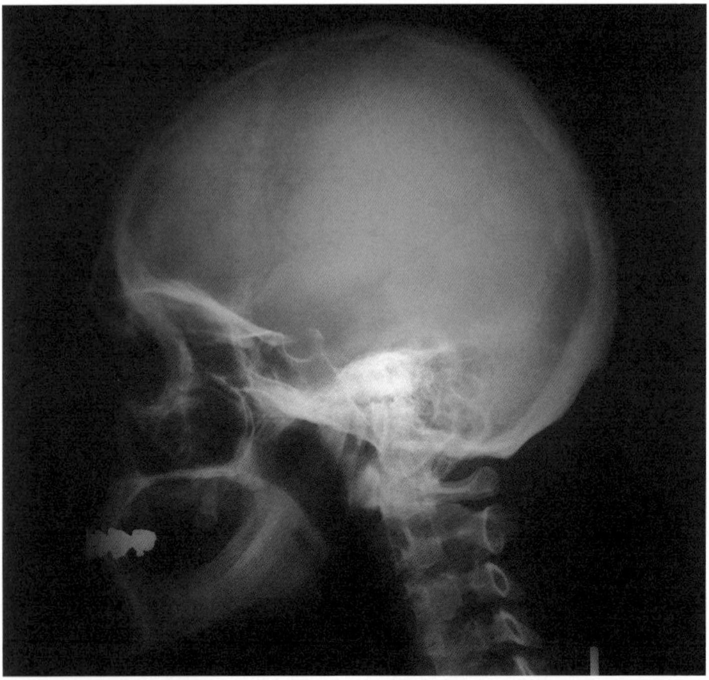

頭部

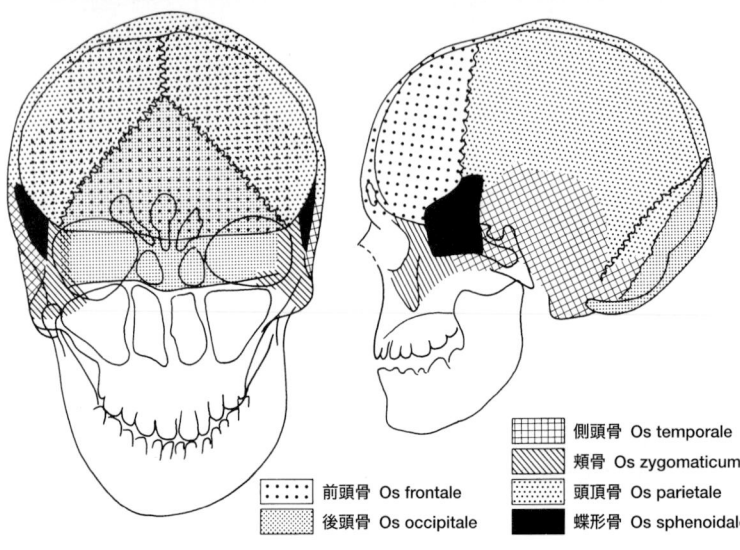

側頭骨 Os temporale
頬骨 Os zygomaticum
前頭骨 Os frontale
頭頂骨 Os parietale
後頭骨 Os occipitale
蝶形骨 Os sphenoidale

頭蓋骨　側面　5

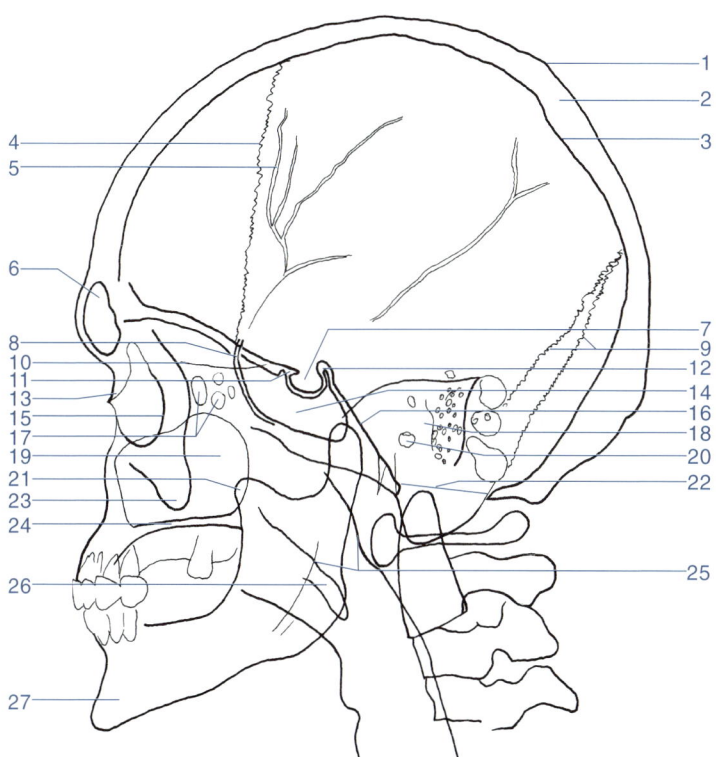

1 頭頂骨外板 Outer table of the parietal bone
2 板間層 Diploe
3 頭頂骨内板 Inner table of the parietal bone
4 冠状縫合 Coronal suture
5 中硬膜動脈溝 Groove of the middle meningeal artery
6 前頭洞 Frontal sinus
7 下垂体窩 Pituitary fossa
8 蝶形骨大翼 Greater wing of the sphenoid
9 ラムダ縫合 Lambdoid suture
10 篩板 Cribriform plate
11 前床突起 Anterior clinoid process
12 後床突起 Posterior clinoid process
13 鼻骨 Nasal bone
14 蝶形骨洞 Sphenoid sinus
15 頬骨 Zygomatic bone 眼窩外側壁
16 斜台 Clivus
17 篩骨洞 Ethmoid sinus
18 側頭骨岩様部 Petrous portion of the temporal bone
19 上顎洞 Maxillary sinus
20 外耳孔 Opening of the external auditory canal
21 下顎骨筋突起 Coronoid process of the mandible
22 大後頭孔 Foramen magnum
23 頬骨突起 Zygomatic process
24 硬口蓋 Hard palate
25 鼻咽頭 Nasopharynx
26 軟口蓋 Soft palate
27 下顎骨 Mandible

頭部

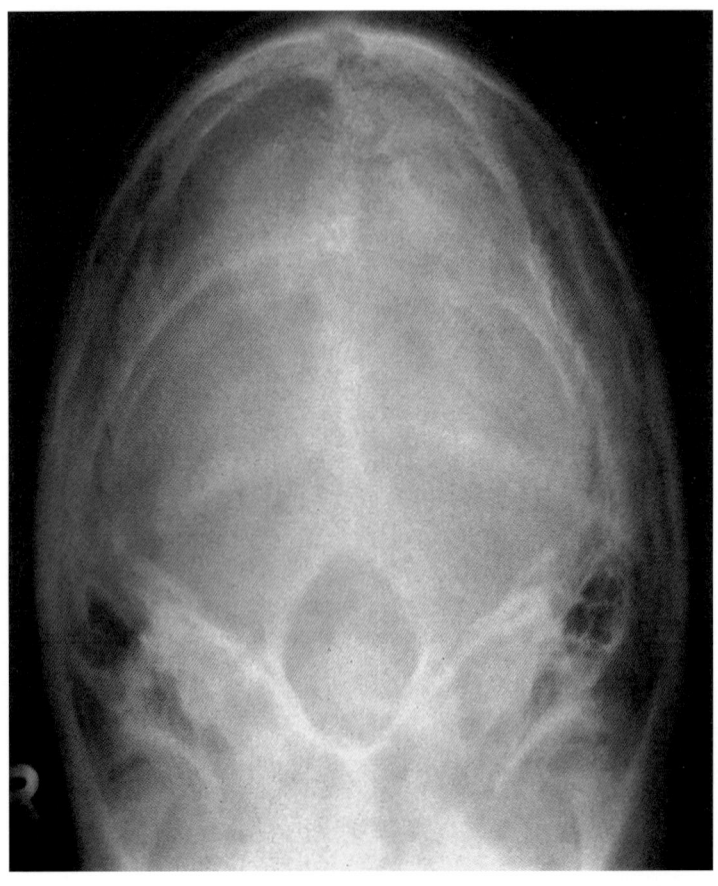

後頭蓋 Towne法

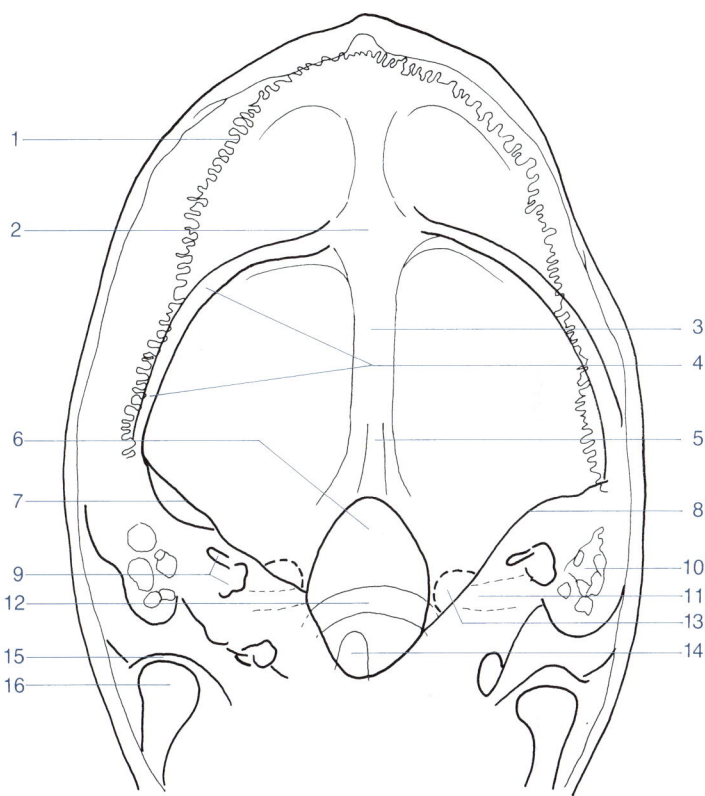

1	ラムダ縫合 Lambdoid suture	9	半規管 Semicircular canals
2	（内および外）後頭隆起 Occipital protuberances（external and internal）	10	乳突蜂巣 Mastoid air cells
		11	内耳道 Internal auditory canal
3	後頭骨 Occipital bone	12	環椎後弓 Posterior arch of the atlas
4	横洞溝 Sulcus of the transverse sinus	13	頸静脈孔 Jugular foramen
5	後頭稜 Occipital crest	14	歯突起 Dens
6	大後頭孔 Foramen magnum	15	顎関節 Temporomandibular joint
7	錐体骨 Petrous bone	16	下顎頭（関節突起） Condyle of the mandible
8	弓状隆起 Arcuate eminence		

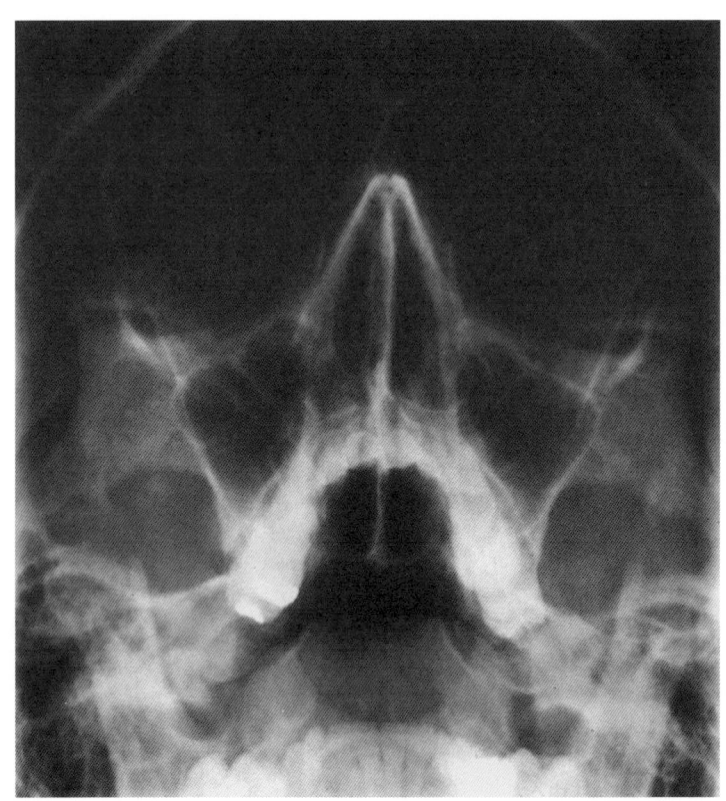

副鼻腔 Waters法

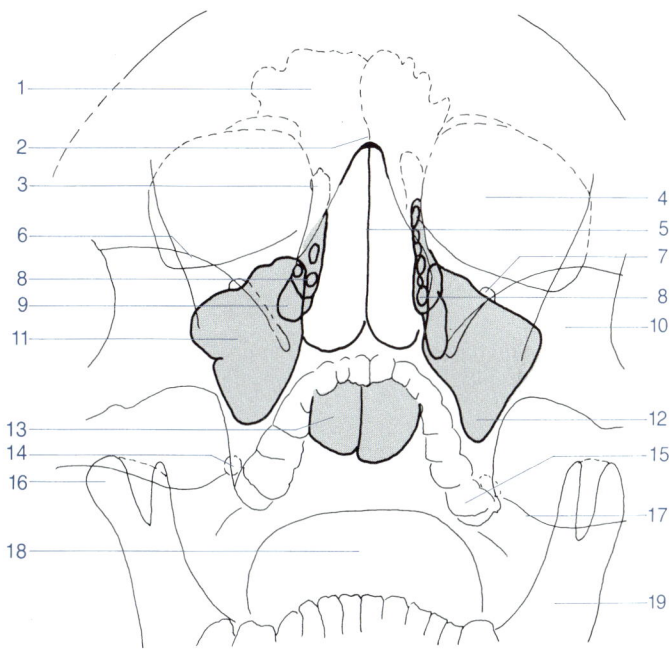

1 前頭洞 Frontal sinus
2 鼻骨 Nasal bone
3 前篩骨洞 Anterior ethmoid sinus
4 眼窩 Orbit
5 鼻中隔 Nasal septum
6 蝶形骨大翼 Greater wing of the sphenoid
7 眼窩下孔 Infraorbital foramen
8 正円孔 Foramen rotundum
9 後篩骨洞 Posterior ethmoid sinus
10 頬骨 Zygomatic bone
11 上顎洞 Maxillary sinus
12 上顎洞歯槽陥凹 Alveolar recess of the maxillary sinus
13 蝶形骨洞 Sphenoid sinus
14 卵円孔 Foramen ovale
15 上顎骨歯槽突起 Alveolar process of the maxilla
16 下顎頭（関節突起）Condyle of the mandible
17 錐体縁 Petrous ridge
18 舌 Tongue
19 下顎骨 Mandible

頭 部

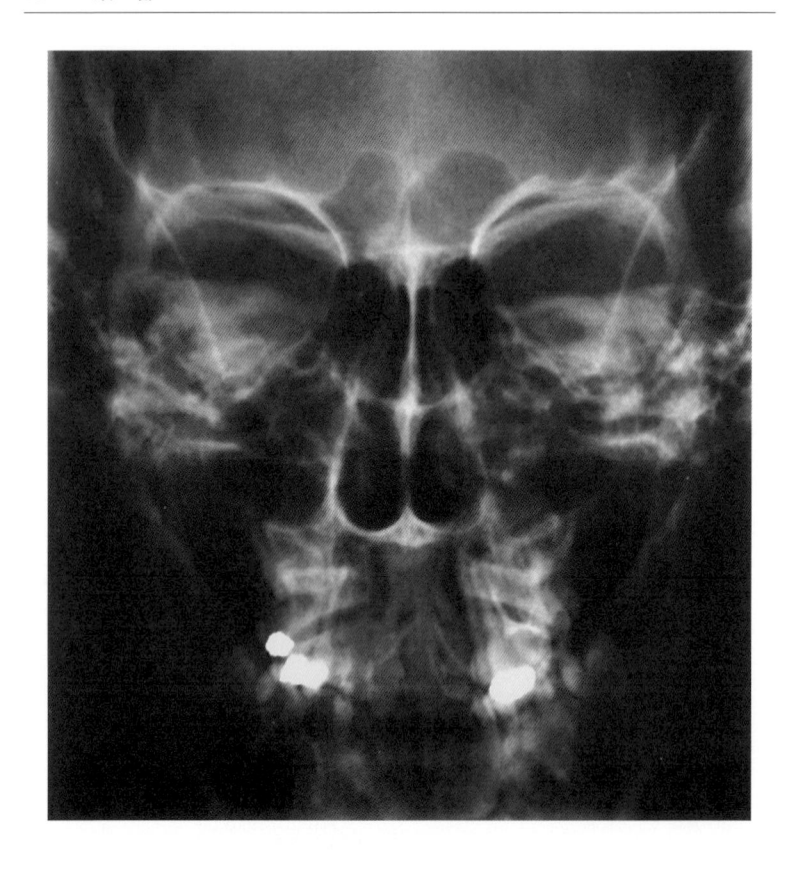

副鼻腔 正面(後前)

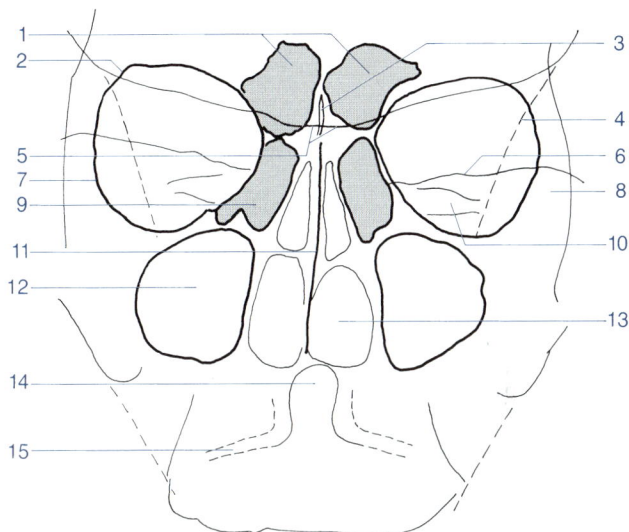

1 前頭洞 Frontal sinus
2 眼窩上壁 Roof of the orbit
3 鶏冠 Crista galli
4 無名線 Innominate line
5 蝶形骨 Sphenoid
6 錐体縁 Petrous ridge
7 眼窩外側壁 Lateral wall of the orbit
8 頬骨 Zygomatic bone
9 前篩骨洞 Anterior ethmoid sinus
10 内耳道 Internal auditory canal
11 鼻中隔 Nasal septum
12 上顎洞 Maxillary sinus
13 鼻腔 Nasal cavity
14 歯突起 Dens
15 環軸関節 Atlantoaxial joint

12　頭　部

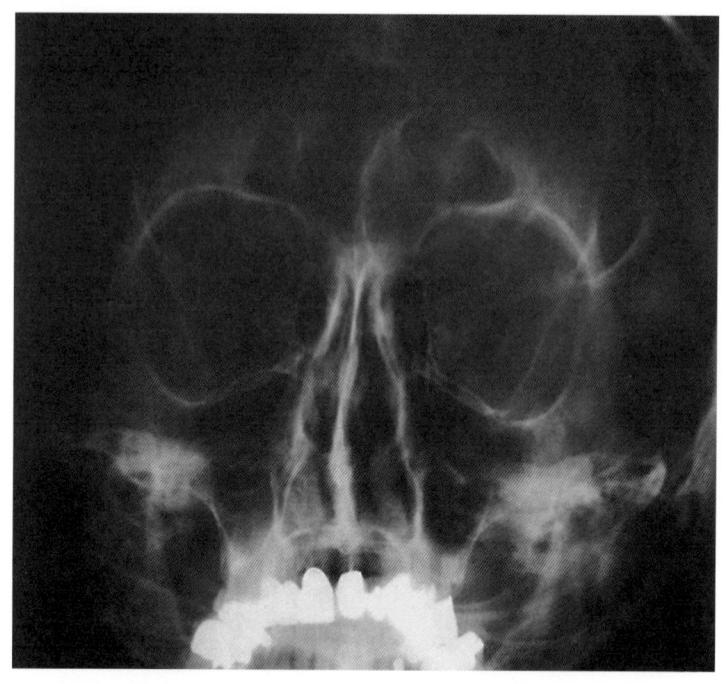

眼窩　正面(後前)　13

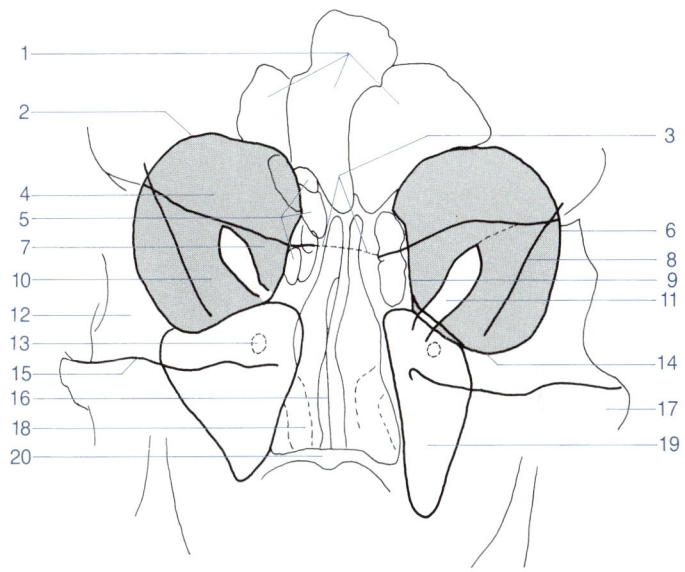

1　前頭洞　Frontal sinus
2　眼窩上壁　Roof of the orbit
3　蝶形骨　Sphenoid
4　眼窩　Orbit 図の灰色部分
5　篩骨洞　Ethmoid sinus
6　眼窩外側壁　Lateral wall of the orbit
7　蝶形骨小翼　Lesser wing of the sphenoid
8　無名線　Innominate line
9　眼窩板　Orbital plate
10　蝶形骨大翼　Greater wing of the sphenoid
11　上眼窩裂　Superior orbital fissure
12　頬骨前頭突起　Frontal process of the zygomatic bone
13　正円孔　Foramen rotundum
14　眼窩底　Floor of the orbit
15　錐体縁　Petrous ridge
16　鼻中隔　Nasal septum
17　頬骨弓　Zygomatic arch
18　下鼻甲介　Inferior turbinate
19　上顎洞　Maxillary sinus
20　硬口蓋　Hard palate

14　頭　部

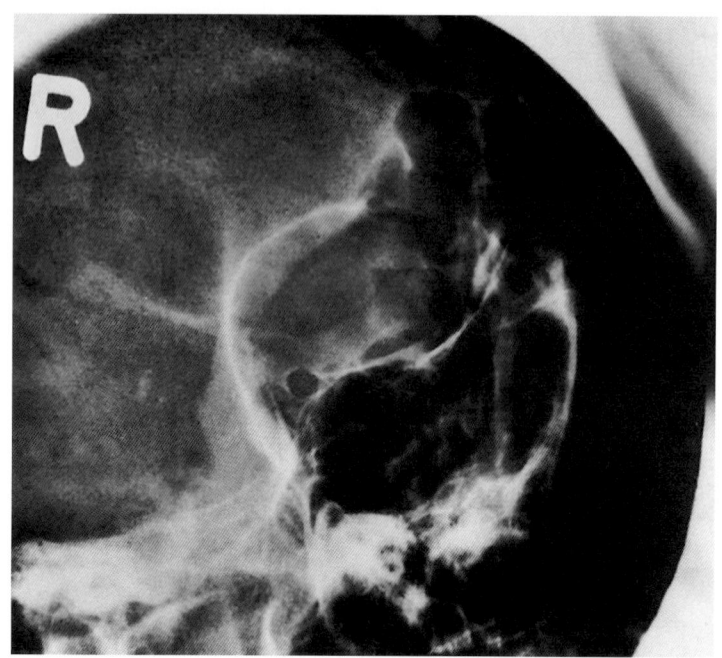

眼窩 Rhese法

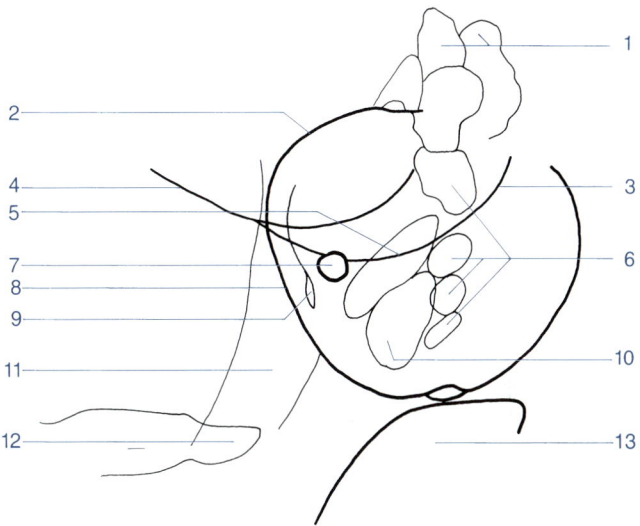

1 前頭洞 Frontal sinus
2 眼窩上壁 Roof of the orbit
3 左蝶形骨小翼 Left lesser wing of the sphenoid
4 右蝶形骨小翼 Right lesser wing of the sphenoid
5 蝶形骨 Sphenoid
6 篩骨洞 Ethmoid sinus
7 視神経管 Optic canal
8 眼窩外側壁 Lateral wall of the orbit
9 上眼窩裂 Superior orbital fissure
10 蝶形骨洞 Sphenoid sinus
11 頬骨弓 Zygomatic arch
12 側頭骨岩様部 Petrous portion of the temporal bone
13 上顎洞 Maxillary sinus

16 頭部

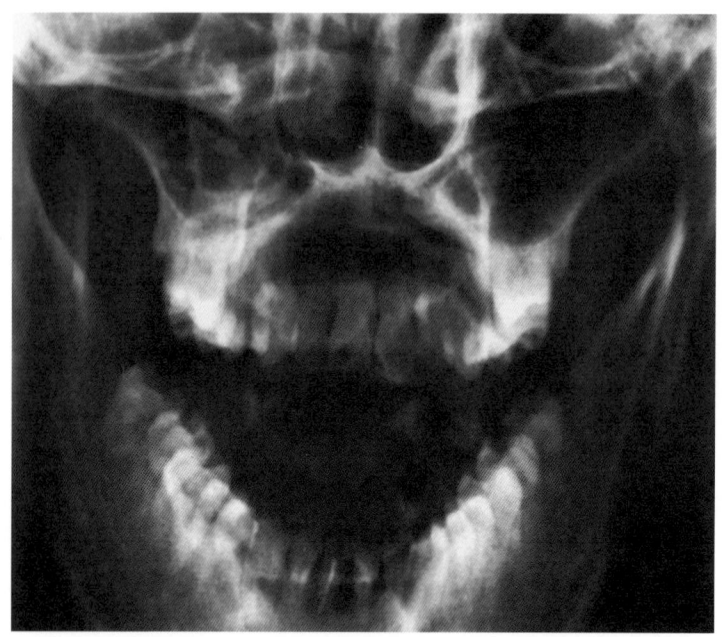

上顎骨　17

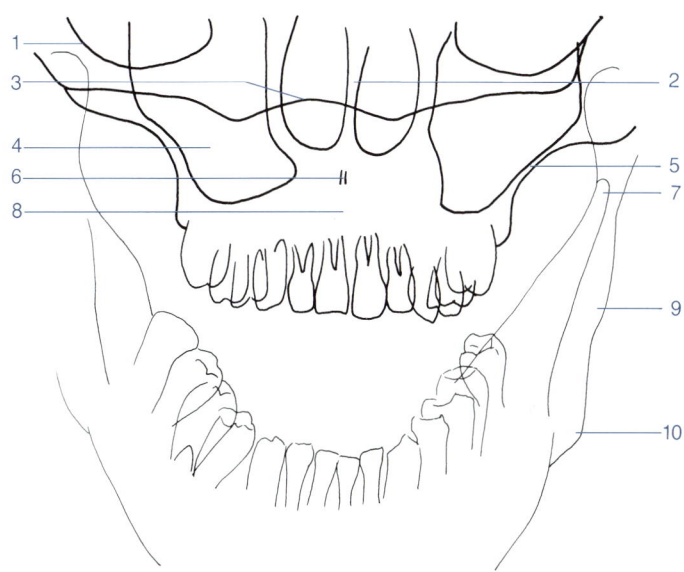

1	眼窩底 Floor of the orbit		6	前鼻棘 Anterior nasal spine
2	鼻中隔 Nasal septum		7	筋突起 Coronoid process
3	頭蓋底 Base of the skull		8	上顎骨 Maxilla
4	上顎洞 Maxillary sinus		9	下顎枝 Ramus of the mandible
5	上顎洞外側壁 Lateral wall of the maxillary sinus		10	下顎角 Angle of the mandible

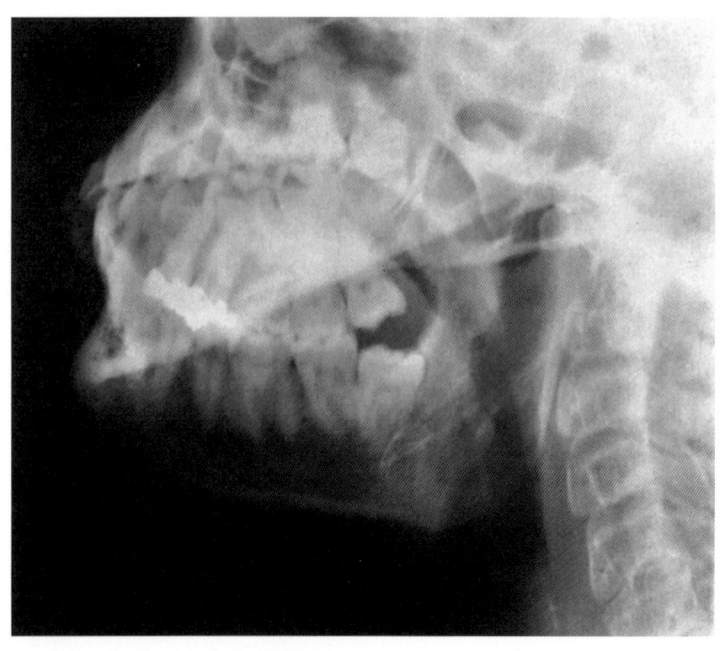

下顎枝 **19**

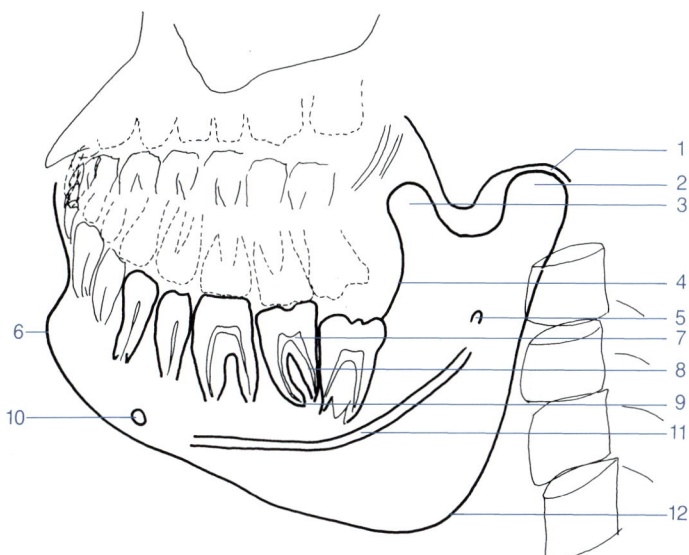

1	顎関節 Temporomandibular joint	6	オトガイ隆起 Mental protuberance
2	下顎頭(関節突起) Condyle of the mandible	7	歯髄腔 Pulp cavity
3	筋突起 Coronoid process	8	歯根管 Root canal
4	下顎枝の骨皮質 Cortex of ramus of the mandible	9	歯根尖孔 Apical foramen of the tooth
5	下顎孔 Mandibular foramen	10	オトガイ孔 Mental foramen
		11	下顎管 Mandibular canal
		12	下顎角 Angle of the mandible

頭 部

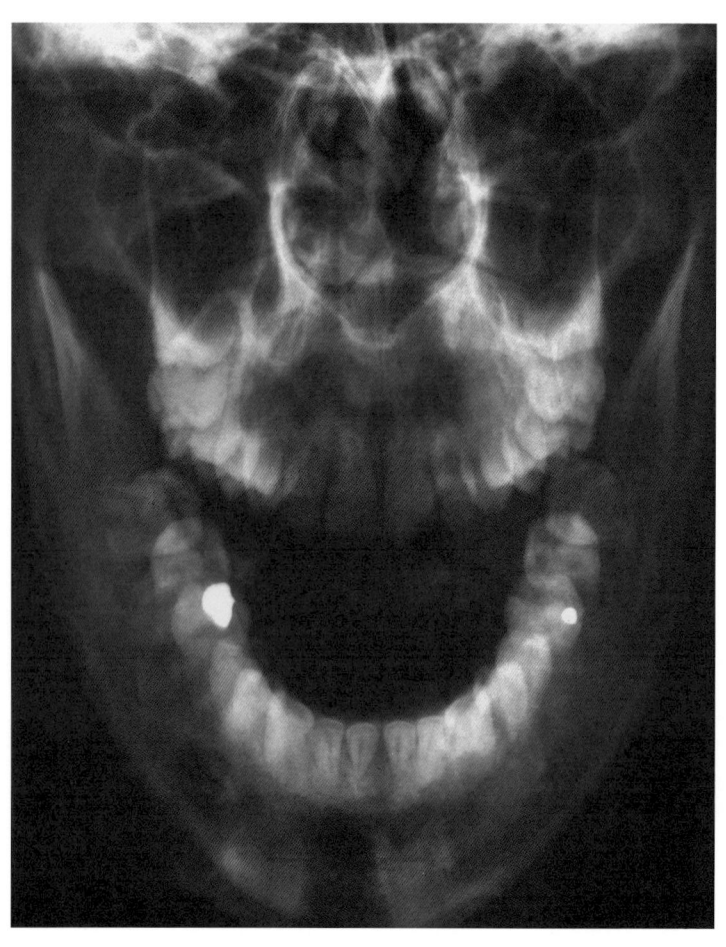

下顎骨 Clementschitsh法

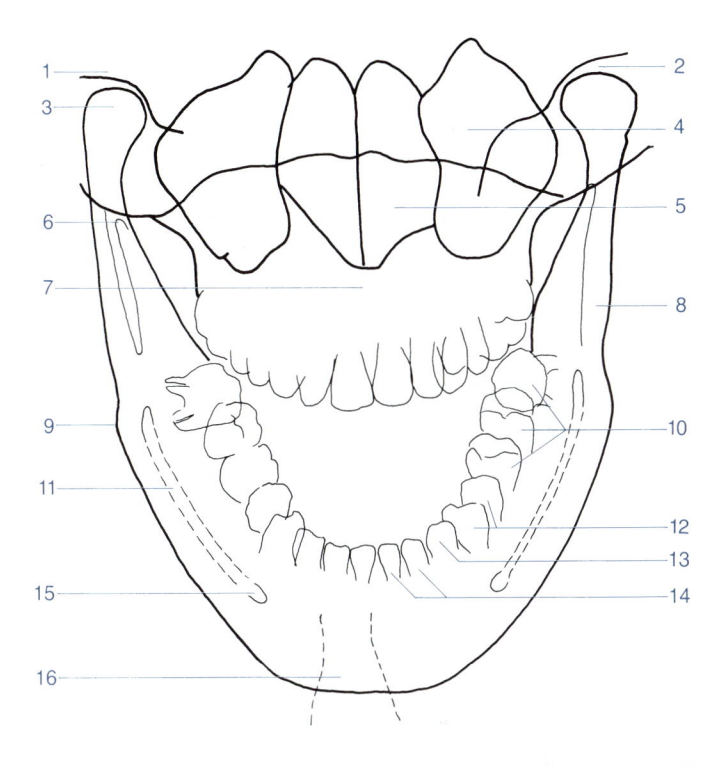

1 側頭骨 Temporal bone
2 顎関節（側頭下顎関節）Temporomandibular joint
3 下顎頭（関節突起）Condyle of the mandible
4 上顎洞 Maxillary sinus
5 鼻腔 Nasal cavity
6 筋突起 Coronoid process
7 上顎骨 Maxilla
8 下顎枝 Ramus of the mandible
9 下顎角 Angle of the mandible
10 大臼歯 Molars
11 下顎管 Mandibular canal
12 小臼歯 Premolars
13 犬歯 Canines
14 切歯 Incisors
15 オトガイ孔 Mental foramen
16 オトガイ隆起 Mental protuberance
気管が透亮像として重なっている

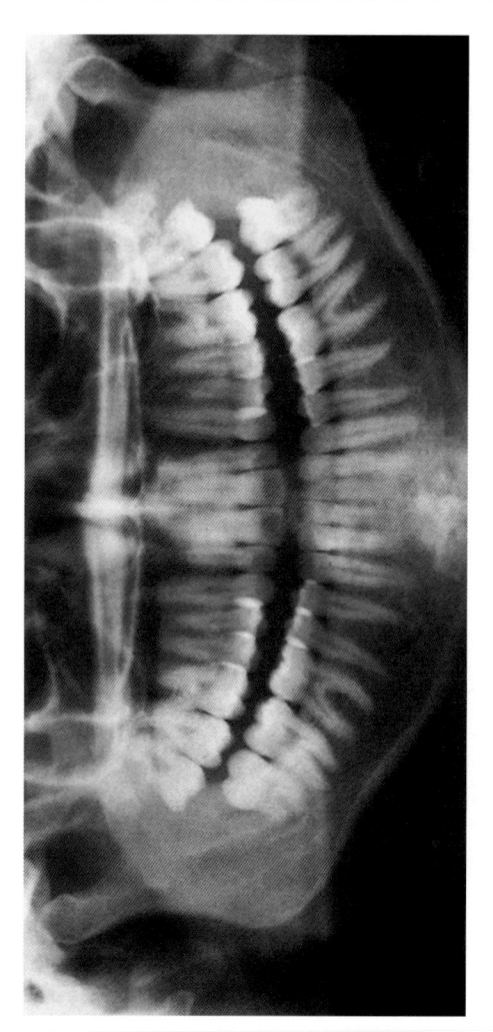

1 茎状突起 Styloid process
2 軟口蓋 Soft palate
3 下顎頭 (関節突起) Condyle of the mandible
4 関節突起 Condylar process
5 頬骨弓 Zygomatic arch
6 筋突起 Coronoid process
7 眼窩底 Floor of the orbit
8 鼻腔 Nasal cavity
9 硬口蓋 Hard palate
10 上顎洞歯槽陥凹 Alveolar recess of the maxillary sinus
11 上顎洞 Maxillary sinus
12 翼口蓋窩 Pterygopalatine fossa
13 翼状突起 Pterygoid process
14 下顎角 Angle of the mandible
15 舌の陰影 Shadow of the tongue
16 下顎管 Mandibular canal
17 舌骨 Hyoid bone
18 歯根尖孔 Apical foramen of the tooth
19 歯根管 Root canal
20 歯髄腔 Pulp cavity
21 象牙質 Dentin
22 エナメル質 Enamel
23 オトガイ孔 Mental foramen
24 歯根 Root of the tooth
25 切歯 Incisor
26 犬歯 Canine
27 小臼歯 Premolar
28 大臼歯 Molar

顎・顔面骨 パントモ撮影   23

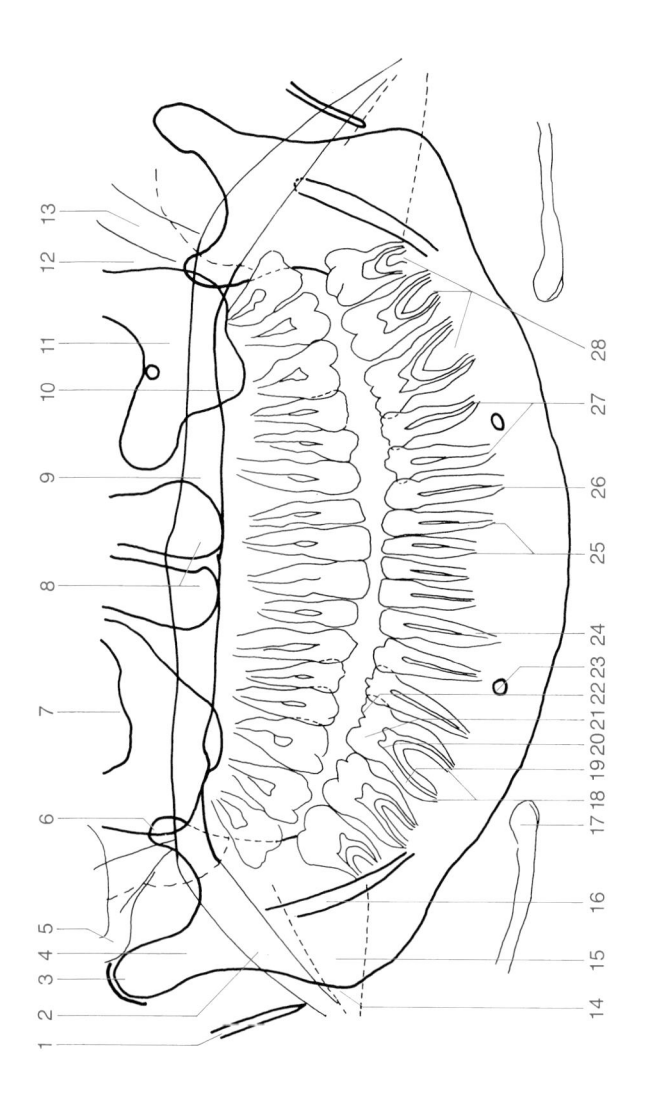

24 頭 部

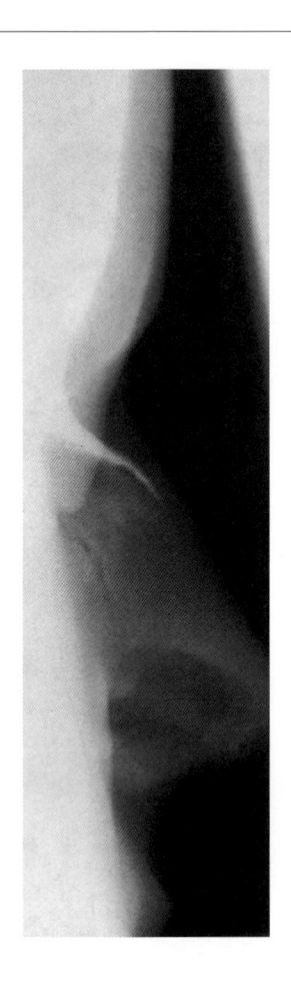

鼻骨 側面 25

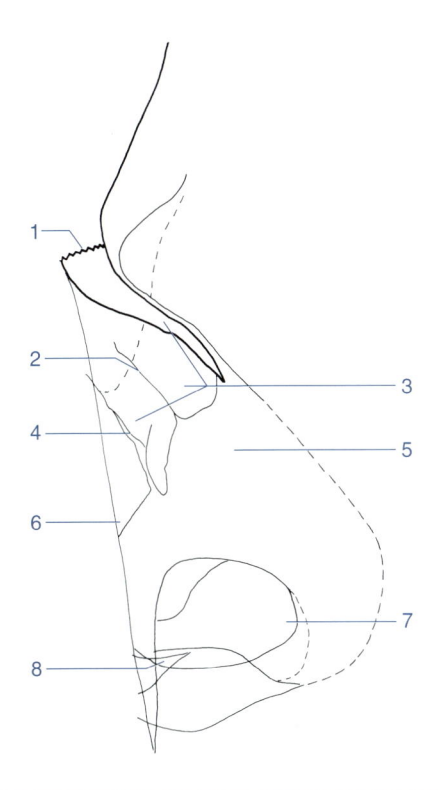

1	前頭鼻骨縫合 Frontonasal suture	5	鼻軟骨 Nasal cartilage
2	篩骨神経溝 Ethmoidal groove	6	上顎骨 Maxilla
3	鼻骨 Nasal bone	7	鼻前庭 Vestibule of nose
4	鼻骨上顎縫合 Nasomaxillary suture	8	前鼻棘 Anterior nasal spine

頭部

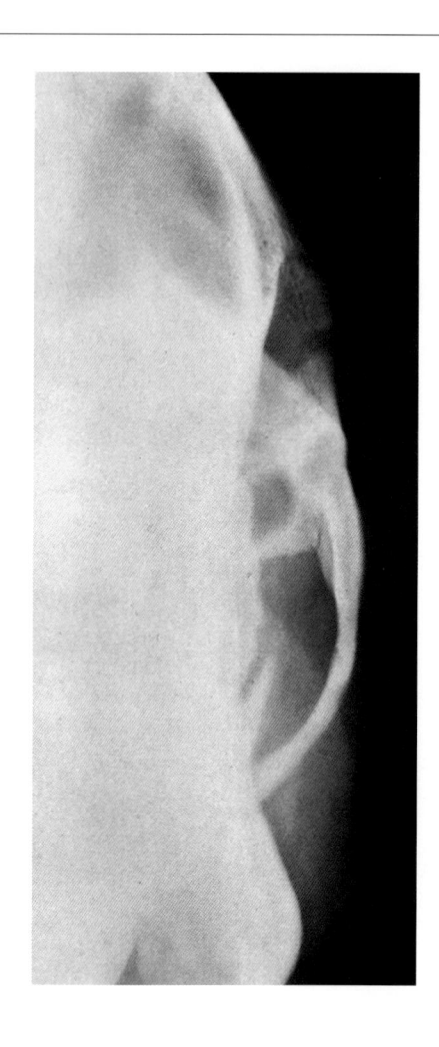

頬骨弓　**27**

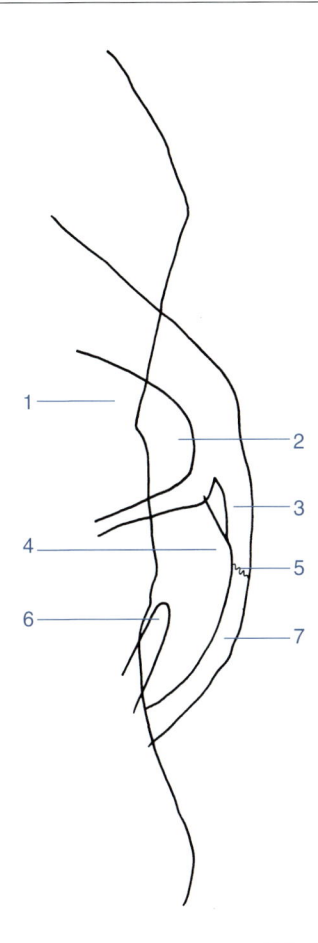

1 上顎洞　Maxillary sinus
2 （上顎洞）頬骨陥凹　Zygomatic recess (of the Maxillary sinus)
3 頬骨弓　Zygomatic arch
4 側頭窩　Temporal fossa
5 側頭頬骨縫合　Temporozygomatic suture
6 筋突起　Coronoid process
7 側頭骨頬骨突起　Zygomatic process of the temporal bone

28　頭　部

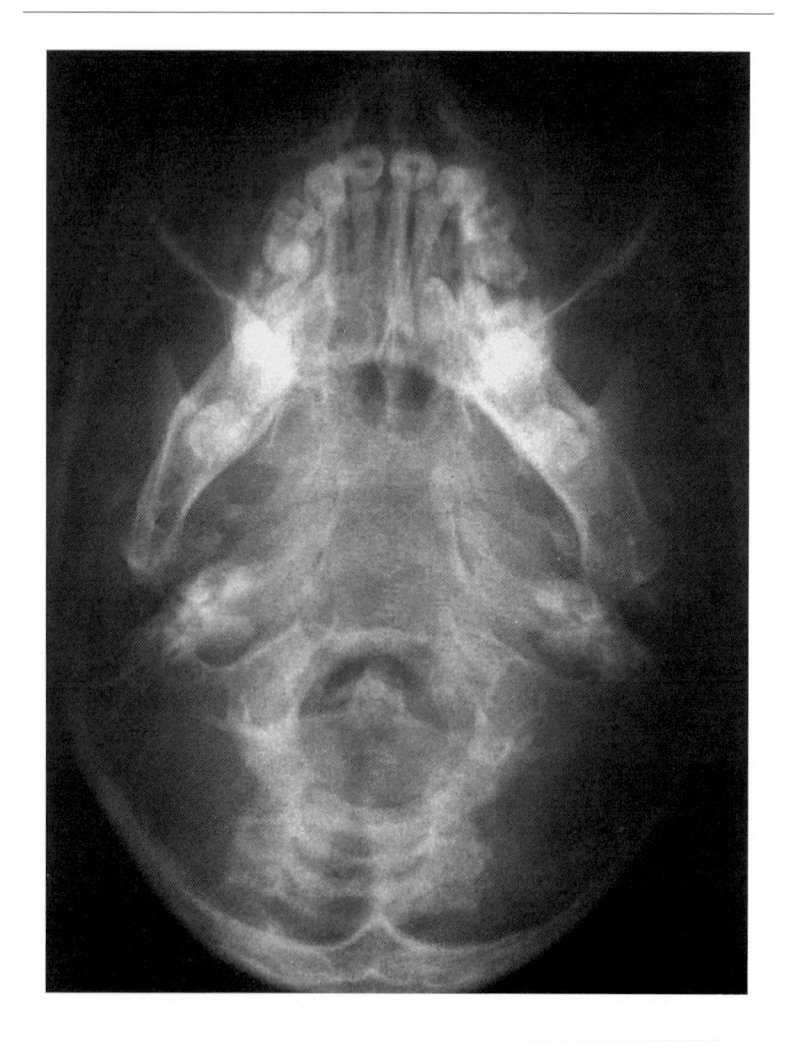

頭蓋底　29

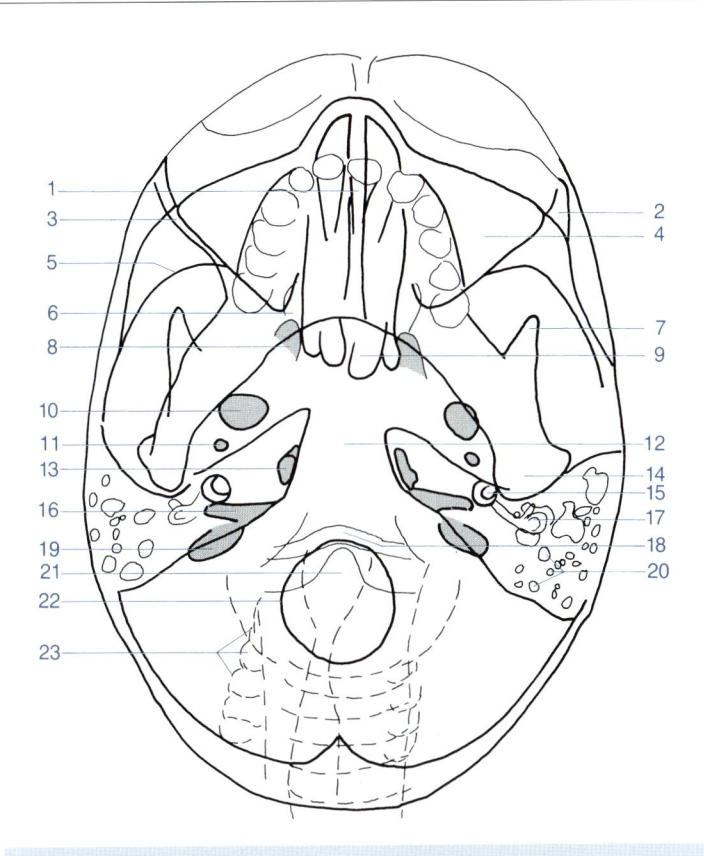

1	鼻中隔 Nasal septum
2	頬骨 Zygomatic bone
3	上顎洞後壁 Posterior wall of maxillary sinus
4	上顎洞 Maxillary sinus 一部，眼窩と重なっている
5	中頭蓋窩 Middle cranial fossa 大翼 Greater wing 中頭蓋窩前壁
6	翼口蓋窩 Pterygopalatine fossa
7	筋突起 Coronoid process
8	翼突窩 Pterygoid fossa
9	蝶形骨洞 Sphenoid sinus
10	卵円孔 Foramen ovale
11	棘孔 Foramen spinosum
12	斜台 Clivus
13	破裂孔 Foramen lacerum
14	下顎頭（関節突起）Condyle of the mandible
15	蝸牛 Cochlea
16	内耳道 Internal auditory canal
17	半規管 Semicircular canals
18	環椎前弓 Anterior arch of the atlas
19	頸静脈孔 Jugular foramen
20	乳突蜂巣 Mastoid air cells
21	軸椎歯突起 Dens of the axis
22	大後頭孔 Foramen magnum
23	頸椎 Cervical spine

30　頭　部

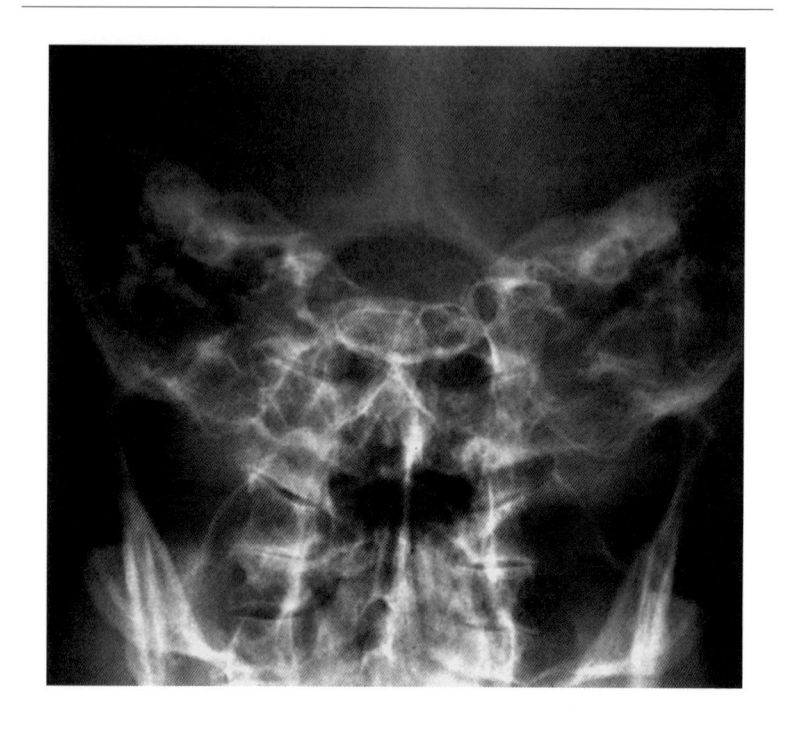

側頭骨（錐体） Altschul法

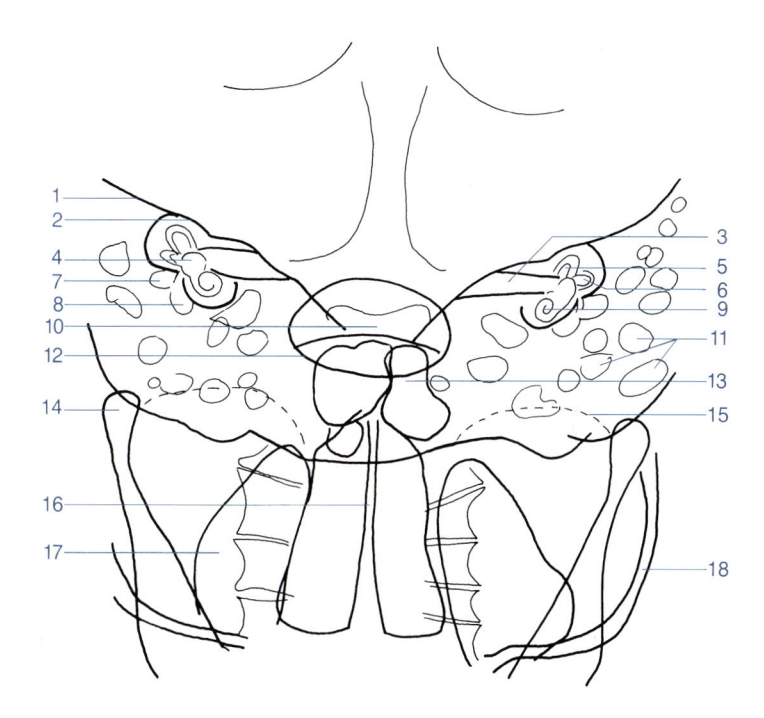

1 錐体縁 Petrous ridge
2 弓状隆起 Arcuate eminence
3 内耳道 Internal auditory canal
4 前庭 Vestibule
5 前（上）半規管 Anterior (superior) semicircular canal
6 外側半規管 Lateral semicircular canal
7 乳突洞 Antrum of the mastoid
8 鼓室 Tympanic cavity
9 蝸牛 Cochlea
10 鞍背 Dorsum sellae
11 乳突蜂巣 Mastoid air cells
12 大後頭孔 Foramen magnum
13 前頭洞 Frontal sinus
14 下顎頭（関節突起） Condyle of the mandible
15 眼窩上壁 Roof of the orbit
16 鼻中隔 Nasal septum
   鼻腔 Nasal cavities
17 上顎洞 Maxillary sinus
18 頬骨弓 Zygomatic arch

32 頭 部

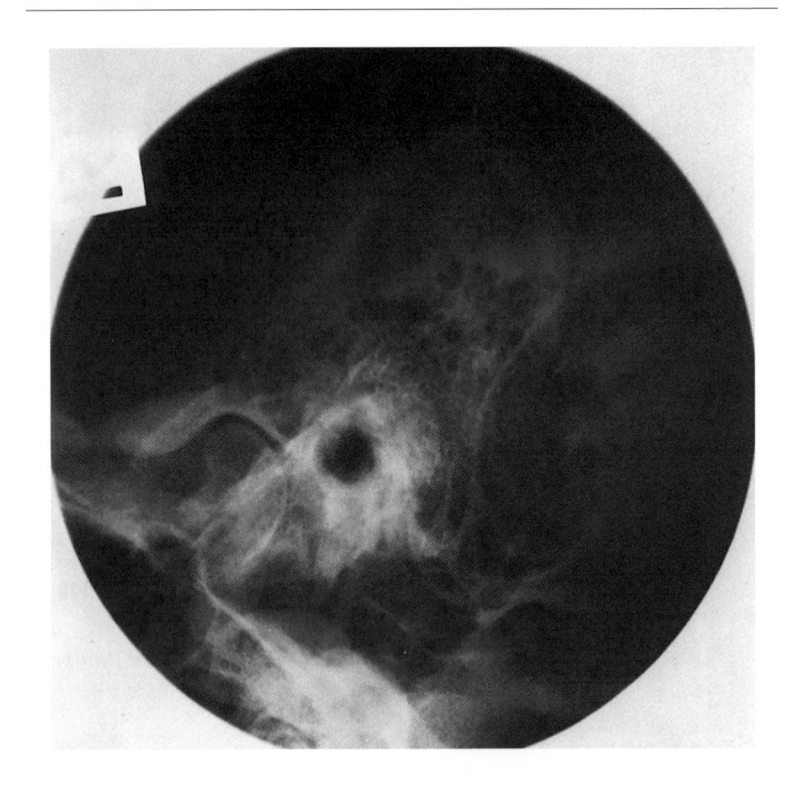

側頭骨（錐体）　Schüller法　*33*

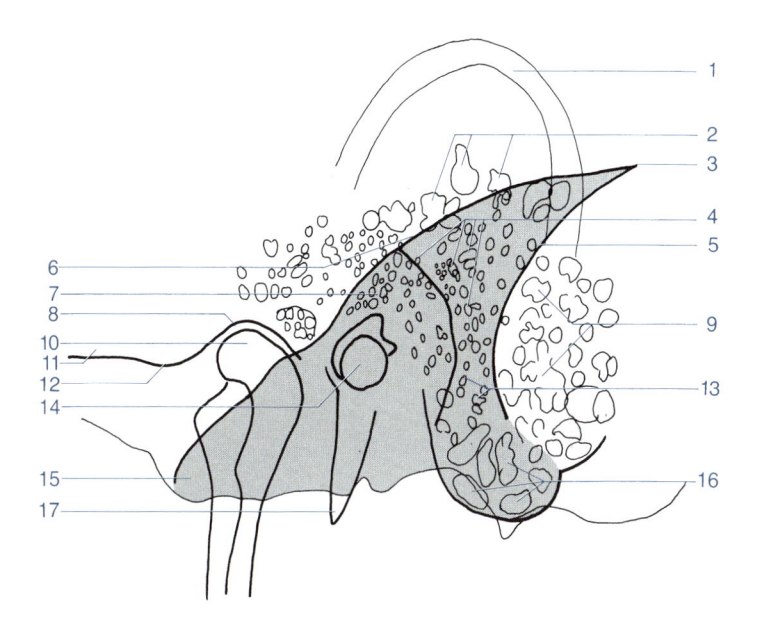

1　外耳　Outer ear	10　下顎頭（関節突起）　Condyle of the mandible
2　鱗部蜂巣　Squamous air cells	11　側頭骨頬骨突起　Zygomatic process of the temporal bone
3　Citelli角　Angle of Citelli	12　関節結節　Articular tubercle
4　乳突洞周囲部蜂巣　Periantral air cells	13　顔面神経後部蜂巣　Retrofacial air cells
5　S状洞溝　Sulcus of the sigmoid sinus	14　内耳道および外耳道　Internal and external auditory canal
6　錐体前縁　Anterior margin of the petrous bone	15　錐体尖　Apex of the Petrous bone
7　乳突洞　Antrum of the mastoid	16　乳様突起先端の蜂巣　Air cells in the tip of the Mastoid process
8　顎関節関節窩　Temporomandibular joint fossa	17　茎状突起　Styloid process
9　辺縁部蜂巣　Marginal air cells	

34 頭　部

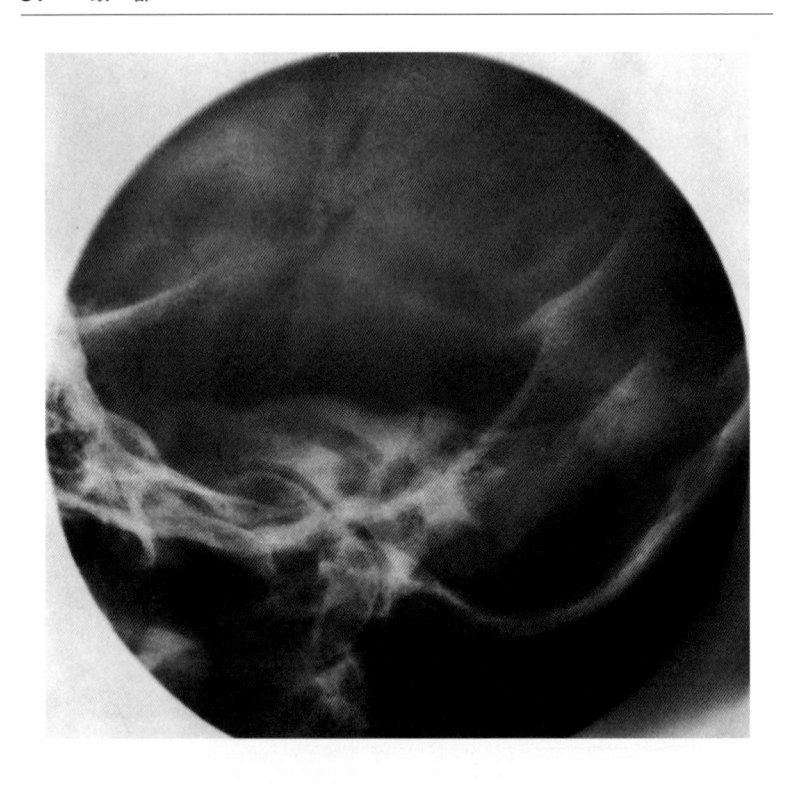

側頭骨（錐体） Stenvers法

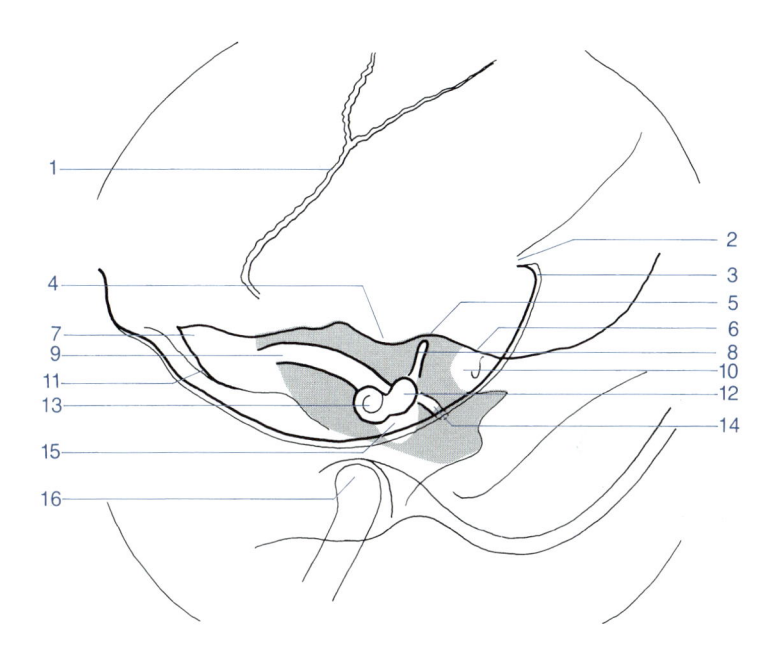

1 蝶鱗縫合 Sphenosquamous suture
2 内後頭隆起 Internal occipital protuberance
3 内後頭稜 Internal occipital crest
4 弓下窩 Subarcuate fossa
5 弓状隆起 Arcuate eminence
6 鼓室蓋 Roof of the tympanic cavity
7 錐体尖 Apex of the petrous pyramid
8 前(上)半規管 Anterior (superior) semicircular canal
9 内耳道 Internal auditory canal
10 乳突洞 Antrum
11 蝶錐体裂 Sphenopetrosal fissure
12 前庭 Vestibule
13 蝸牛 Cochlea
14 外側半規管 Lateral semicircular canal
15 鼓室 Tympanic cavity
16 下顎頭（関節突起）Condyle of the mandible

36　頭　部

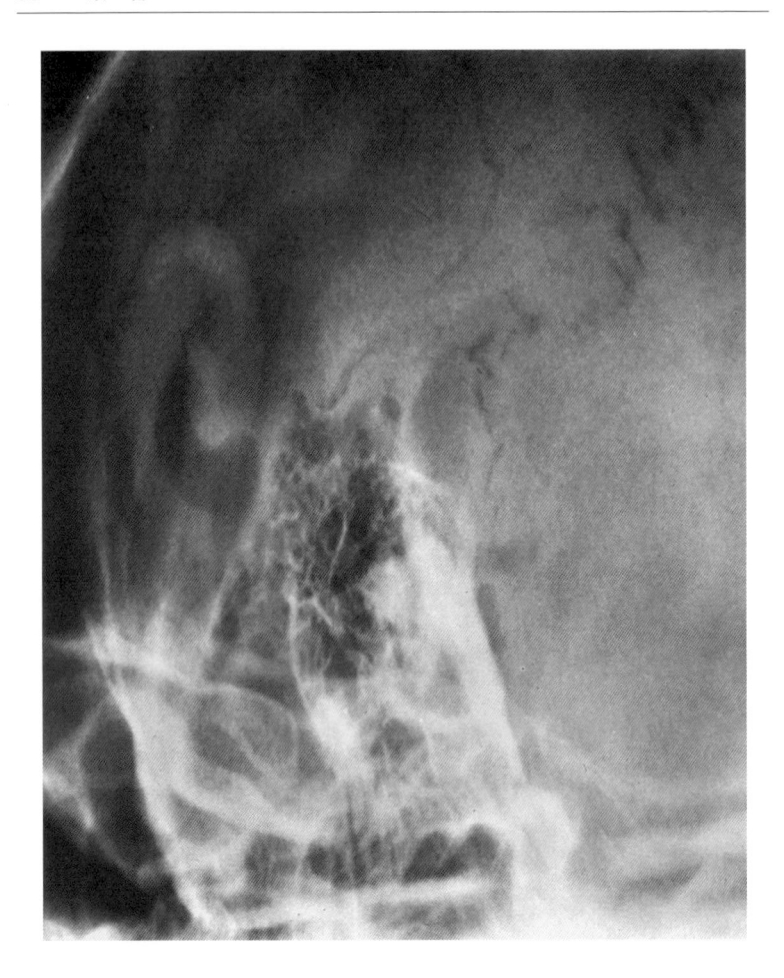

側頭骨(錐体) Mayer法

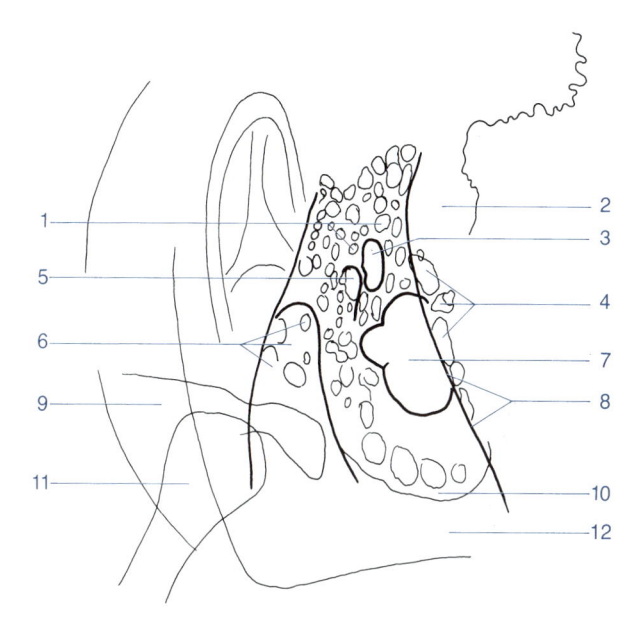

1 乳突洞周囲部蜂巣 Periantral air cells
2 S状静脈洞 Sigmoid sinus
3 乳突洞 Antrum
4 副鼻腔後部蜂巣 Retrosinus air cells
5 乳突洞口 Aperture of mastoid antrum
6 外耳道 External auditory canal
　鼓室 Tympanic cavity
7 骨迷路 Osseous labyrinth
8 錐体後縁 Posterior wall of the petrous bone
9 頬骨 Zygomatic bone
10 乳様突起尖端 Apex of the mastoid
11 下顎頭(関節突起) Condyle of the mandible
12 錐体尖 Apex of the Petrous bone

38 頭 部

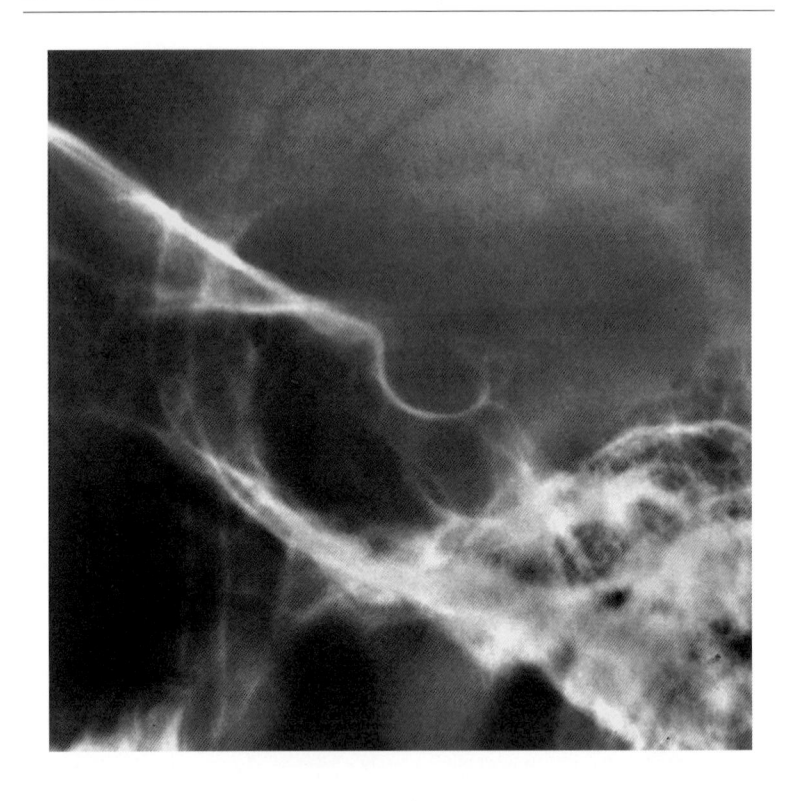

トルコ鞍　側面　39

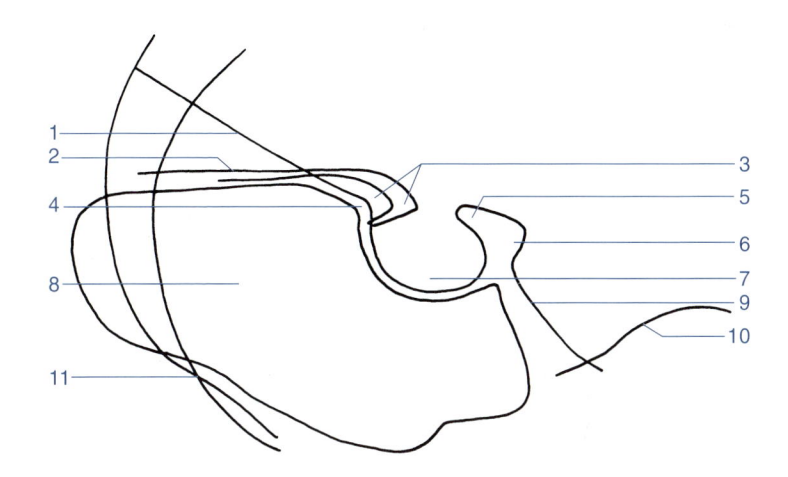

1	前頭蓋底 Floor of anterior cranial fossa	6	鞍背 Dorsum sellae
	眼窩上壁 Roof of orbits	7	下垂体窩 Pituitary fossa
2	蝶形骨 Sphenoid	8	蝶形骨洞 Sphenoid sinus
3	前床突起 Anterior clinoid process	9	斜台 Clivus
4	鞍結節 Tuberculum sellae	10	錐体縁 Petrous ridge
5	後床突起 Posterior clinoid process	11	蝶形骨大翼 Greater wing of the sphenoid

40 頭 部

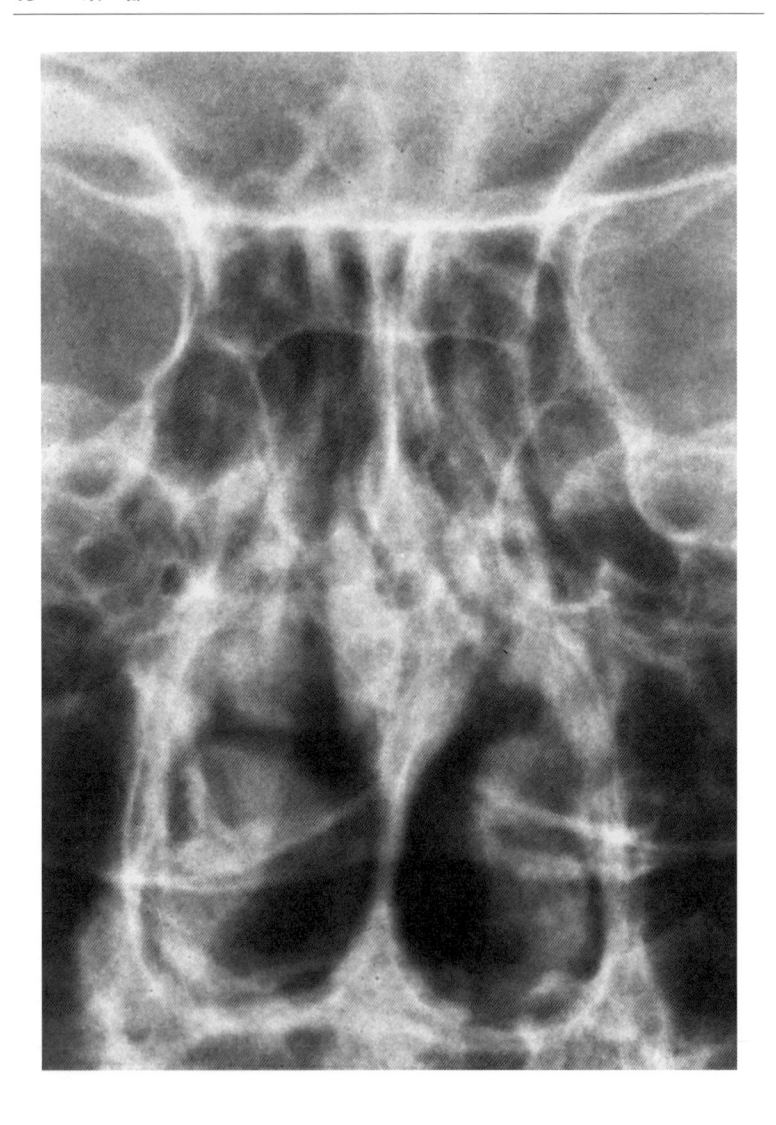

トルコ鞍　正面（前後）

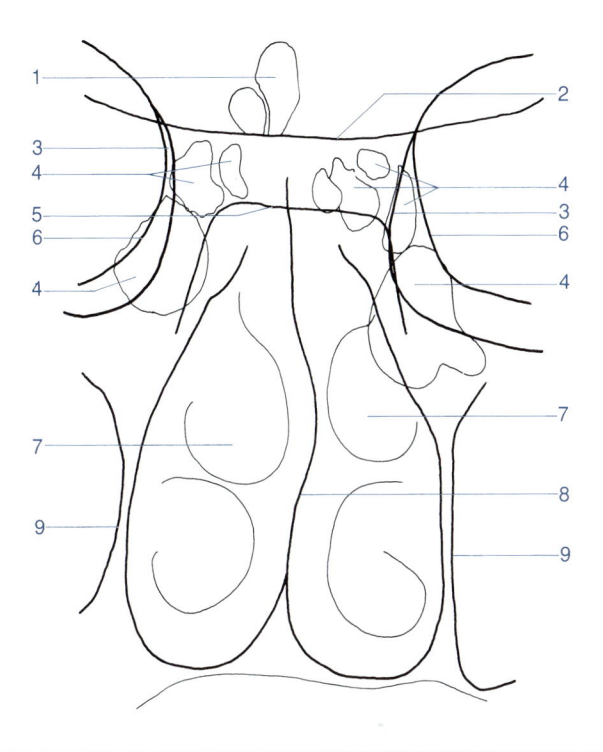

1 前頭洞　Frontal sinuses
2 蝶形骨　Sphenoid
3 眼窩内側壁　Medial wall of Orbit
4 篩骨洞　Ethmoid sinus
5 下垂体窩　Pituitary fossa
　（トルコ鞍底　Floor of the sella turcica）
6 眼窩板　Orbital plate
7 鼻甲介　Nasal turbinates
8 鼻中隔　Nasal septum
9 上顎洞内側壁　Medial wall of the maxillary sinus

42 脊 椎

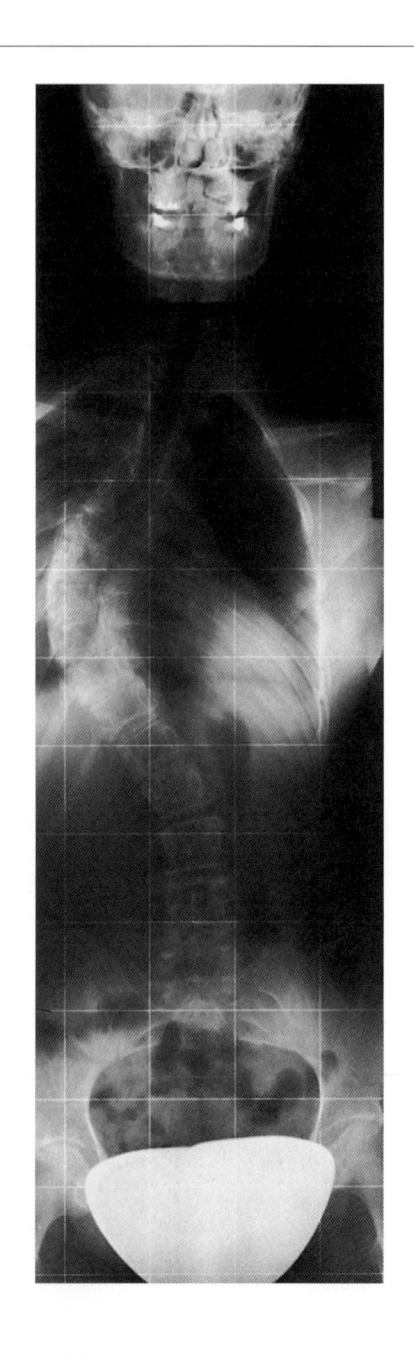

全脊椎　正面（前後）

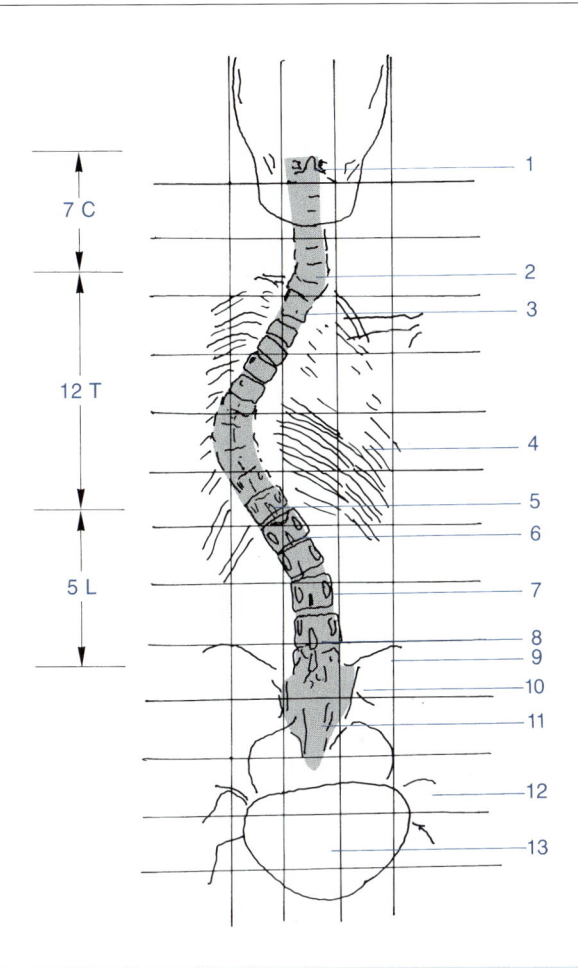

1	軸椎歯突起 Dens of the axis
2	第7頸椎 C7
3	第2胸椎 Th2
4	胸郭 Rib cage
5	第12胸椎 Th12
6	第1腰椎 L1
7	第3腰椎椎弓根 Pedicle, L3
8	第6腰椎棘突起 Spinous process, L6
9	腸骨 Ilium
10	仙腸関節 Sacroiliac joint
11	仙骨 Sacrum
12	股関節 Hip joint
13	生殖腺防護 Gonad shield

44　脊椎

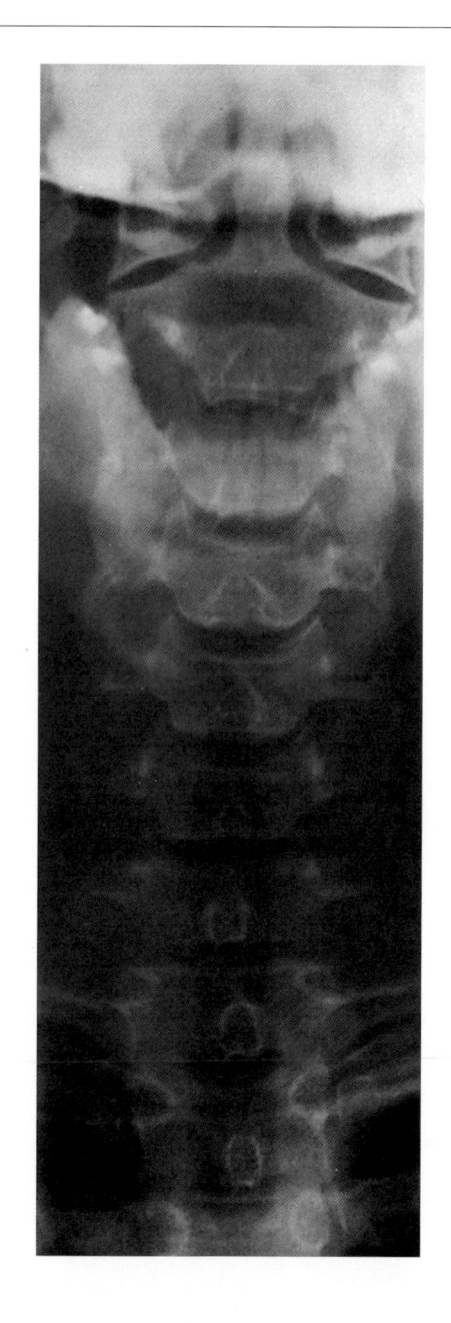

頸椎　正面（前後）

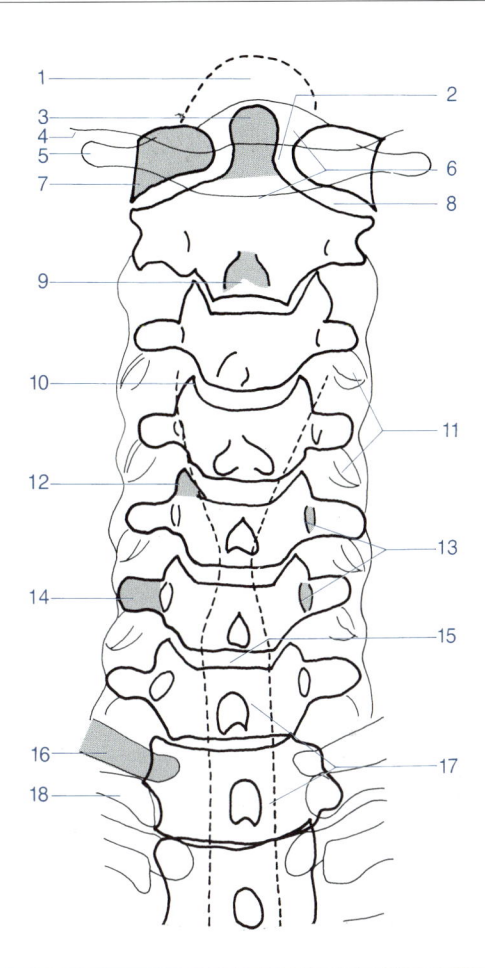

1	大後頭孔　Foramen magnum
2	環軸関節　Atlantoaxial joint
3	軸椎歯突起　Dens of the axis
4	後頭骨　Occipital bone
5	横突起　Transverse process
6	椎弓　Vertebral arch
7	第1頸椎外側塊　Lateral mass of C1
8	環軸関節　Atlantoaxial joint
9	棘突起　Spinous process　二分している
10	鈎椎関節（ルシュカ関節）Uncovertebral joint
11	関節突起の重なり　Overlapping articular processes
12	鈎状突起　Uncinate process
13	椎弓根　Pedicle
14	横突起　Transverse process
15	椎間板腔　Intervertebral disk space
16	第1胸椎横突起　Transverse process of Th1
17	気管の透亮像　Radiolucent band of the trachea
18	第1肋骨　First rib

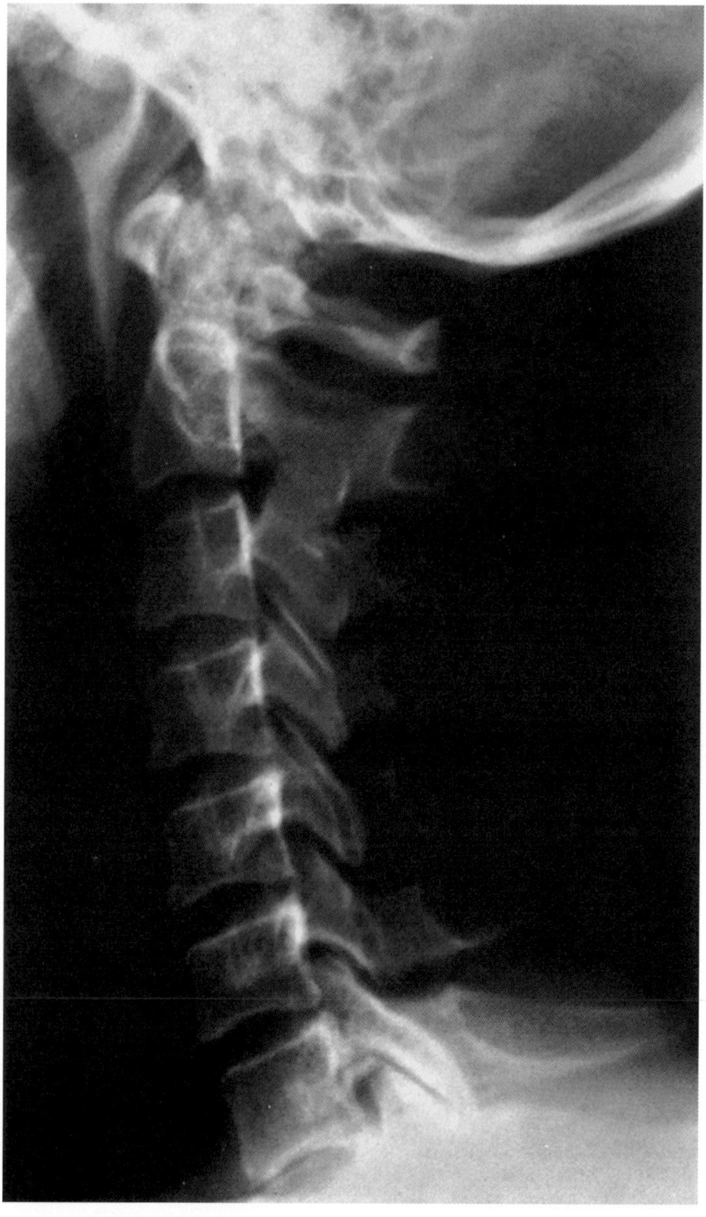

頸椎　側面

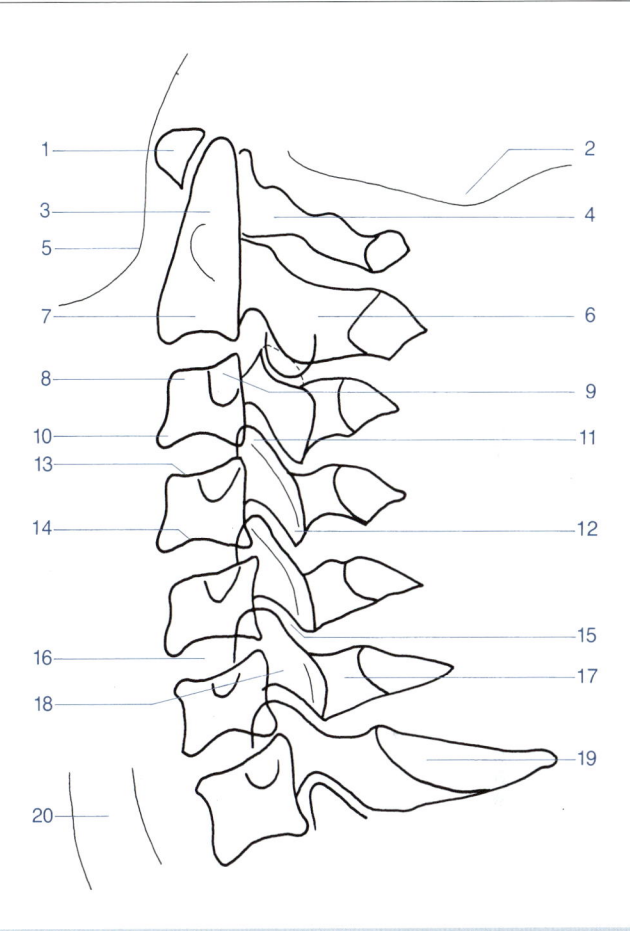

1　環椎前弓 Anterior arch of the atlas	11　上関節突起 Superior articular process
2　頭蓋底 Base of the skull	12　下関節突起 Inferior articular process
3　歯突起 Odontoid process	13　椎体上面 Superior vertebral end plate
4　環椎後弓 Posterior arch of the atlas	14　椎体下面 Inferior vertebral end plate
5　下顎骨 Mandible	15　椎間関節 Intervertebral facet joint
6　棘突起 Spinous process	16　椎間板腔 Intervertebral disk space
7　軸椎椎体 Body of the axis	17　椎弓板 Lamina
8　椎体前上縁 Anterior superior margin of the vertebra	18　椎間関節柱 Articular pillar
9　横突起 Transverse process	19　棘突起 Spinous process
10　椎体前下縁 Anterior inferior margin of the vertebra	20　気管 Trachea

48　脊　椎

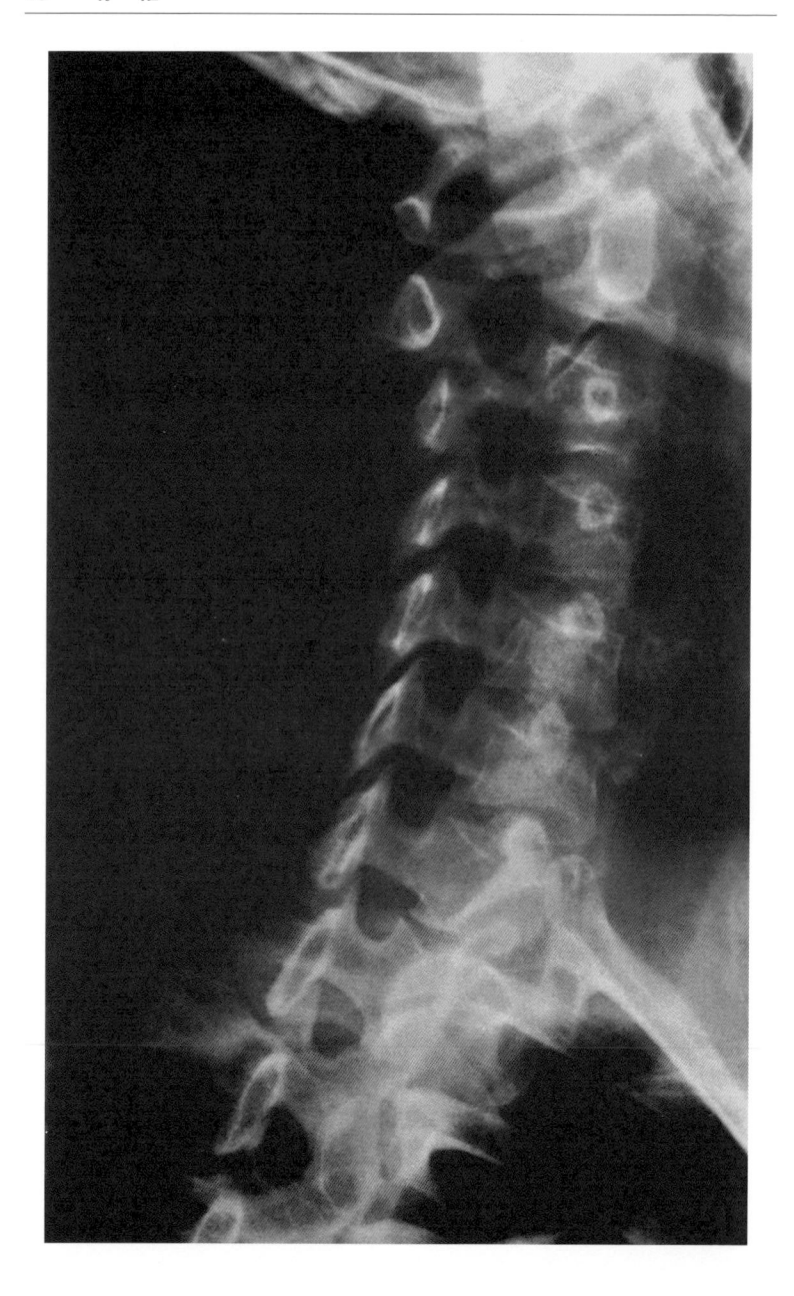

頸椎 斜位

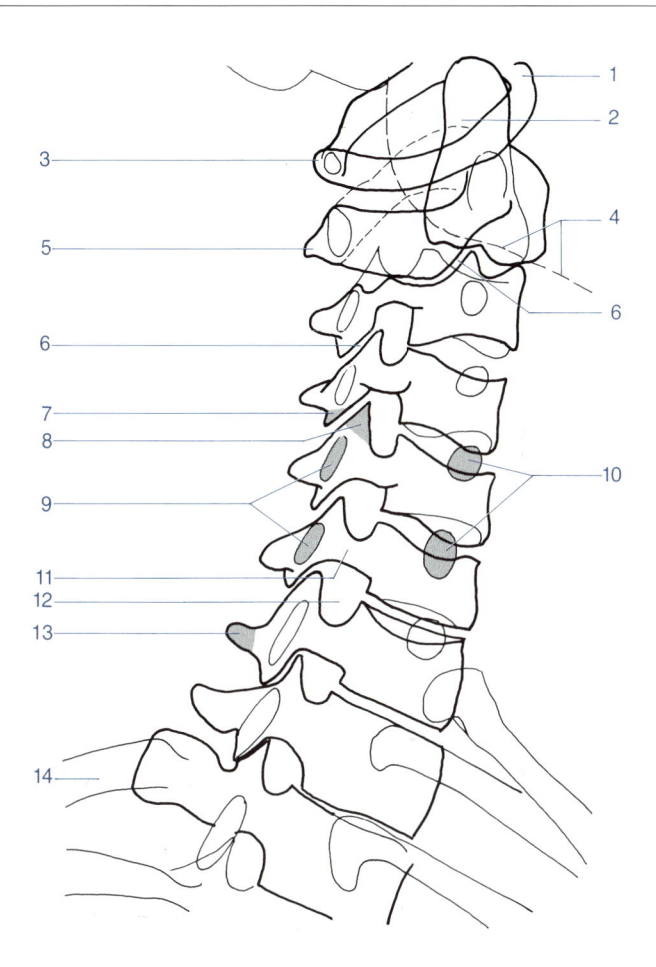

1 前弓 Anterior arch	8 上関節突起 Superior articular process
2 歯突起 Odontoid process	9 横突起 Transverse process
3 環椎 Atlas	10 対側の椎弓根 Contralateral pedicle
4 下顎骨 Mandible	11 椎弓根 Pedicle
5 第2頸椎椎体 Body of C2	12 椎間孔 Intervertebral foramen
6 椎間関節 Facet joint	13 棘突起 Spinous process
7 下関節突起 Inferior articular process	14 肋骨 Ribs

50　脊　椎

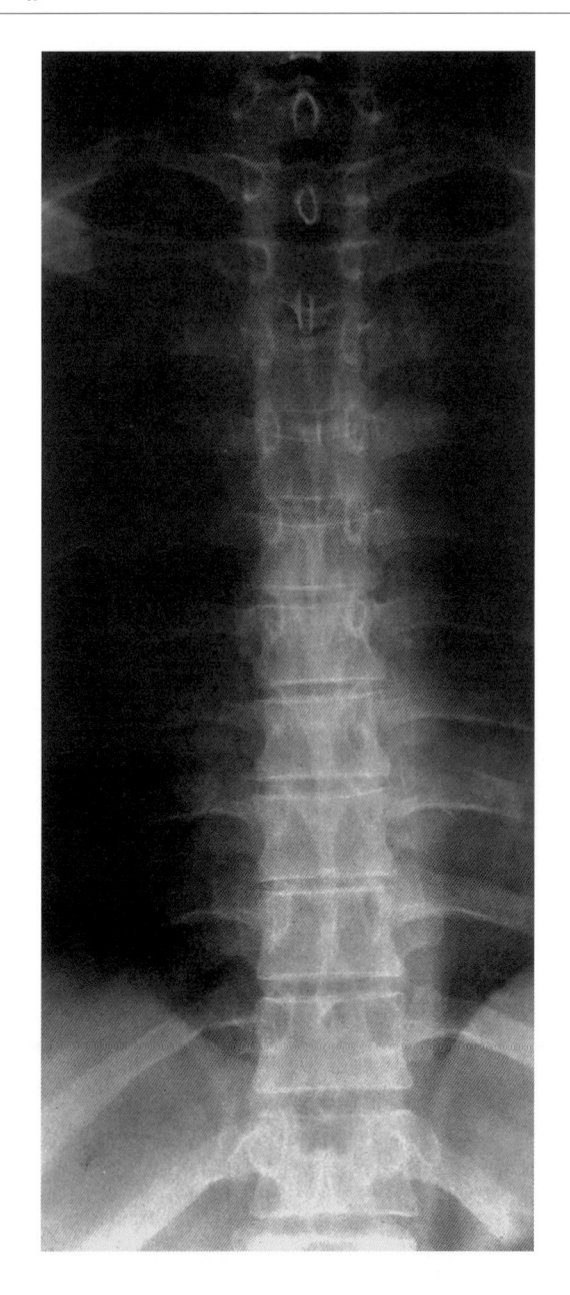

胸椎　正面（前後）

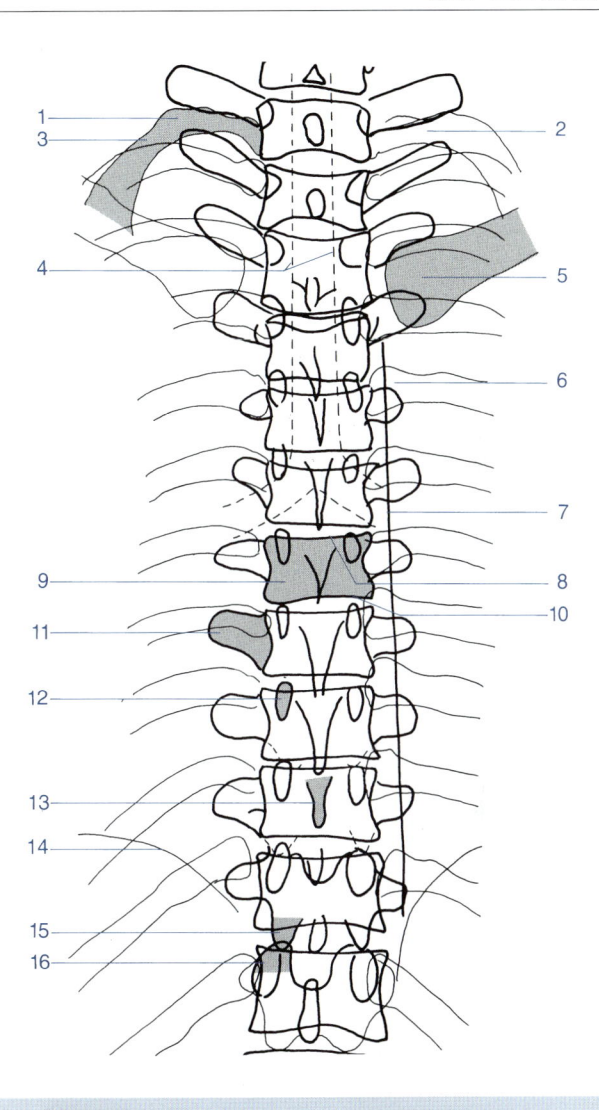

1　第1肋骨肋骨結節　Tubercle of first rib	9　椎体　Body of vertebra
2　肋骨頸　Neck of the rib	10　椎体下面　Inferior vertebral end plate
3　第1肋骨　First rib	11　横突起　Transverse process
4　気管　Trachea	12　椎弓根　Pedicle
5　鎖骨　Clavicle	13　棘突起　Spinous process
6　肋骨頭　Head of the rib	14　横隔膜　Diaphragm
7　椎骨傍線　Paravertebral line	15　下関節突起　Inferior articular process
8　椎体上面　Superior vertebral end plate	16　上関節突起　Superior articular process

52　脊　椎

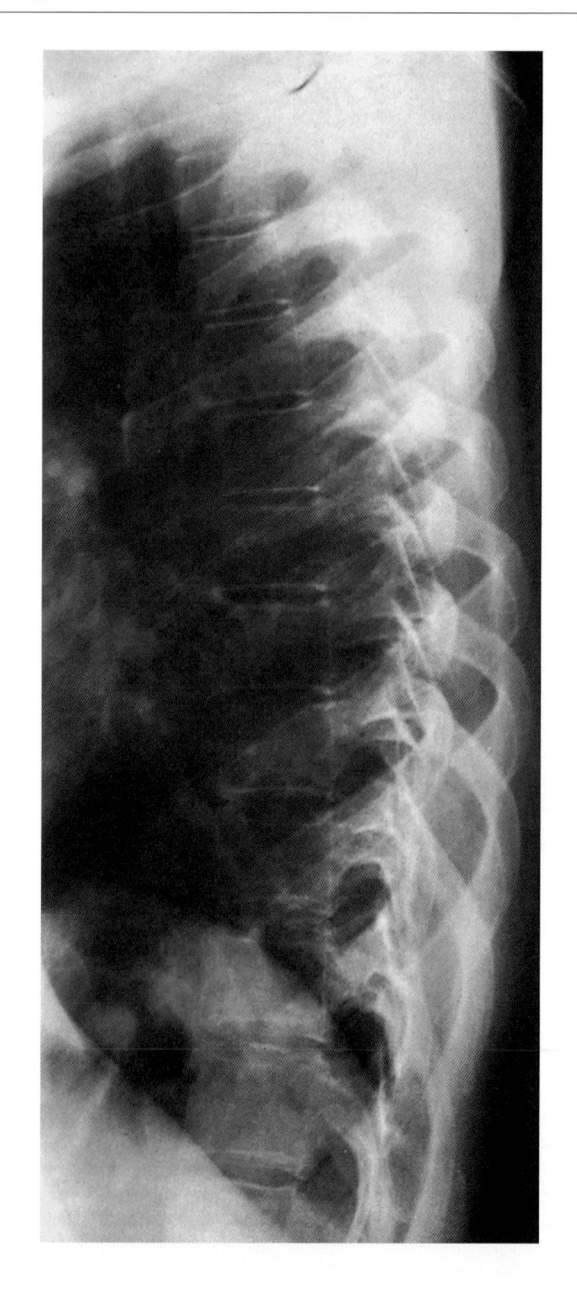

胸椎 側面 53

1 肩甲骨 Scapula	10 椎体下面 Inferior vertebral end plate
2 前上縁 Anterior superior margin	11 肋骨頭 Head of the rib
3 後上縁 Posterior superior margin	12 椎間板腔 Intervertebral disk space
4 前下縁 Anterior inferior margin	13 椎間孔 Intervertebral foramen
5 後下縁 Posterior inferior margin	14 横突起 Transverse process
6 椎体 Body of vertebra	15 棘突起 Spinous process
7 上関節突起 Superior articular process	16 横隔膜 Diaphragm
8 下関節突起 Inferior articular process	17 椎間関節 Facet joint
9 椎体上面 Superior vertebral end plate	

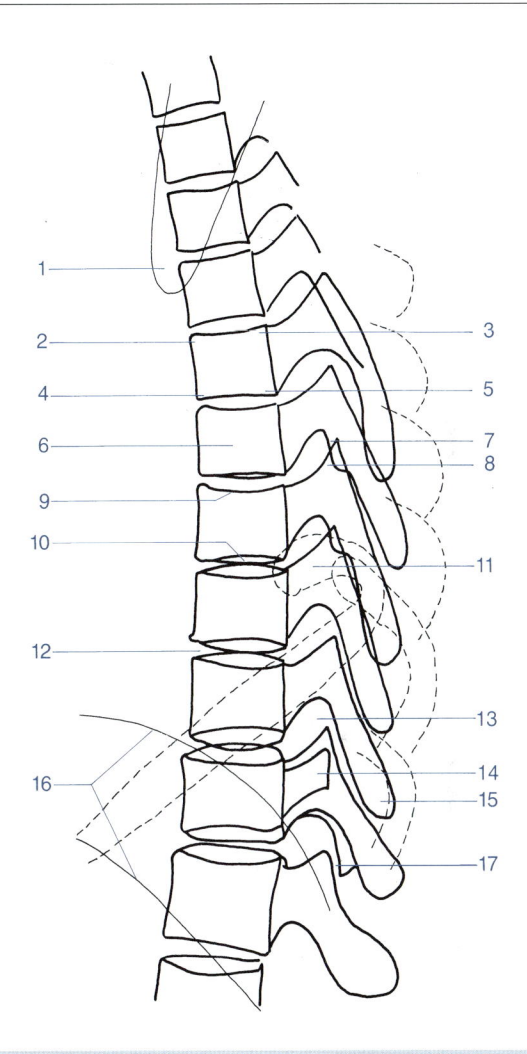

54　脊　椎

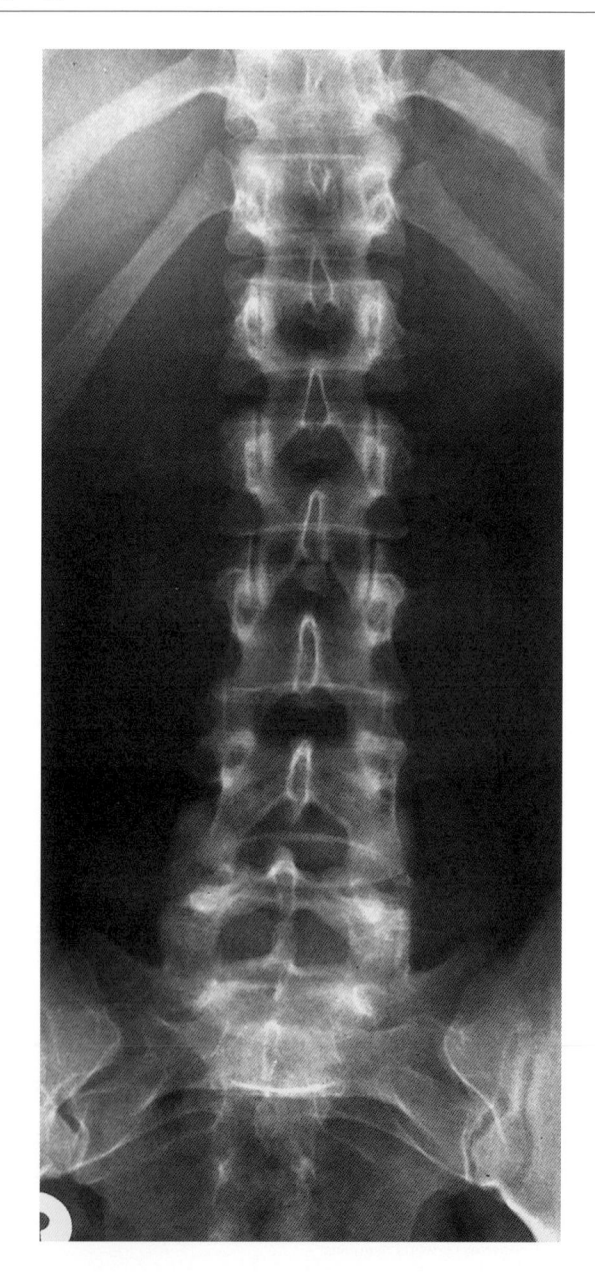

腰椎　正面(前後)

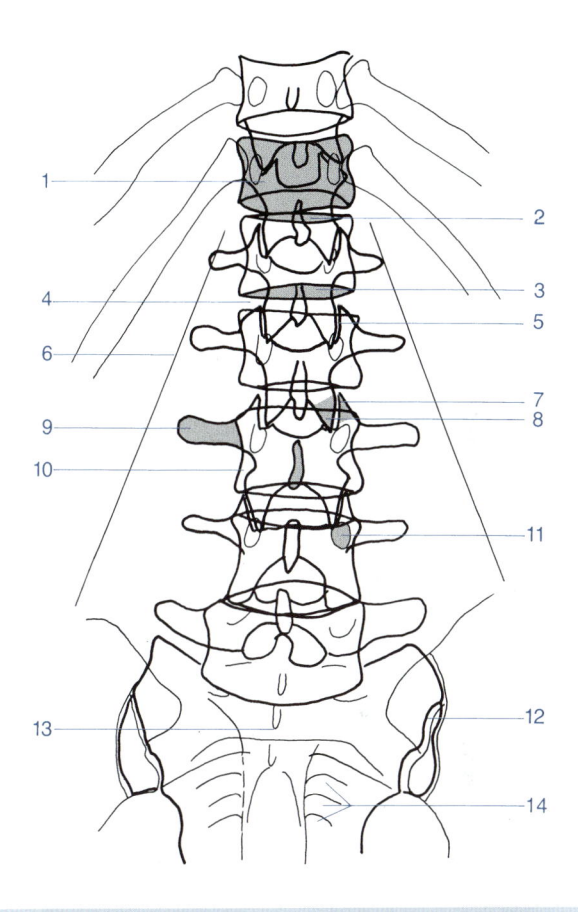

1	椎体 Body of vertebra
2	椎体上面 Superior vertebral end plate
3	椎体下面 Inferior vertebral end plate
4	椎間板腔 Intervertebral disk space
5	椎間関節 Facet joint
6	大腰筋 Psoas muscle
7	上関節突起 Superior articular process
8	下関節突起 Inferior articular process
9	横突起 Transverse process
10	棘突起 Spinous process
11	椎弓根 Pedicle
12	仙腸関節 Sacroiliac joint
13	仙骨 Sacrum
14	仙骨孔 Sacral foramen

56　脊　椎

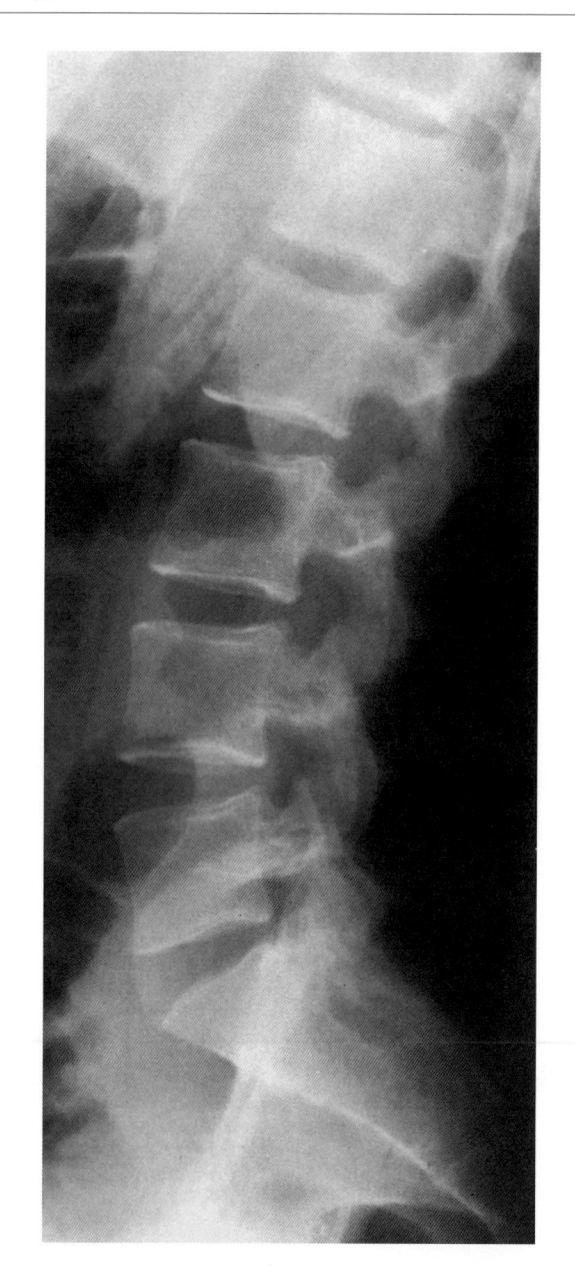

腰椎　側面　**57**

1 椎体上面 Superior vertebral end plate	**7** 上関節突起 Superior articular process
2 椎体下面 Inferior vertebral end plate	**8** 下関節突起 Inferior articular process
3 椎間孔 Intervertebral foramen	**9** 腸骨稜 Iliac crest
4 棘突起 Spinous process	**10** 岬角 Promontory
5 横突起 Transverse process	**11** 仙骨 Sacrum
6 椎間板腔 Intervertebral disk space	

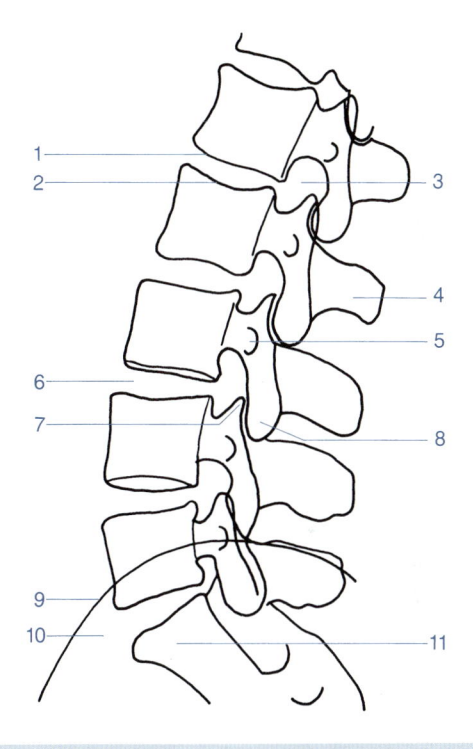

58 脊 椎

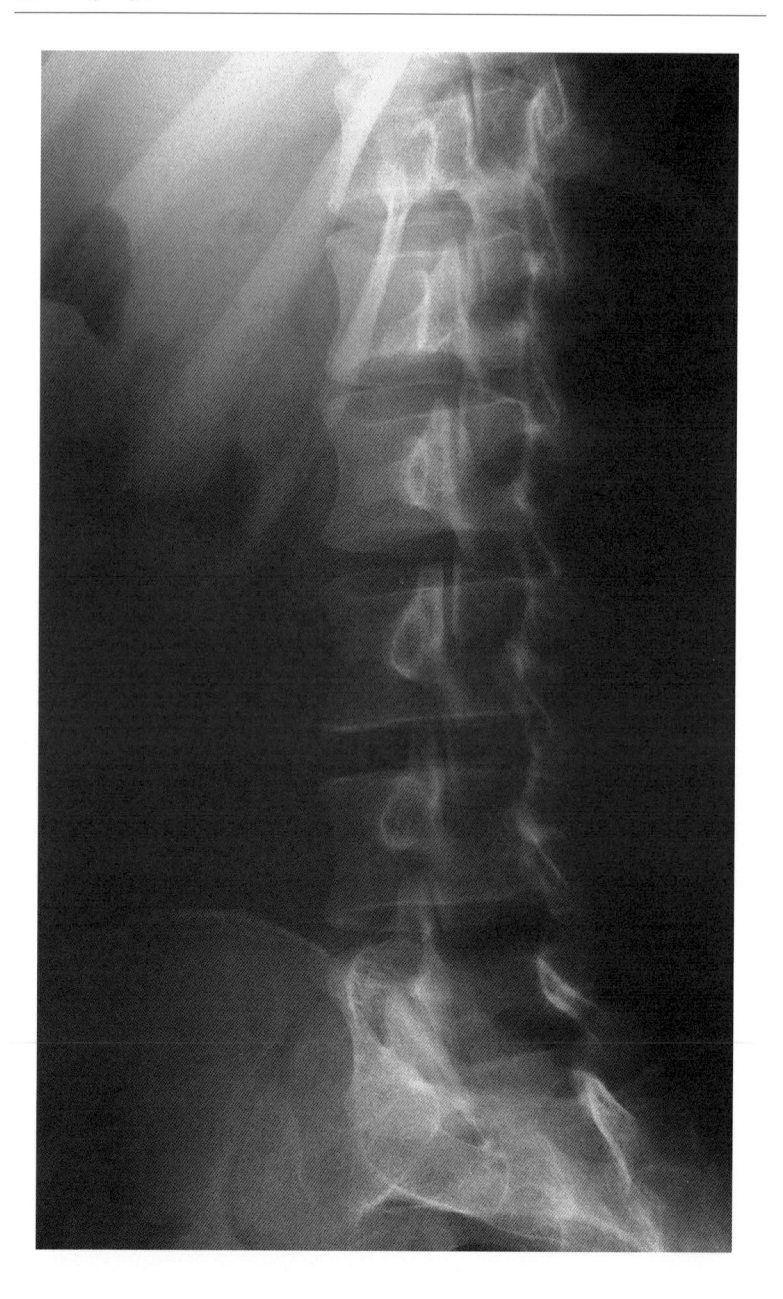

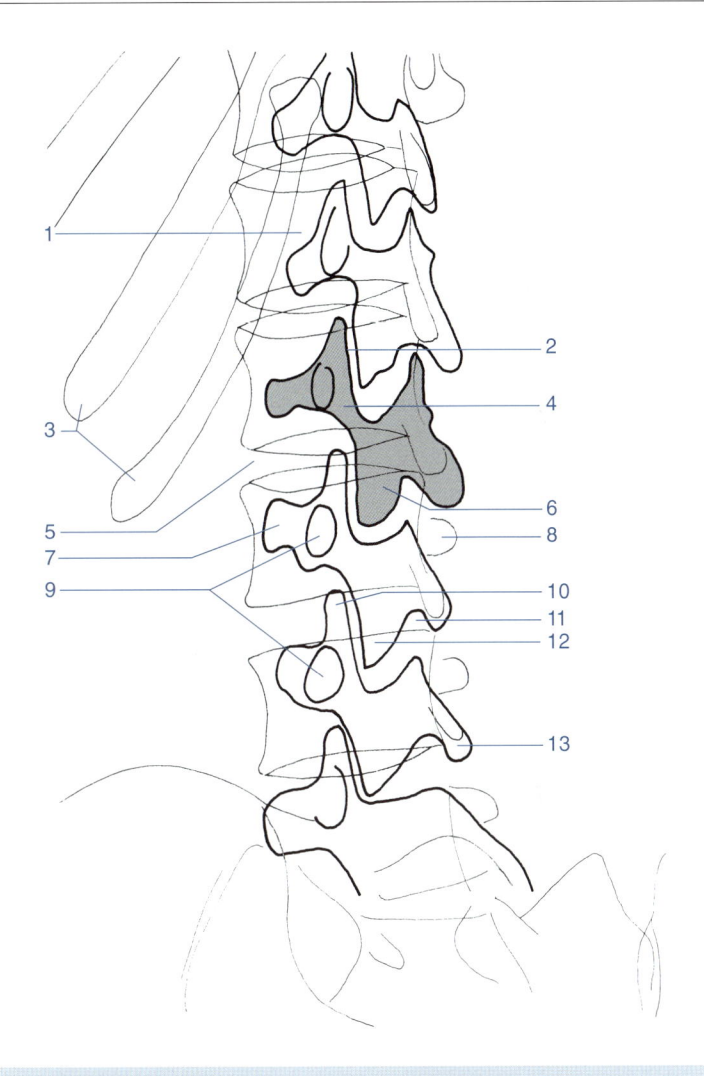

腰椎　斜位

1 椎体 Body of vertebra
2 椎間板腔 Intervertebral disk space
3 肋骨 Ribs
4 関節突起間部 Interarticular part
5 椎間板腔 Intervertebral disk space
6 椎弓板 Lamina
7 同側の横突起 Ipsilateral transverse process
8 対側の横突起 Contralateral transverse process
9 椎弓根 Pedicle
10 上関節突起 Superior articular process
11 椎間孔 Intervertebral foramen
12 下関節突起 Inferior articular process
13 棘突起 Spinous process

60　脊　椎

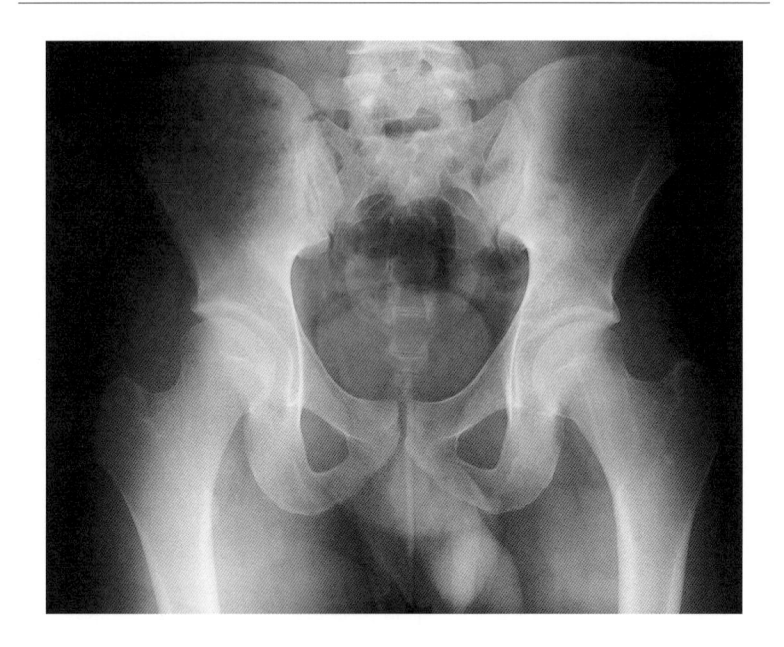

骨盤　正面（前後）

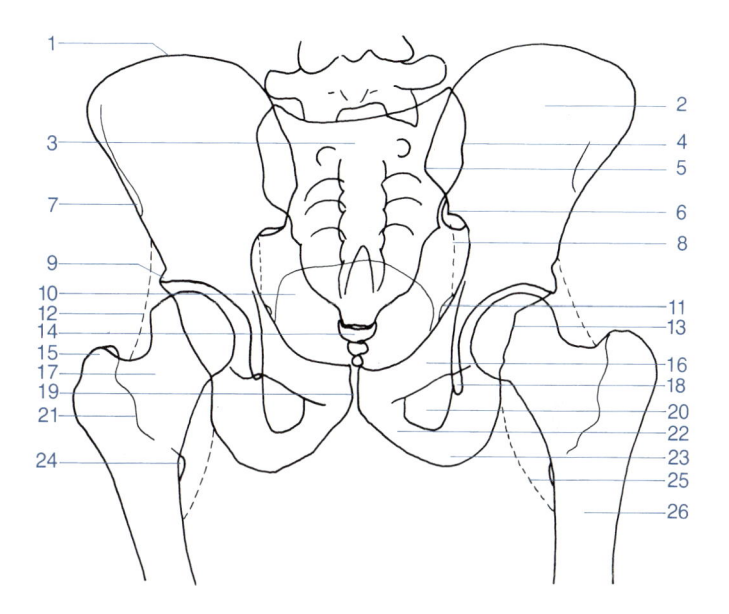

1	腸骨稜 Iliac crest
2	腸骨翼 Iliac wing
3	仙骨 Sacrum
4	仙腸関節 Sacroiliac joint
5	上後腸骨棘 Posterior superior iliac spine
6	下後腸骨棘 Posterior inferior iliac spine
7	上前腸骨棘 Anterior superior iliac spine
8	内閉鎖筋 Internal obturator muscle
9	寛骨臼蓋 Acetabular convexity（白蓋嘴 Promontory）
10	膀胱 Urinary bladder
11	坐骨棘 Spine of the ischium
12	小殿筋内側の脂肪線 Fat stripe medial to the gluteus minimus
13	寛骨臼後縁 Posterior acetabular rim
14	尾骨 Coccyx
15	大転子 Greater trochanter
16	恥骨上枝 Superior pubic ramus
17	大腿骨頸 Femoral neck
18	寛骨涙痕 Acetabular teardrop
19	恥骨結合 Pubic symphysis
20	閉鎖孔 Obturator foramen
21	転子間稜 Intertrochanteric crest
22	恥骨下枝 Inferior pubic ramus
23	坐骨結節 Ischial tuberosity
24	小転子 Lesser trochanter
25	腸腰筋内側の脂肪線 Fat stripe medial to the iliopsoas
26	大腿骨 Femur

62　脊　椎

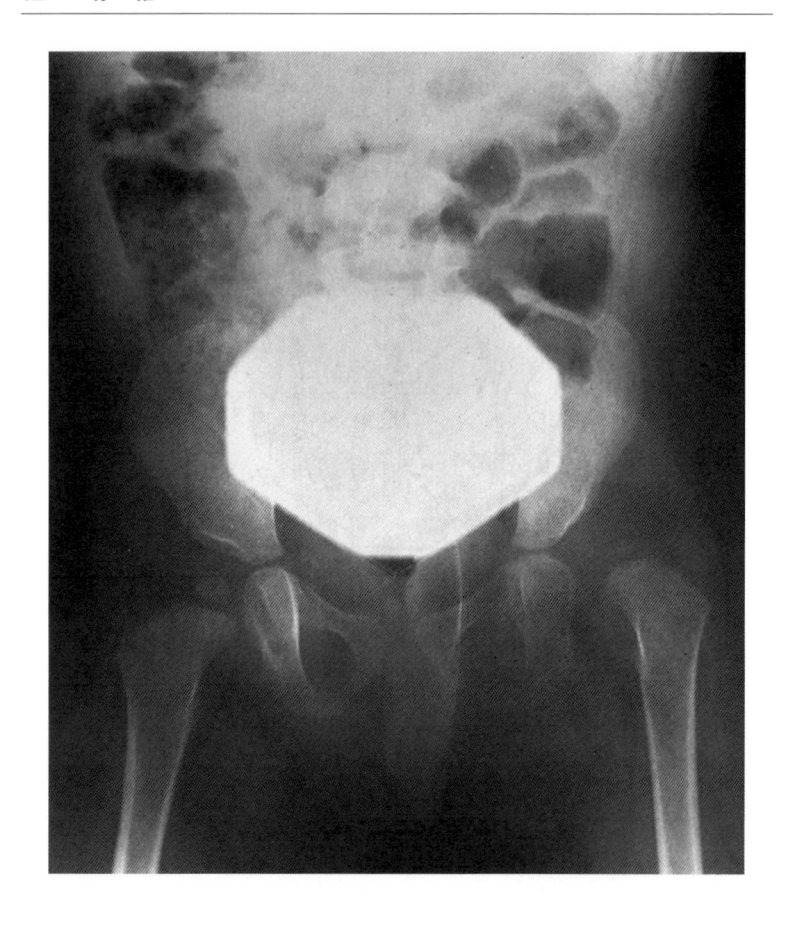

小児骨盤　正面（前後）

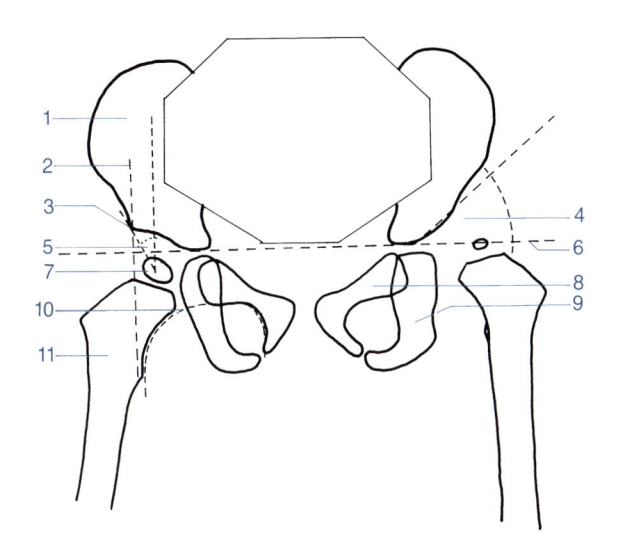

1 腸骨 Ilium
2 **Perkin線** Perkin's line
　臼蓋嘴から Hilgenreiner 線におろした垂線
3 **寛骨臼蓋** Acetabular convexity
　（臼蓋嘴 Promontory）
4 **臼蓋傾斜角** Angle of acetabular inclination
5 **WibergのCE角** Wiberg's center-to-corner angle
　骨端中心からおろした垂線と臼蓋と骨端中心を結ぶ線のなす角
6 **Hilgenreiner線** Hilgenreiner's line
　両側の Y 軟骨を結ぶ線
7 **大腿骨骨端** Femoral epiphysis
8 **恥骨** Pubic bone
9 **坐骨** Ischium
10 **Shenton線** Shenton's line
　閉鎖孔の上縁と大腿骨頸部を結ぶ曲線
11 **大腿骨** Femur

64 脊 椎

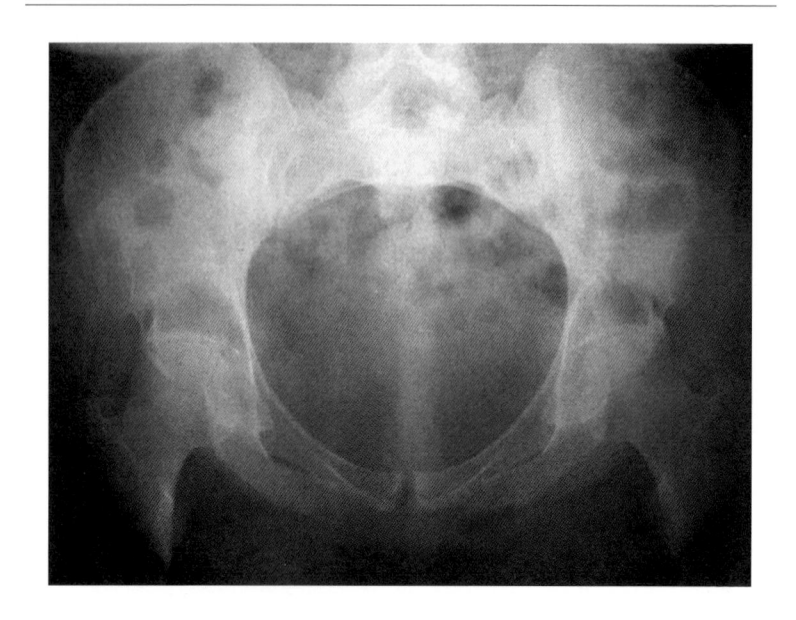

骨盤　入口撮影（インレット）　　**65**

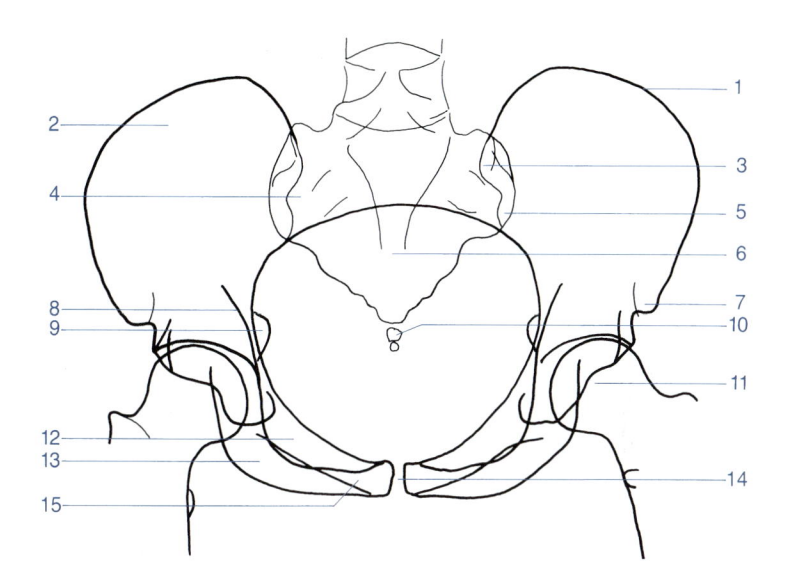

1　腸骨稜　Iliac crest
2　腸骨翼　Iliac wing
3　上後腸骨棘　Posterior superior iliac spine
4　仙骨翼　Sacral wing
5　下後腸骨棘　Posterior inferior iliac spine
6　仙骨　Sacrum
7　上前腸骨棘　Anterior superior iliac spine
8　腸骨恥骨線　Iliopubic line
9　坐骨棘　Spine of the ischium
10　尾骨　Coccyx
11　大腿骨頭　Femoral head
12　恥骨上枝　Superior pubic ramus
13　坐骨結節　Ischial tuberosity
14　恥骨結合　Pubic symphysis
15　恥骨下枝　Inferior pubic ramus

66　脊　椎

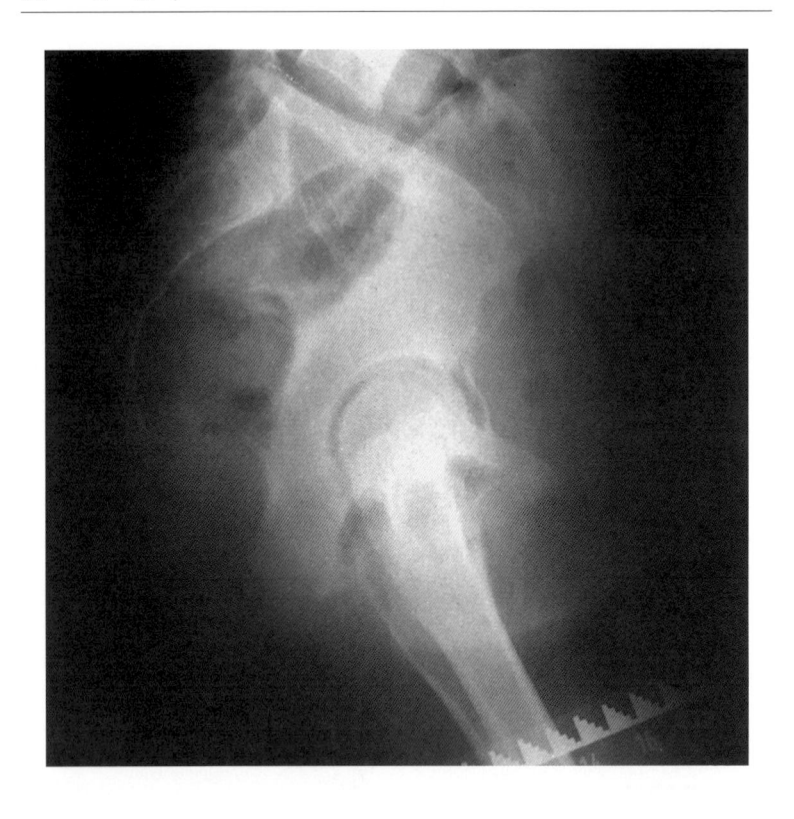

骨盤 Guthmann法

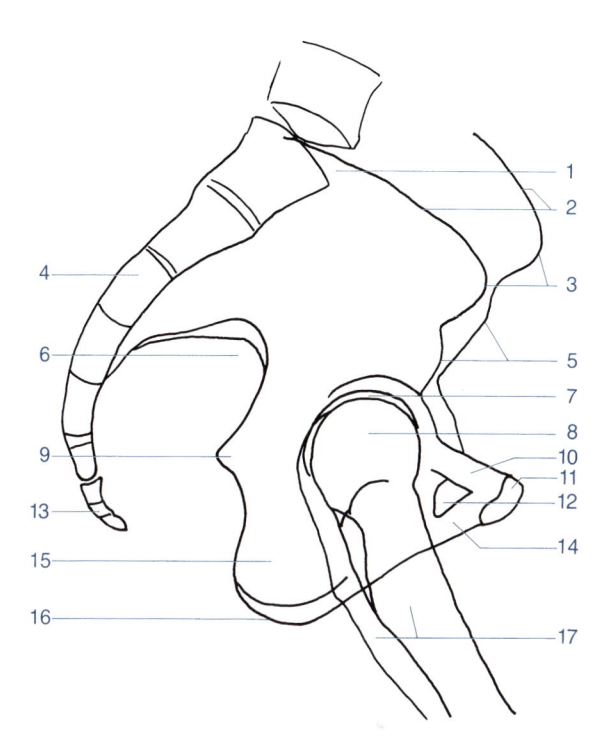

1 岬角 Promontory
2 腸骨稜 Iliac crest
3 上前腸骨棘 Anterior superior iliac spine
4 仙骨 Sacrum
5 下前腸骨棘 Anterior inferior iliac spine
6 大坐骨切痕 Greater sciatic notch
7 股関節腔 Joint space of the hip
8 大腿骨頭 Femoral head
9 坐骨棘 Spine of the ischium
10 恥骨上枝 Superior pubic ramus
11 恥骨結合 Pubic symphysis
12 閉鎖孔 Obturator foramen
13 尾骨 Coccyx
14 恥骨下枝 Inferior pubic ramus
15 坐骨体 Body of the ischium
16 坐骨結節 Ischial tuberosity
17 大腿骨 Femur

68　脊　椎

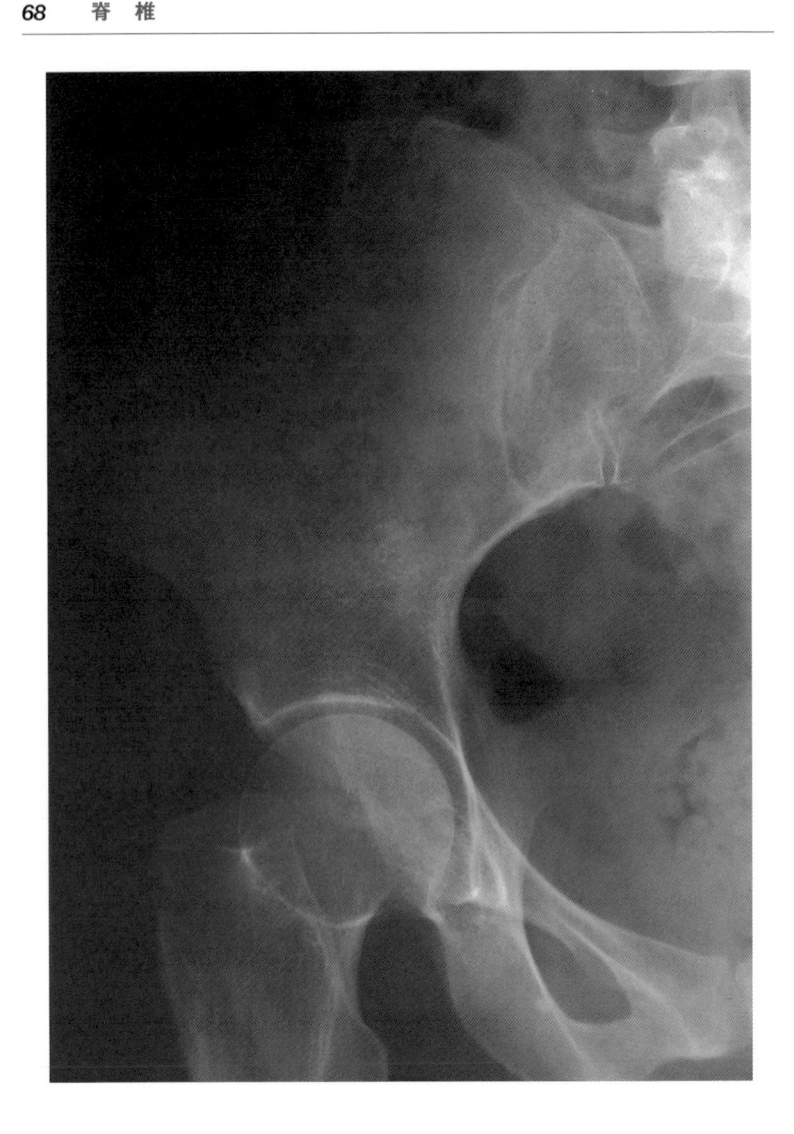

骨盤　腸骨翼斜位

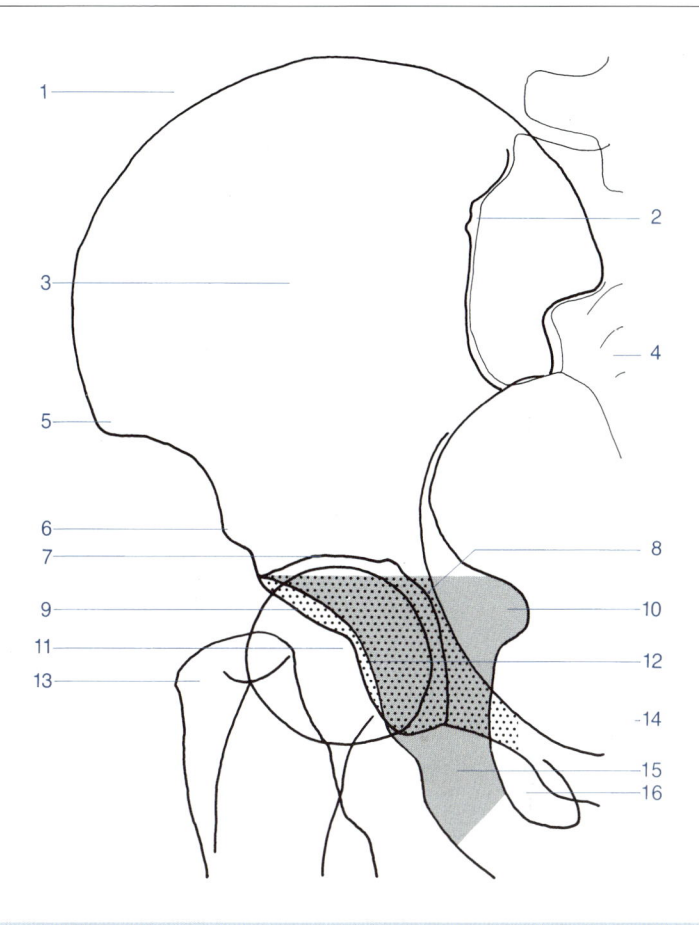

1　腸骨稜 Iliac crest	9　寛骨臼前縁 Anterior acetabular rim
2　仙腸関節 Sacroiliac joint	10　坐骨棘 Spine of the ischium
3　腸骨翼 Iliac wing	11　大腿骨頭 Femoral head
4　仙骨 Sacrum	12　寛骨臼後縁 Posterior acetabular rim
5　上前腸骨棘 Anterior superior iliac spine	13　大転子 Greater trochanter
6　下前腸骨棘 Anterior inferior iliac spine	14　恥骨 Pubis（前柱 Anterior column）
7　臼蓋 Roof of the acetabulum	15　坐骨 Ischium（後柱 Posterior column）
8　臼底 Floor of the acetabulum	16　閉鎖孔 Obturator foramen

70　脊　椎

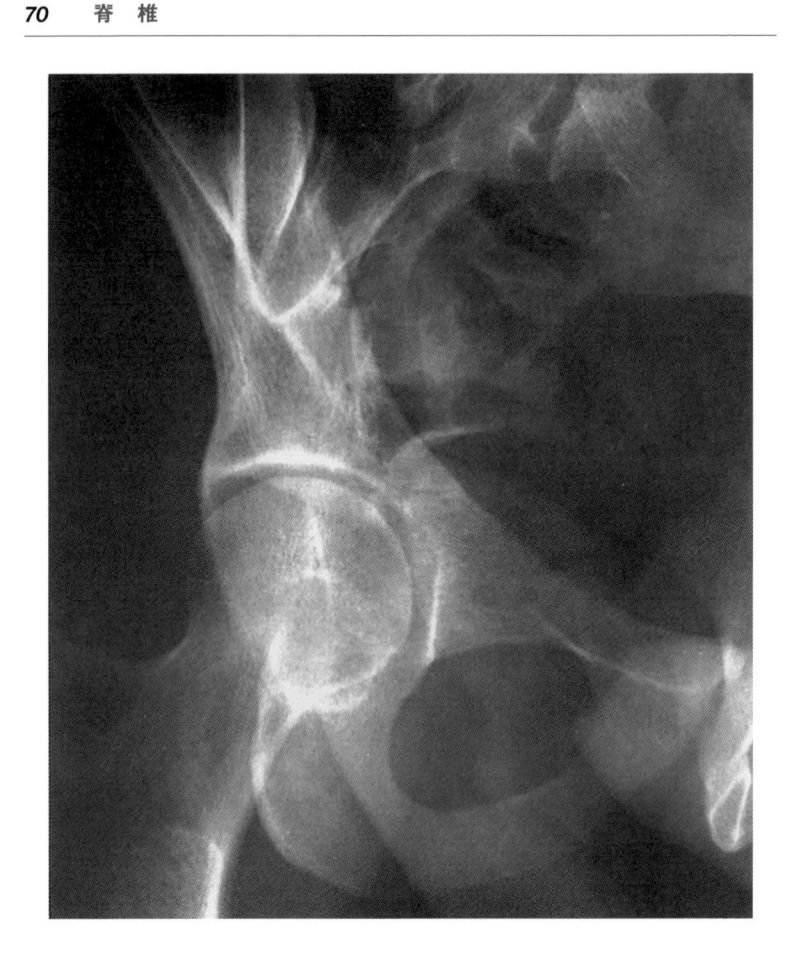

骨盤　閉鎖孔斜位

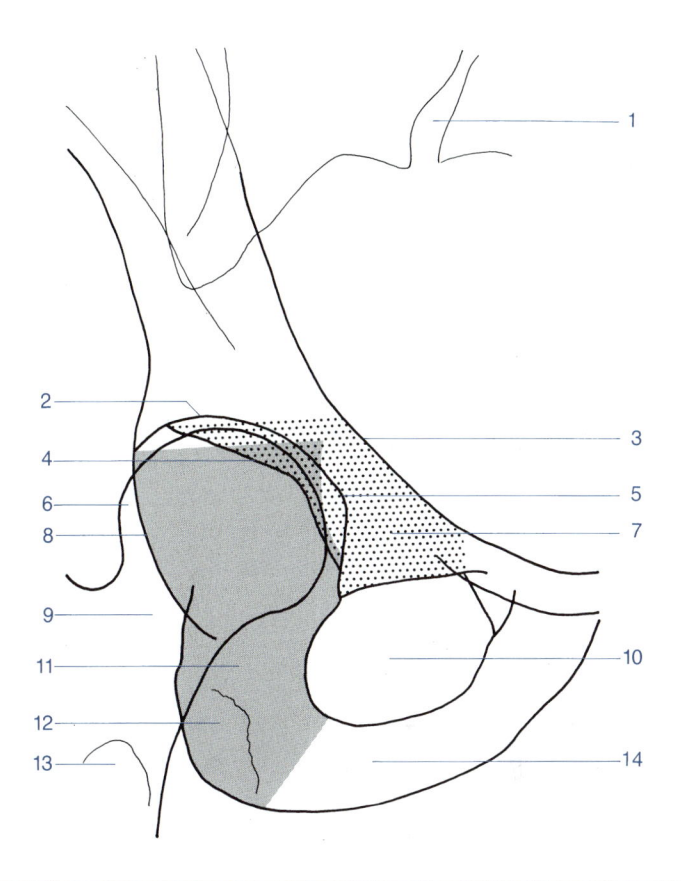

1　仙腸関節 Sacroiliac joint	8　寛骨臼後縁 Posterior acetabular rim
2　臼蓋 Roof of the acetabulum	9　大腿骨頸 Femoral neck
3　腸骨恥骨線 Iliopectineal line	10　閉鎖孔 Obturator foramen
4　寛骨臼前縁 Anterior acetabular rim	11　坐骨 Ischium(後柱 Posterior column)
5　臼底前部 Anterior acetabular floor	12　坐骨結節 Ischial tuberosity
6　大腿骨頭 Femoral head	13　小転子 Lesser trochanter
7　恥骨 Pubis(前柱 Anterior column)	14　恥骨下枝 Inferior pubic ramus

72　脊 椎

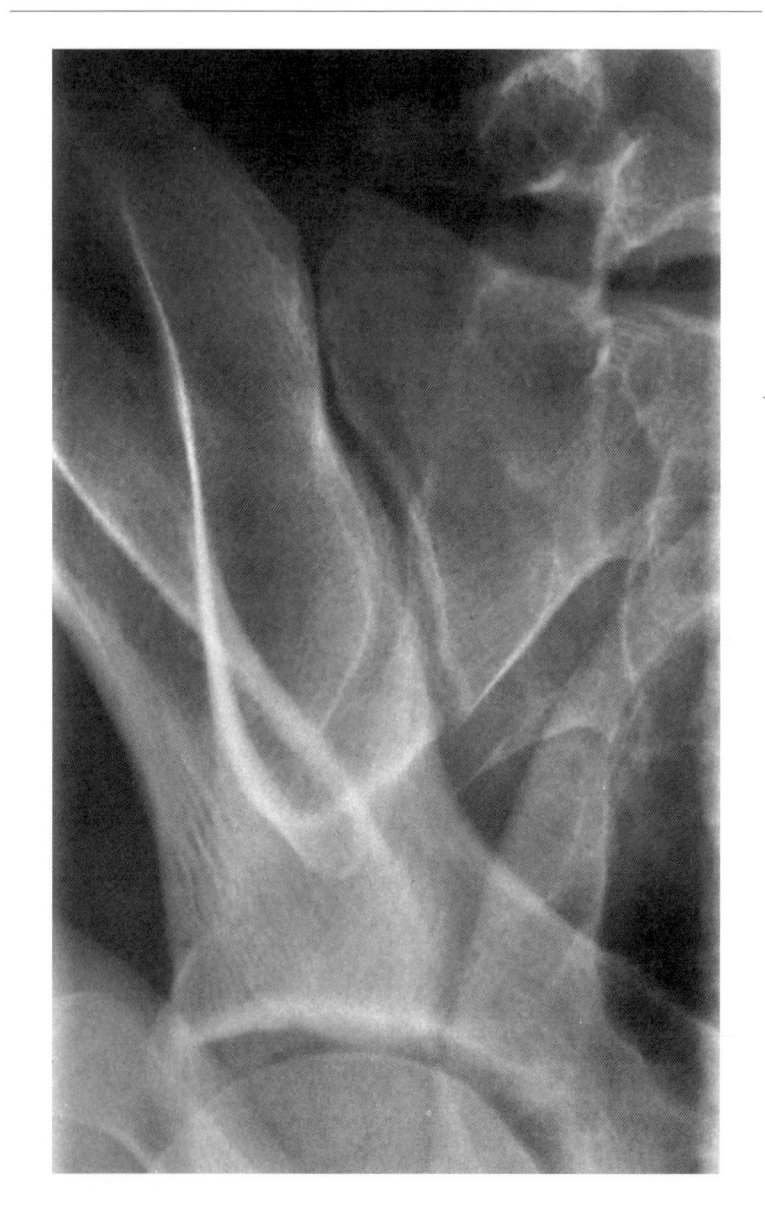

仙腸関節 30°前斜位

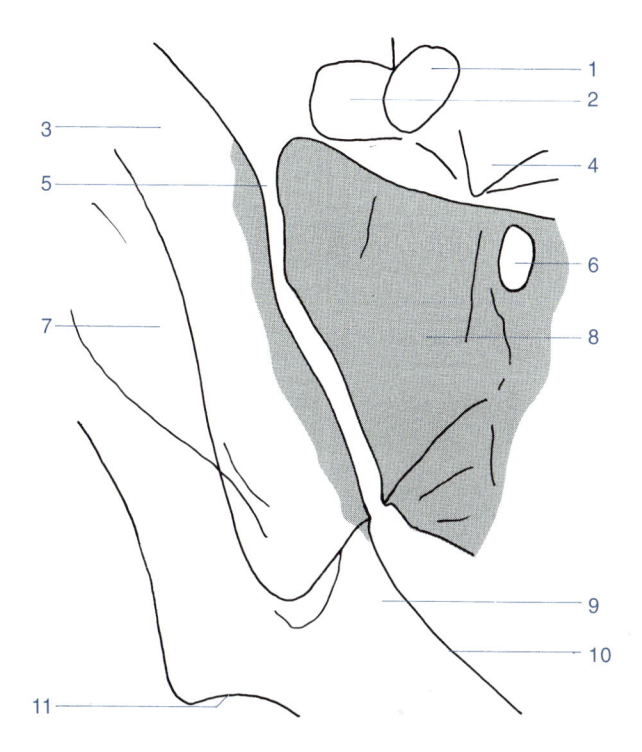

1 第5腰椎椎弓根 Pedicle of L5	7 腸骨翼 Iliac wing
2 第5腰椎横突起 Transverse process of L5	8 仙骨外側部 Lateral part of the sacrum
3 腸骨翼 Iliac wing	9 腸骨 Ilium
4 第5腰椎椎体 Body of vertebra L5	10 弓状線 Arcuate line
5 仙腸関節 Sacroiliac joint	11 臼蓋 Roof of the acetabulum
6 仙骨孔 Sacral foramen	

74　脊　椎

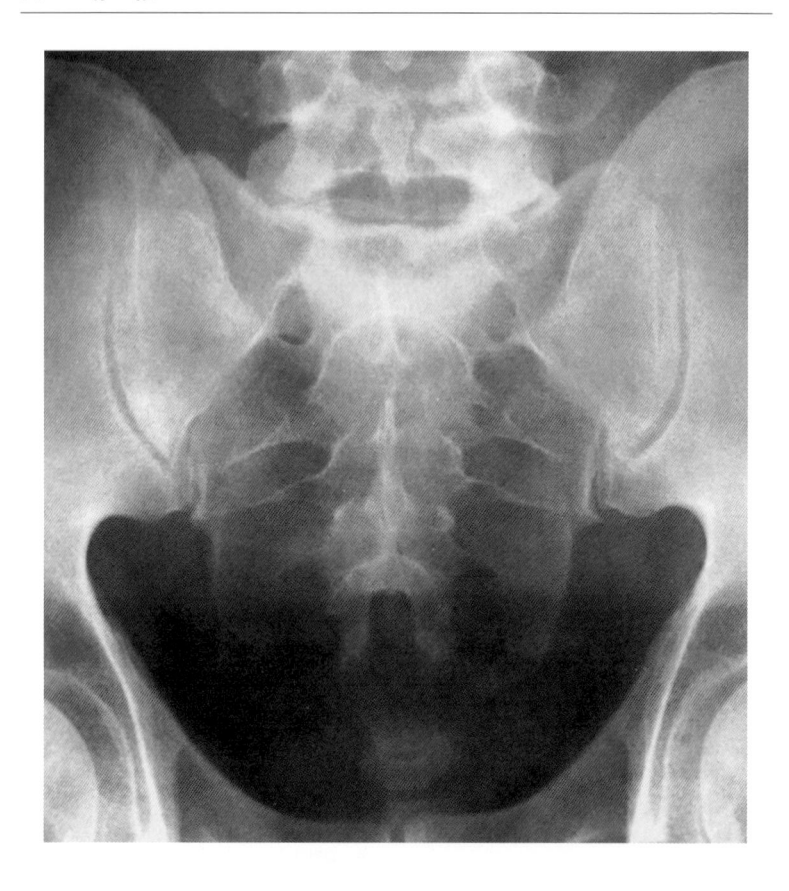

仙骨　正面（前後）

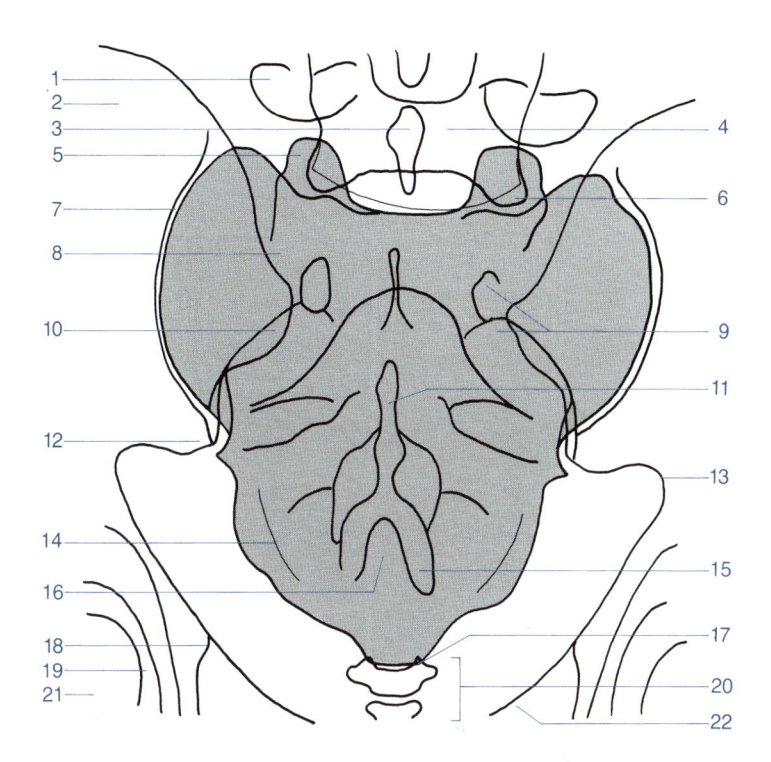

1 横突起　Transverse process
2 腸骨翼　Iliac wing
3 棘突起　Spinous process
4 第5腰椎　L5
5 上関節突起　Superior articular process
6 第5腰椎関節突起　Inferior articular process of L5
7 仙腸関節　Sacroiliac joint
8 仙骨翼　Sacral wing
9 仙骨孔　Sacral foramen
10 上後腸骨棘　Posterior superior iliac spine
11 正中仙骨稜　Median sacral crest
12 下後腸骨棘　Posterior inferior iliac spine
13 大坐骨切痕　Greater sciatic notch
14 外側仙骨稜　Lateral sacral crest
15 仙骨角　Cornu of the sacrum
16 仙骨裂孔　Sacral hiatus
17 尾骨角　Cornu of the coccyx
18 坐骨棘　Spine of the ischium
19 股関節　Hip joint
20 尾骨　Coccyx
21 大腿骨頭　Femoral head
22 恥骨上枝　Superior pubic ramus

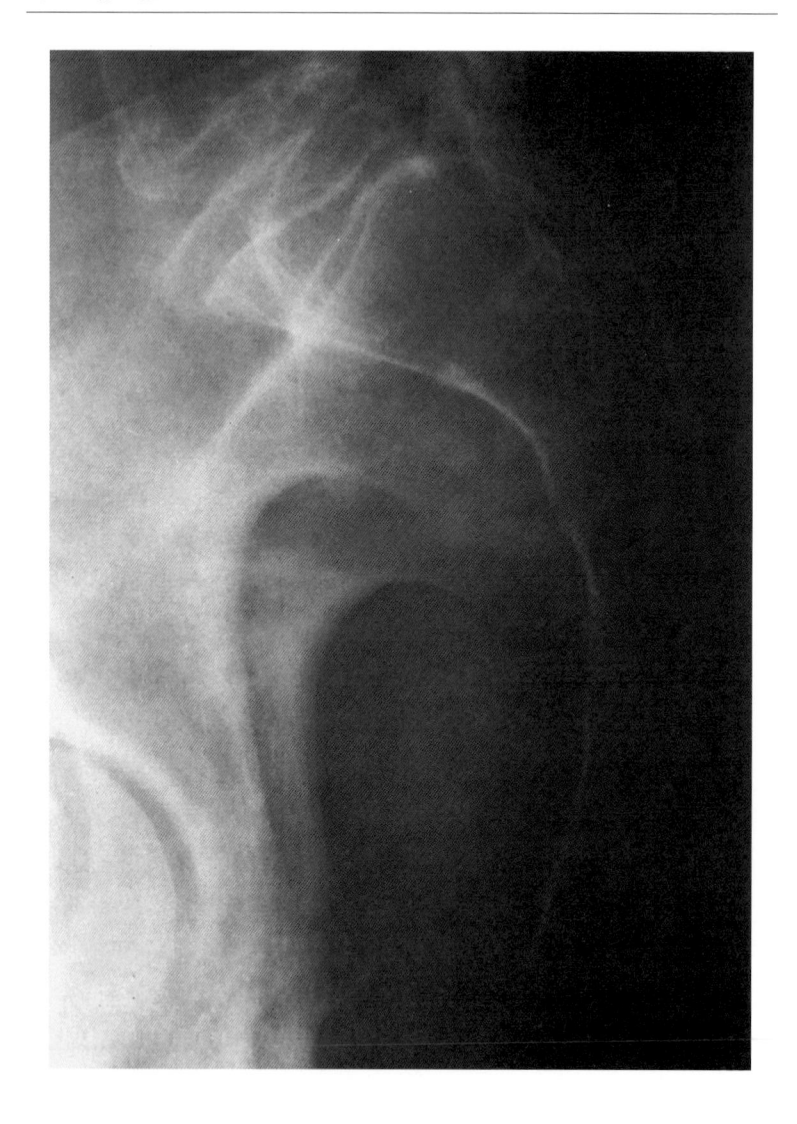

脊 椎

仙骨　側面

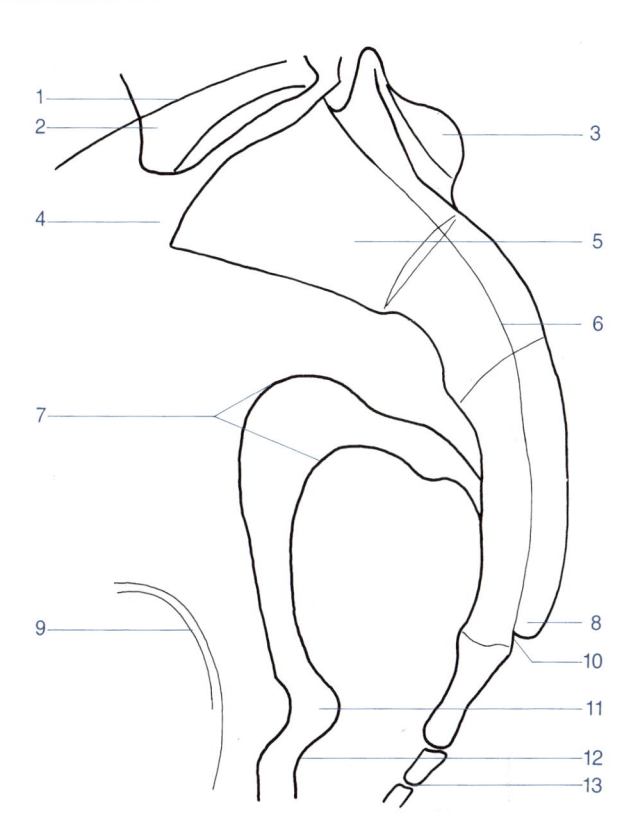

1　腸骨稜　Iliac crest	8　仙骨角　Cornu of the sacrum
2　第5腰椎　L5	9　股関節　Hip joint
3　正中仙骨稜　Median sacral crest	10　仙骨管　Sacral canal
4　岬角　Promontory	11　坐骨棘　Spine of the ischium
5　仙骨　Sacrum	12　小坐骨切痕　Lesser sciatic notch
6　仙骨管　Sacral canal	13　尾骨　Coccyx
7　大坐骨切痕　Greater sciatic notch	

78 脊 椎

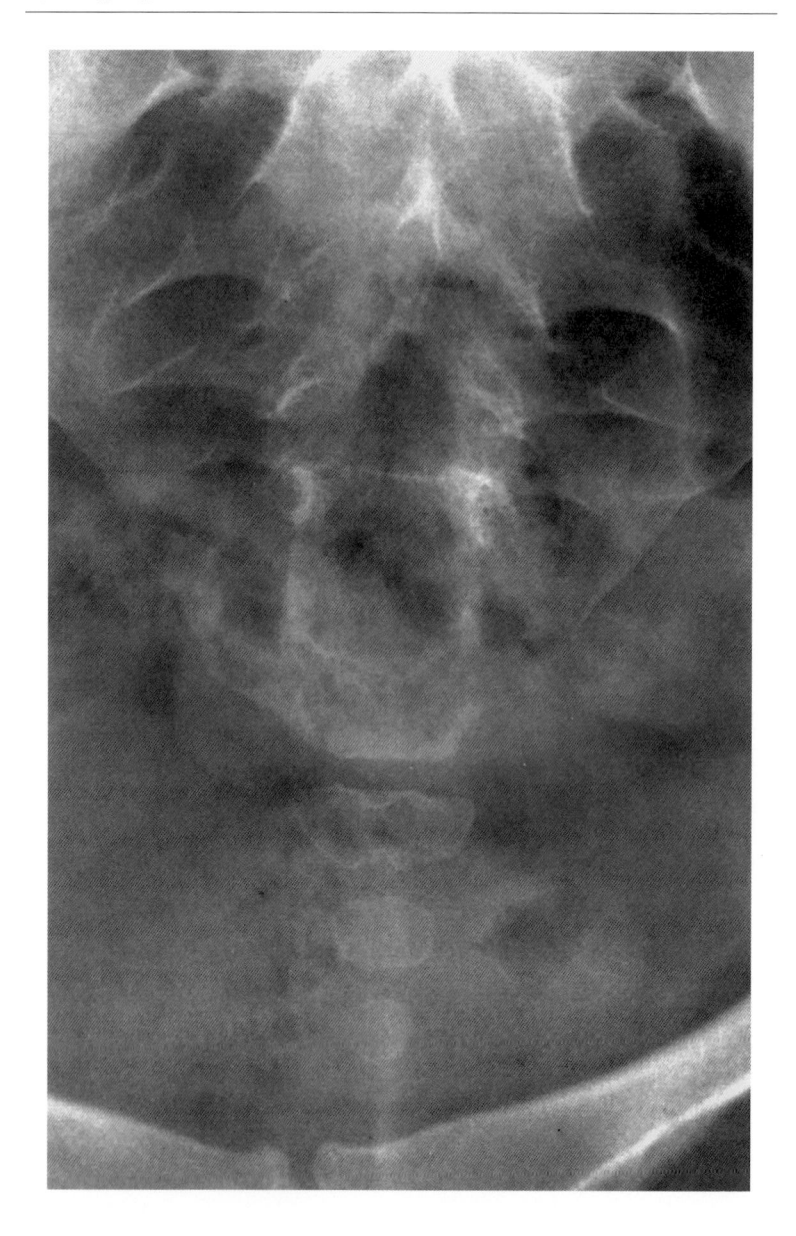

尾骨　正面（前後）　79

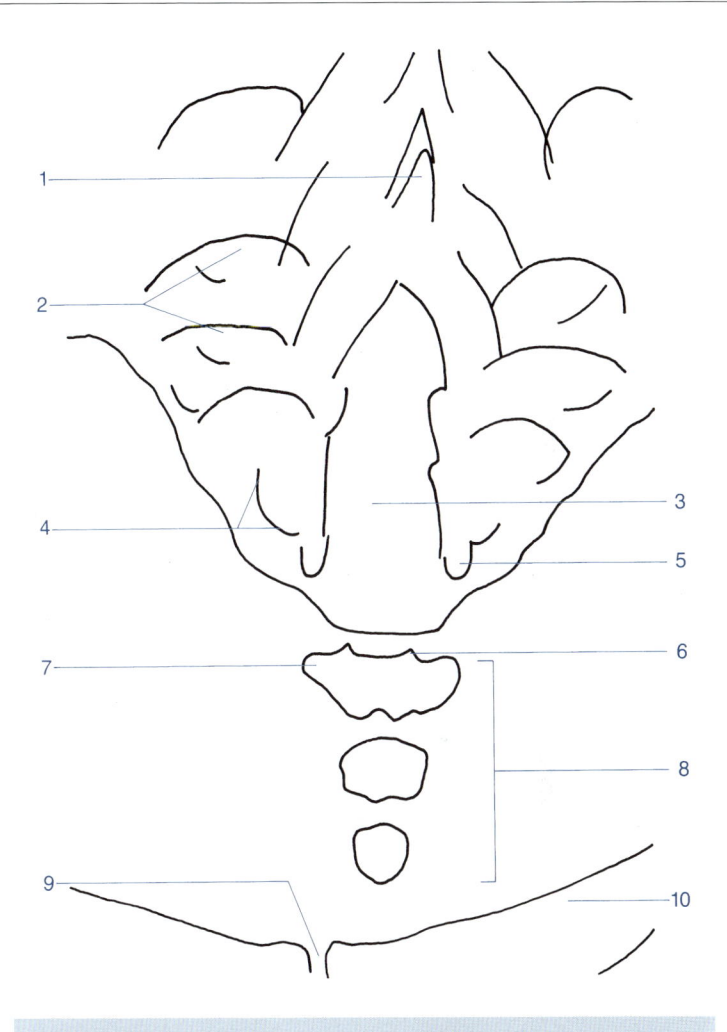

1　正中仙骨稜 Median sacral crest	6　尾骨角 Cornu of the coccyx
2　仙骨孔 Sacral foramen	7　横突起 Transverse process
3　仙骨裂孔 Sacral hiatus	8　尾骨 Coccyx
4　外側仙骨稜 Lateral sacral crest	9　恥骨結合 Pubic symphysis
5　仙骨角 Cornu of the sacrum	10　恥骨上枝 Superior pubic ramus

80 脊 椎

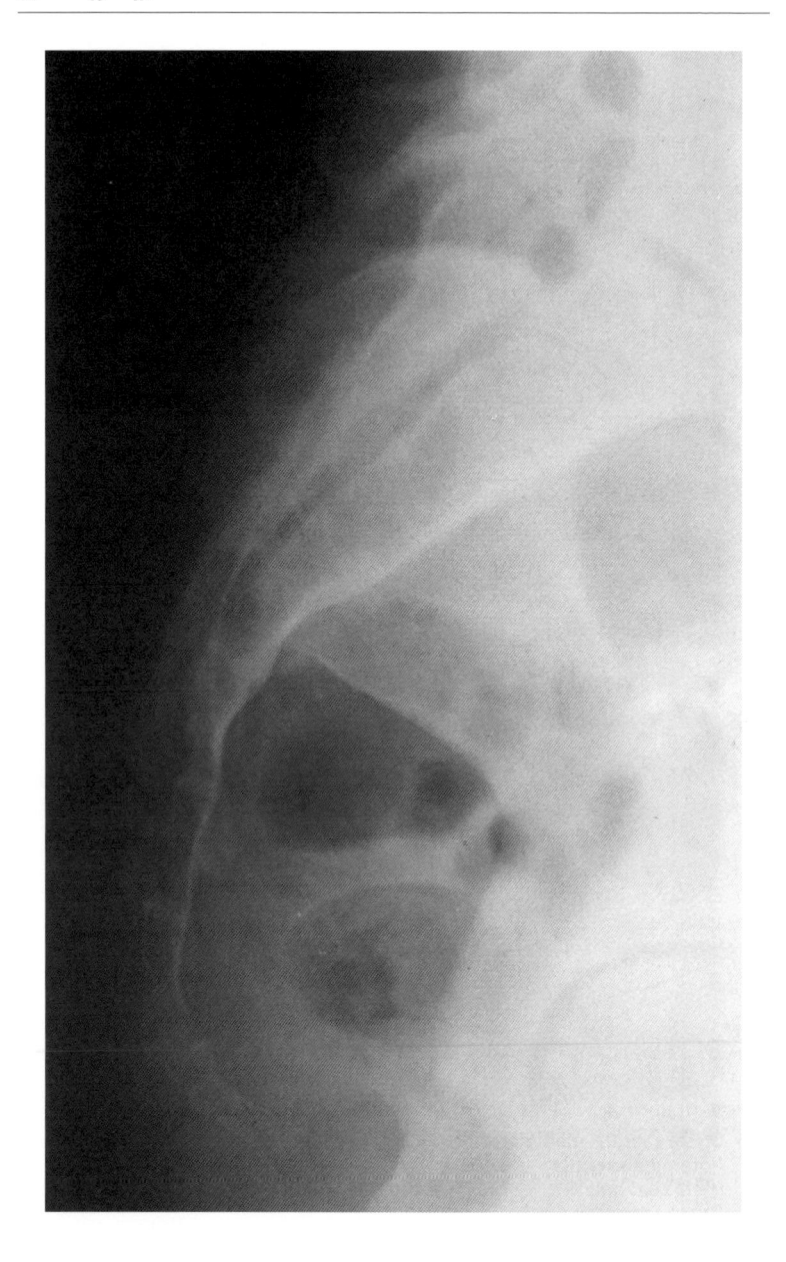

尾骨　側面　81

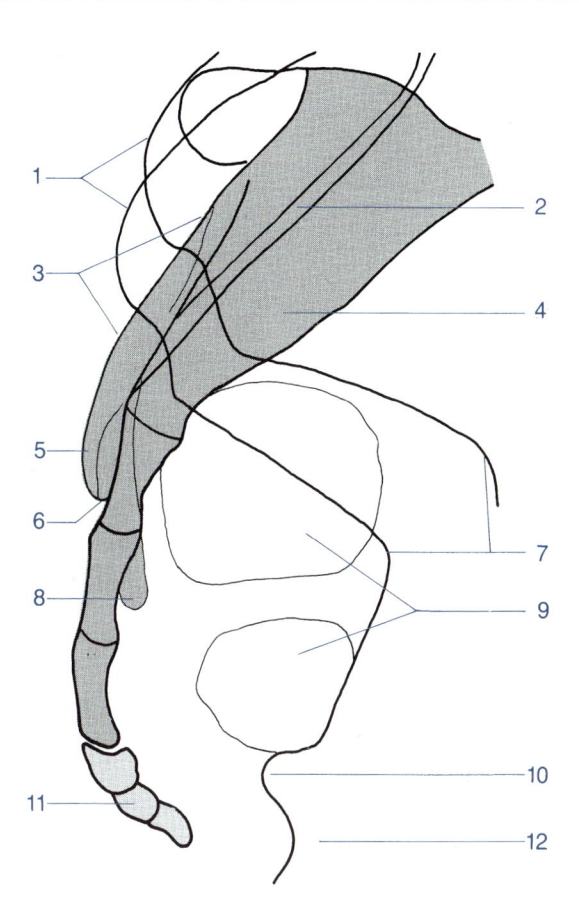

1　腸骨稜　Iliac crest	7　大坐骨切痕　Greater sciatic notch
2　仙骨管　Sacral canal	8　外側仙骨稜　Lateral sacral crest
3　正中仙骨稜　Median sacral crest	9　直腸ガス　Rectal gas
4　仙骨　Sacrum	10　坐骨棘　Spine of the ischium
5　仙骨角　Cornu of the sacrum	11　尾骨　Coccyx
6　仙骨管　Sacral canal	12　坐骨　Ischium

82 上　肢

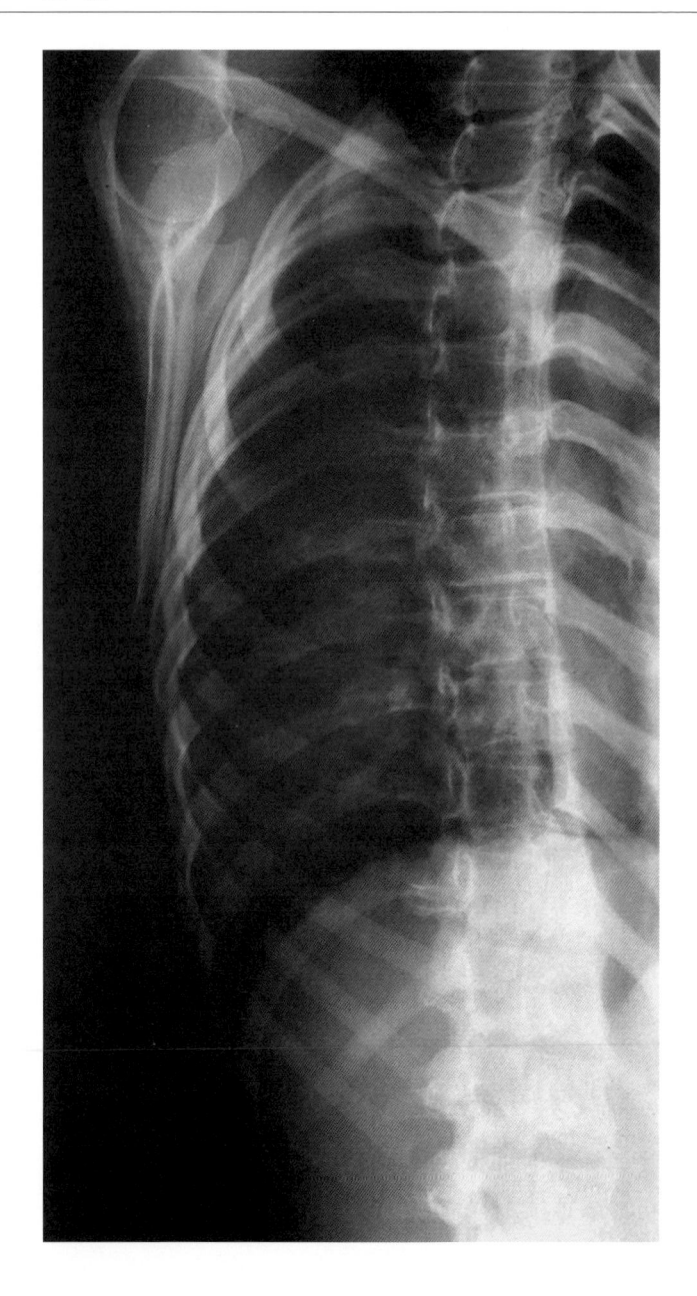

胸　郭　83

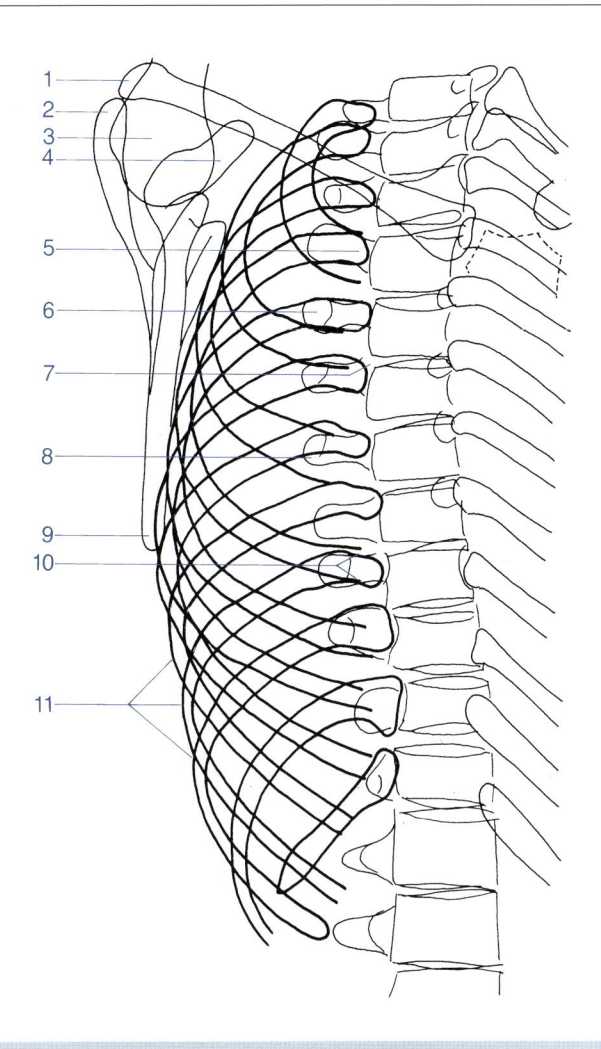

1　鎖骨　Clavicle	7　肋椎関節　Costovertebral joint
2　肩峰　Acromion	8　横突起　Transverse process
3　上腕骨頭　Humeral head	9　肩甲骨下角　Inferior angle of the scapula
4　烏口突起　Coracoid process	10　肋骨頸　Neck of the rib
5　肋骨頭　Head of the rib	11　肋骨　Costal arch
6　肋横突関節　Costotransverse joint	

84　上　肢

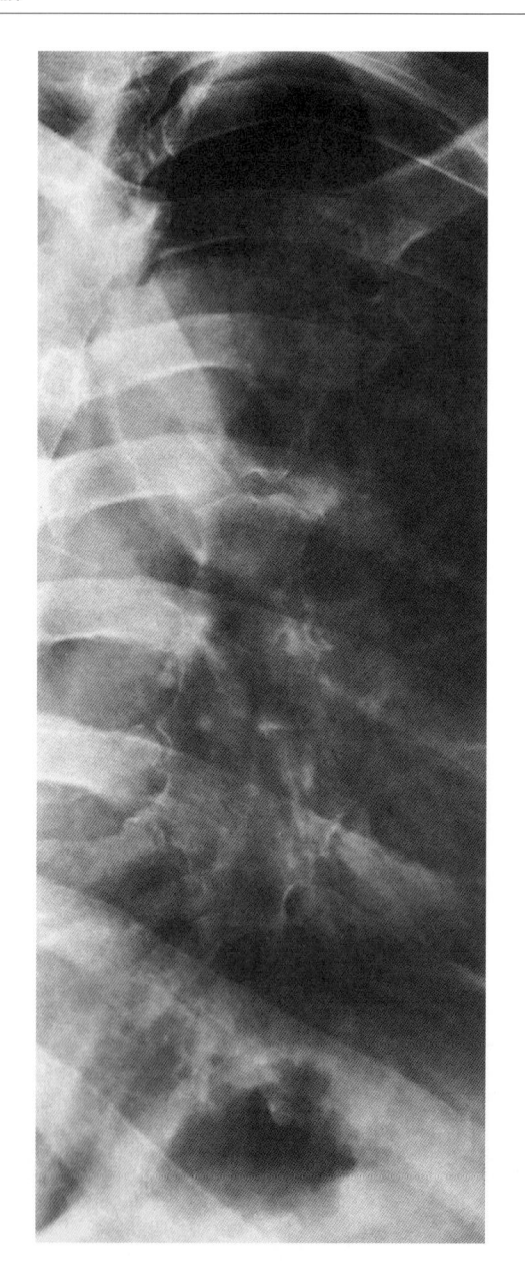

胸骨　正面（前後）

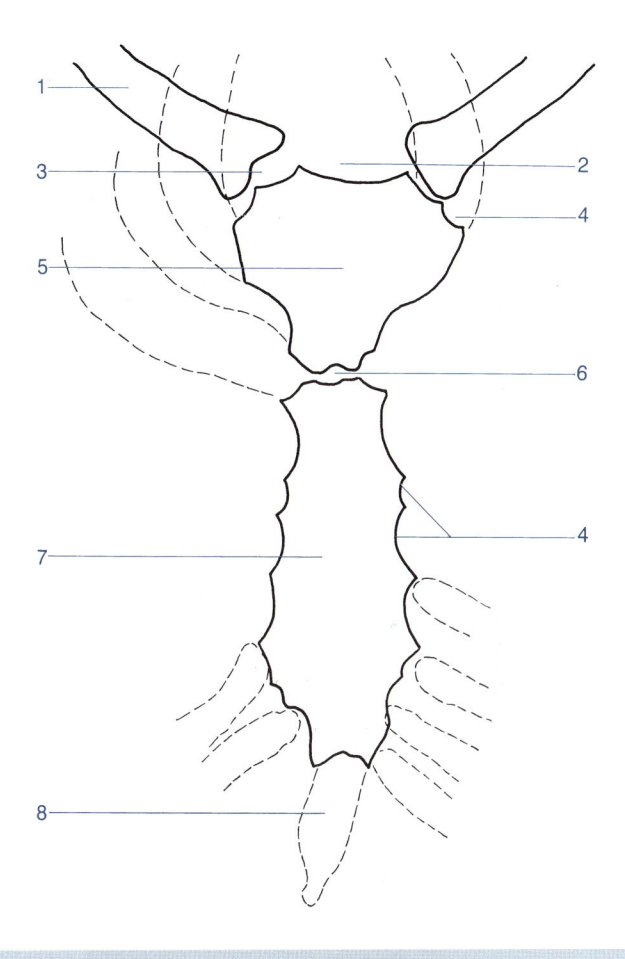

1　鎖骨　Clavicle	5　胸骨柄　Manubrium of the sternum
2　頸切痕　Suprasternal notch	6　胸骨角　Sternal angle
3　胸鎖関節　Sternoclavicular joint	7　胸骨体　Body of the sternum
4　肋骨切痕　Costal notch	8　剣状突起　Xiphoid process

86 上　肢

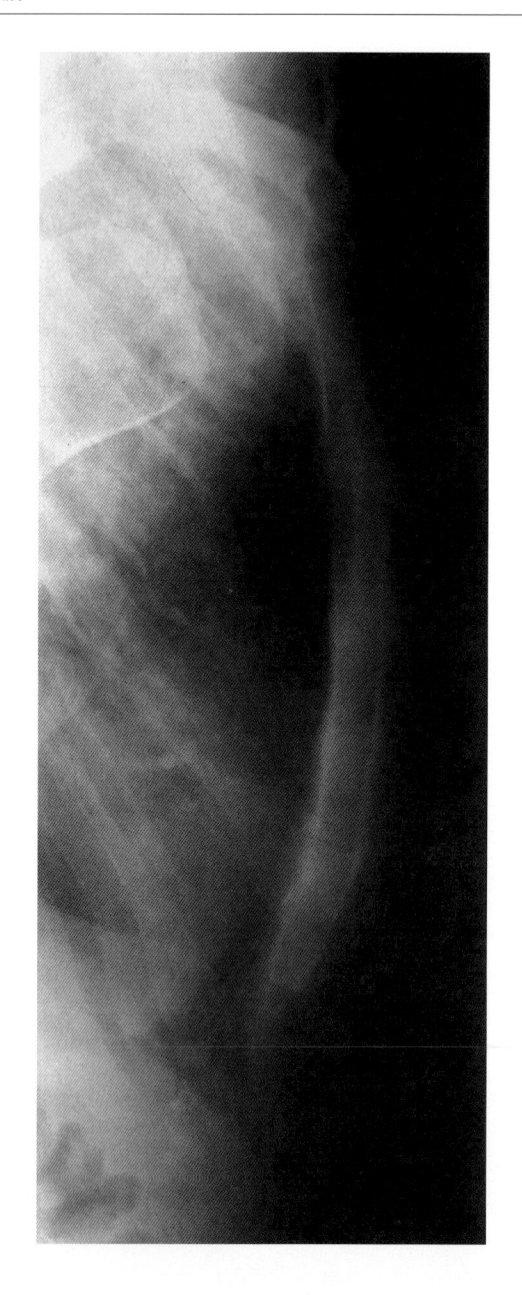

胸骨 側面 87

1	鎖骨 Clavicles	4	胸骨後腔 Retrosternal space
2	胸骨柄 Manubrium of the sternum	5	胸骨体 Body of the sternum
3	胸骨角 Sternal angle	6	剣状突起 Xiphoid process

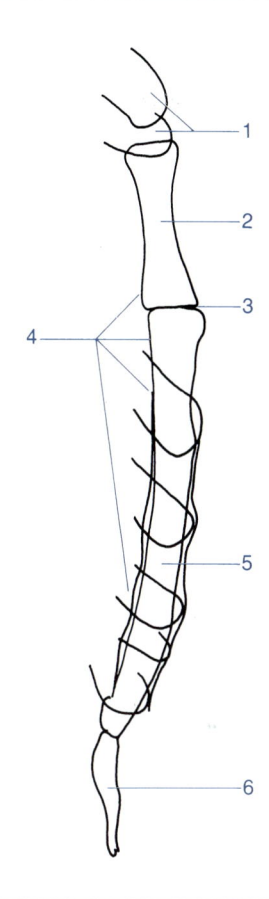

88　上　肢

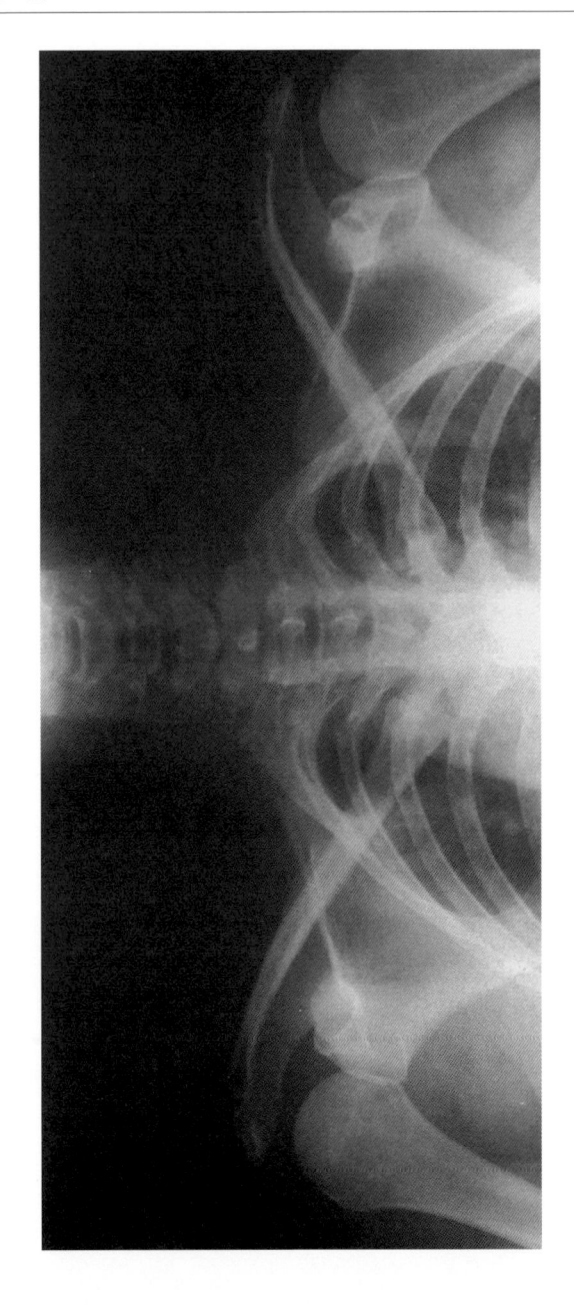

肩関節　ストレス撮影

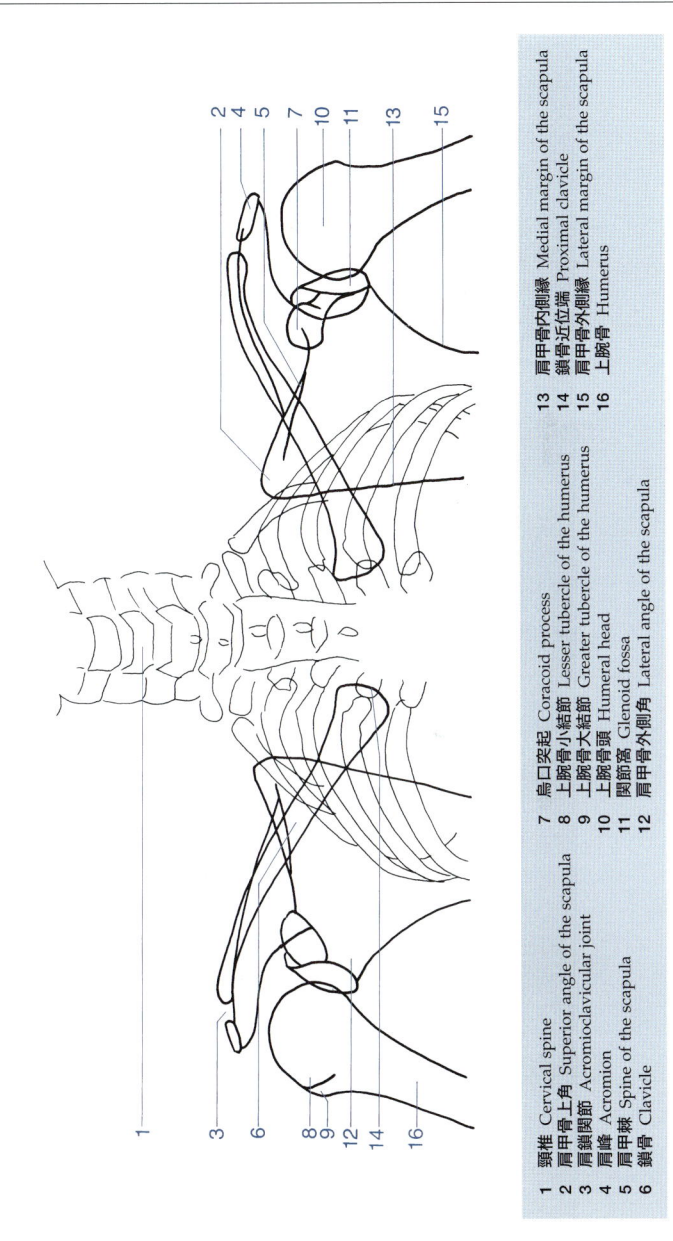

1	頸椎	Cervical spine
2	肩甲骨上角	Superior angle of the scapula
3	肩鎖関節	Acromioclavicular joint
4	肩峰	Acromion
5	肩甲棘	Spine of the scapula
6	鎖骨	Clavicle
7	烏口突起	Coracoid process
8	上腕骨小結節	Lesser tubercle of the humerus
9	上腕骨大結節	Greater tubercle of the humerus
10	上腕骨頭	Humeral head
11	関節窩	Glenoid fossa
12	肩甲骨外側角	Lateral angle of the scapula
13	肩甲骨内側縁	Medial margin of the scapula
14	鎖骨近位端	Proximal clavicle
15	肩甲骨外側縁	Lateral margin of the scapula
16	上腕骨	Humerus

90　上肢

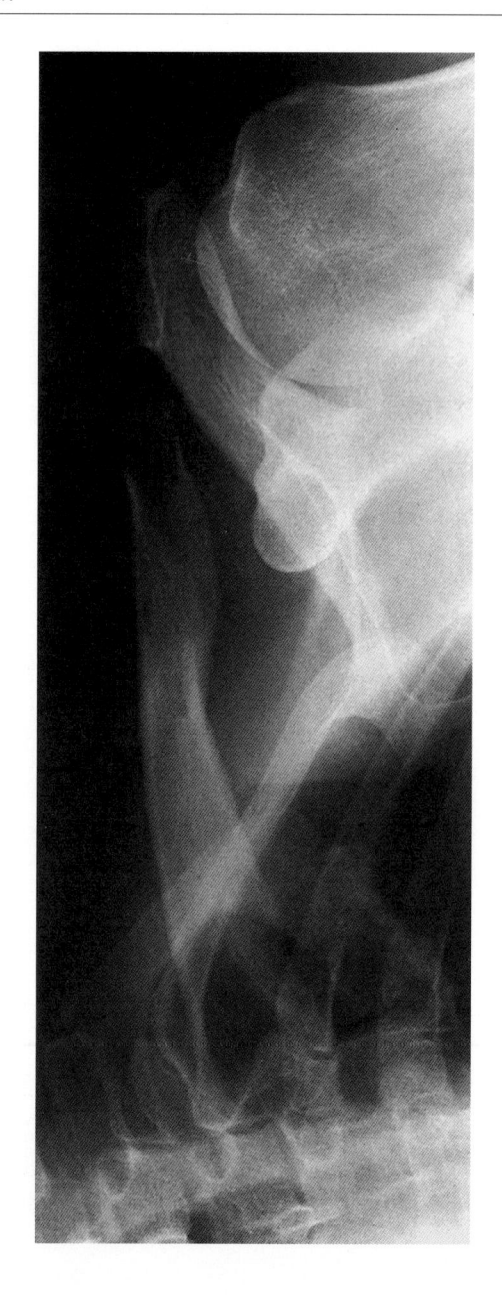

鎖骨　正面（前後）　91

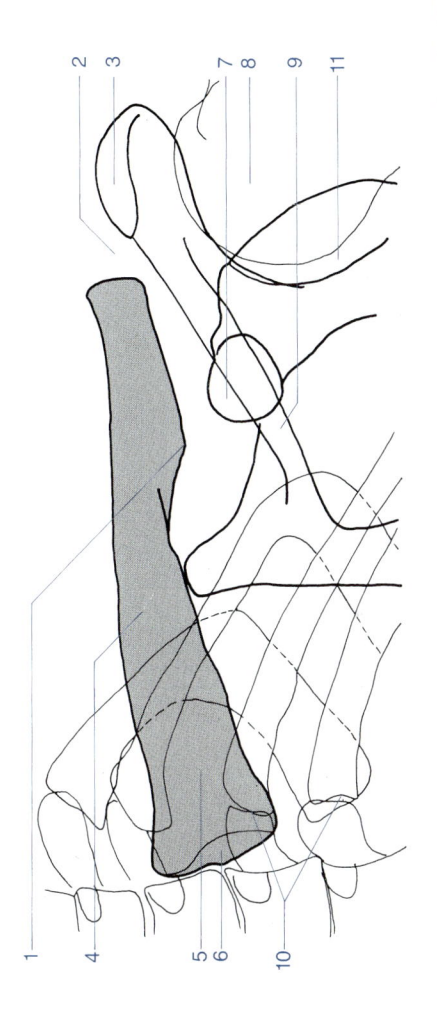

1 鎖骨円錐靭帯結節 Conoid tubercle of the clavicle
2 肩鎖関節 Acromioclavicular joint
3 肩峰 Acromion
4 鎖骨 Clavicle
5 肩甲骨上角 Superior angle of the scapula
6 鎖骨近位端 Proximal clavicle
7 烏口突起 Coracoid process
8 上腕骨頭 Humeral head
9 肩甲棘 Spine of the scapula
10 肋横突関節 Costotransverse joint
11 関節窩 Glenoid fossa

92 上 肢

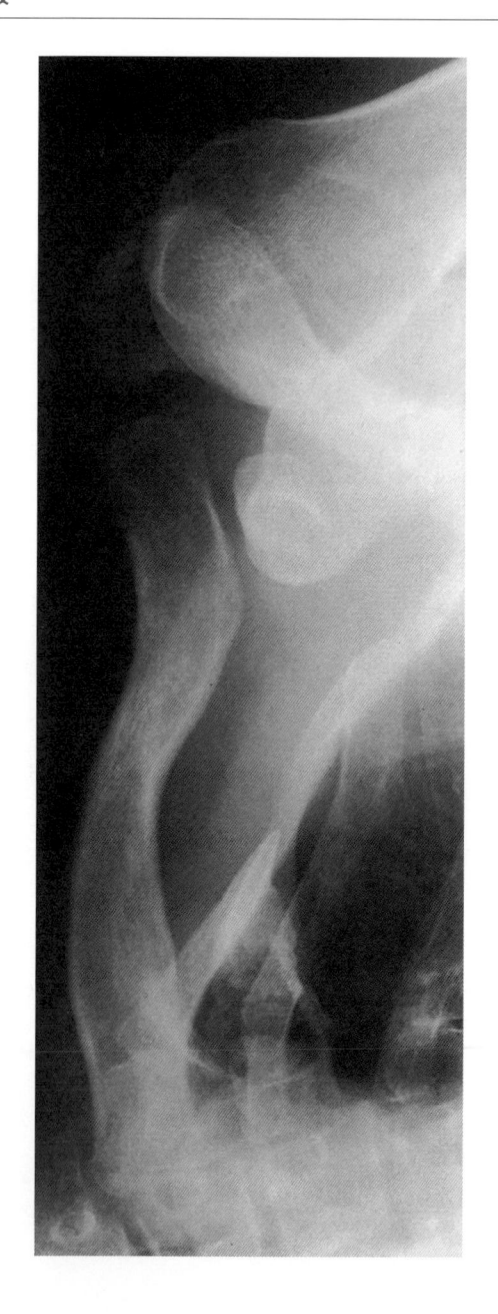

鎖骨　斜位　93

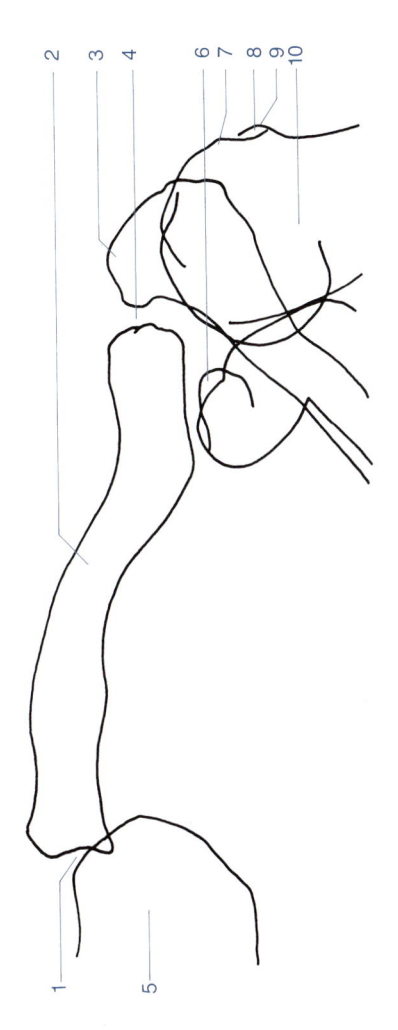

1 胸鎖関節 Sternoclavicular joint
2 鎖骨 Clavicle
3 肩峰 Acromion
4 肩鎖関節 Acromioclavicular joint
5 胸骨(柄) Sternum (manubrium)
6 烏口突起 Coracoid process
7 上腕骨大結節 Greater tubercle of the humerus
8 二頭筋溝 Bicipital groove
9 上腕骨小結節 Lesser tubercle of the humerus
10 上腕骨頭 Humeral head

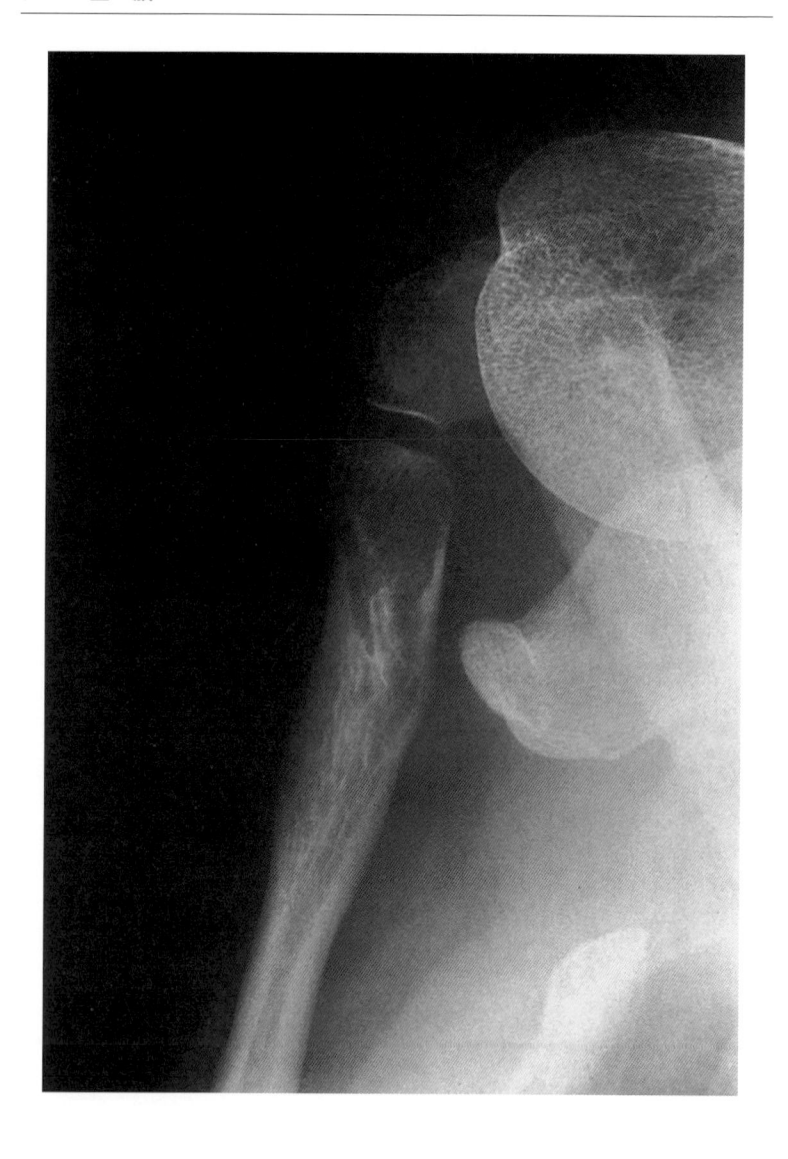

上　肢

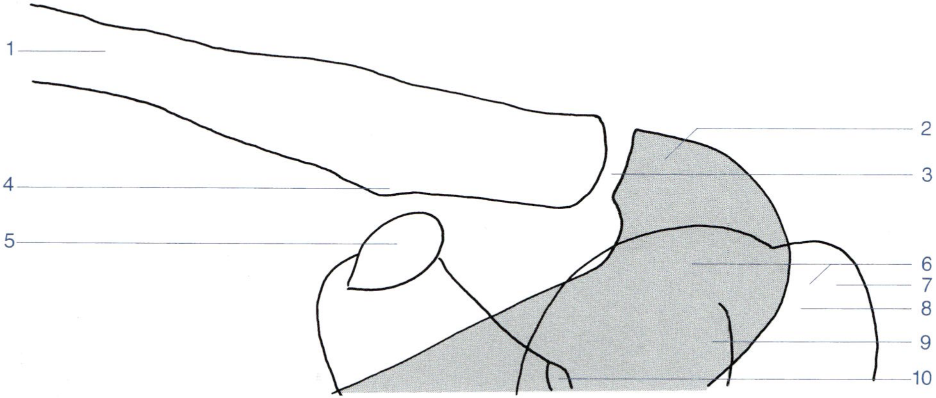

肩鎖関節

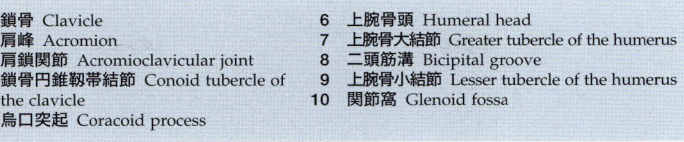

1 鎖骨 Clavicle
2 肩峰 Acromion
3 肩鎖関節 Acromioclavicular joint
4 鎖骨円錐靱帯結節 Conoid tubercle of the clavicle
5 烏口突起 Coracoid process
6 上腕骨頭 Humeral head
7 上腕骨大結節 Greater tubercle of the humerus
8 二頭筋溝 Bicipital groove
9 上腕骨小結節 Lesser tubercle of the humerus
10 関節窩 Glenoid fossa

96　上 肢

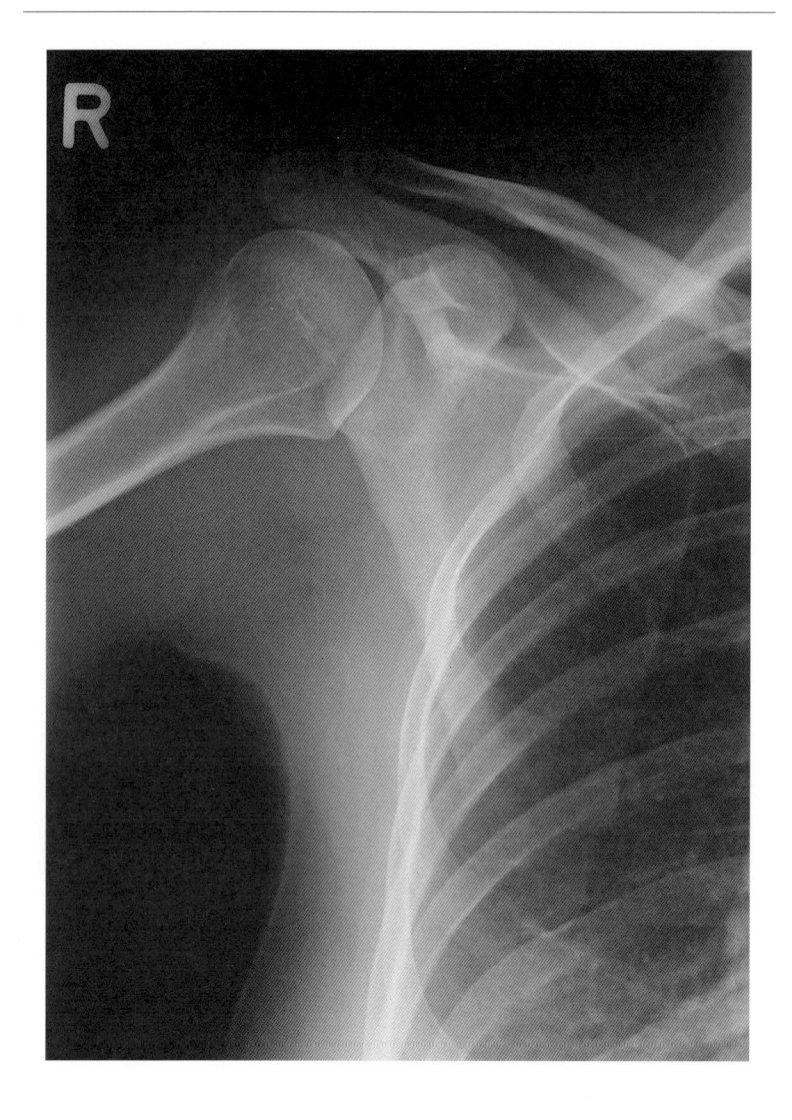

肩甲骨　正面（前後） 97

1　肩鎖関節　Acromioclavicular joint	8　関節面　Articular surface
2　鎖骨　Clavicle	9　肩甲骨外側角（頸）　Lateral angle (neck) of the scapula
3　肩峰　Acromion	10　内側縁　Medial margin
4　烏口突起　Coracoid process	11　外側縁　Lateral margin
5　上角　Superior angle	12　下角　Inferior angle
6　肩甲棘　Spine of the scapula	
7　上腕骨頭　Humeral head	

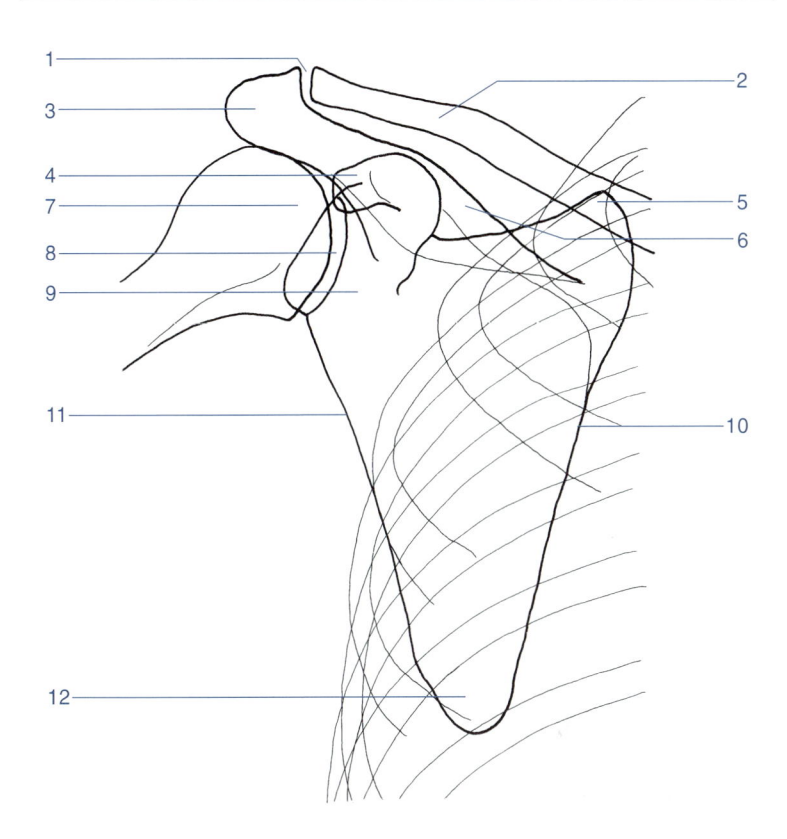

98　上　肢

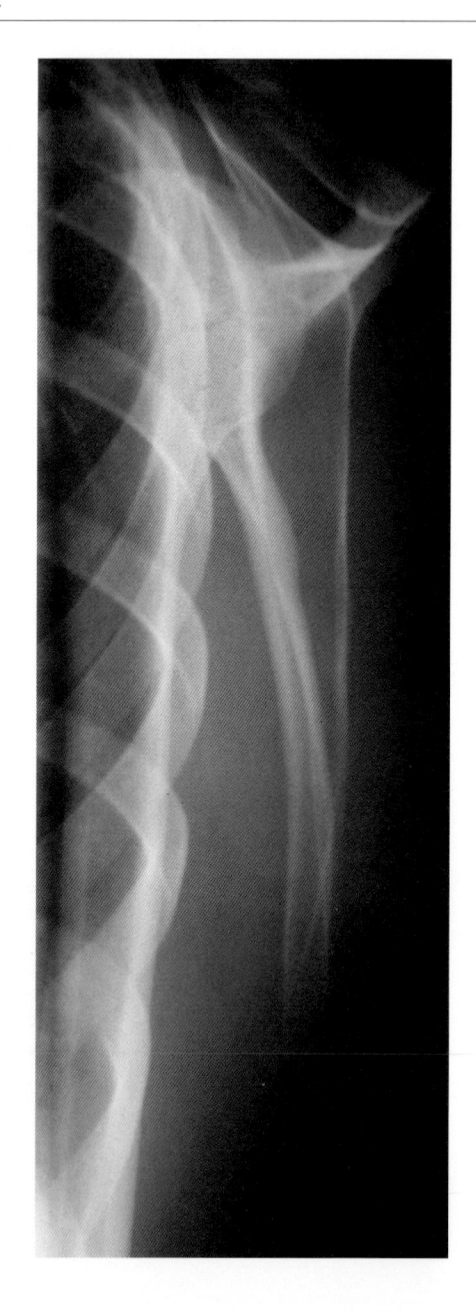

肩甲骨　側面　**99**

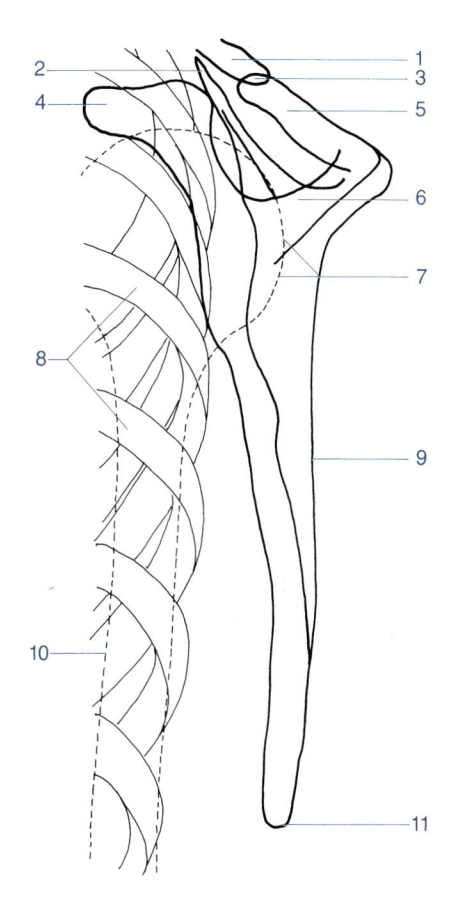

1　鎖骨遠位端 Distal clavicle	7　上腕骨頭 Humeral head
2　肩甲骨上角 Superior angle of the scapula	8　肋骨 Ribs
3　肩鎖関節 Acromioclavicular joint	9　肩甲骨外側縁 Lateral margin of the scapula
4　烏口突起 Coracoid process	10　上腕骨体 Humeral shaft
5　肩峰 Acromion	11　肩甲骨下角 Inferior angle of the scapula
6　肩甲棘 Spine of the scapula	

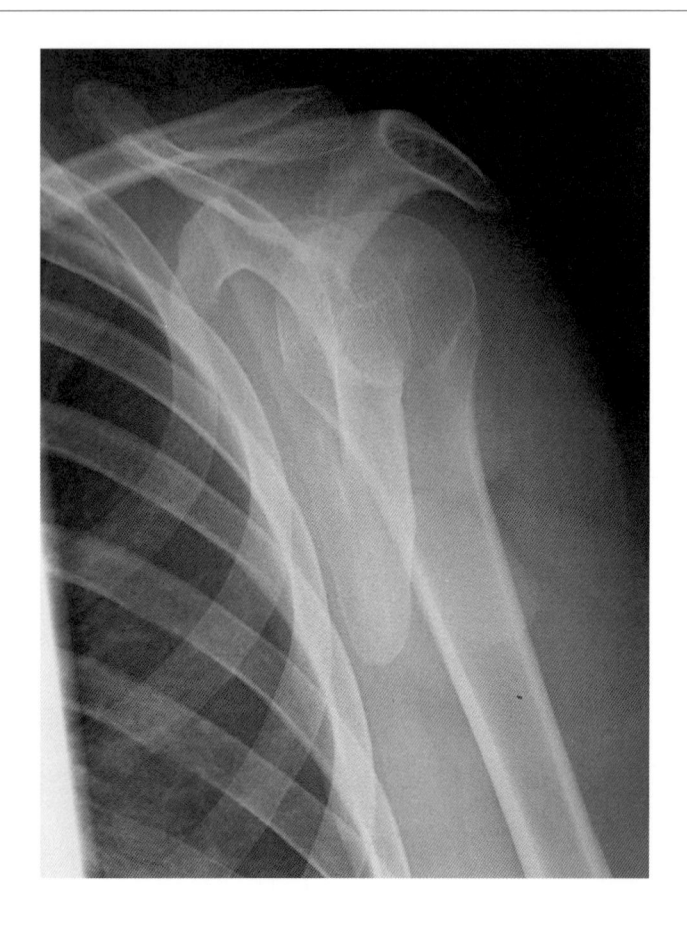

上 肢

肩関節　スカプラY法

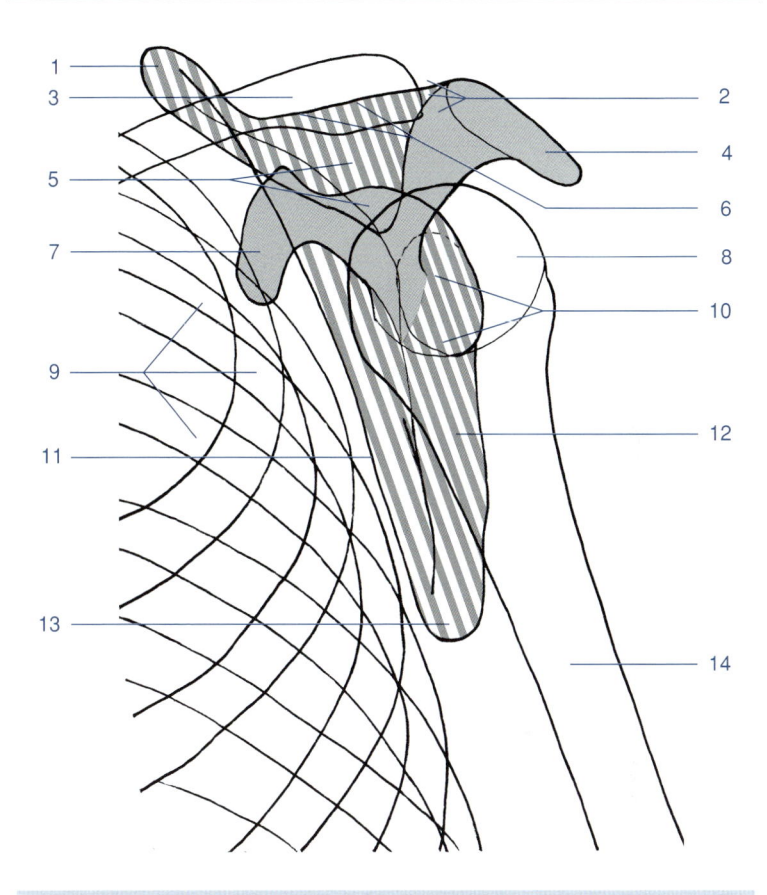

1	肩甲骨上角 Superior angle of the scapula	9	肋骨 Rib
2	肩鎖関節 Acromioclavicular joint	10	関節窩 Glenoid fossa
3	鎖骨 Clavicle	11	肩甲骨肋骨面 Costal surface of the scapula
4	肩峰 Acromion	12	肩甲骨背側面 Posterior surface of the scapula
5	棘上窩 Supraspinatus fossa	13	肩甲骨下角 Inferior angle of the scapula
6	肩甲棘 Spine of the scapula	14	上腕骨体 Humeral shaft
7	烏口突起 Coracoid process		
8	上腕骨頭 Humeral head		

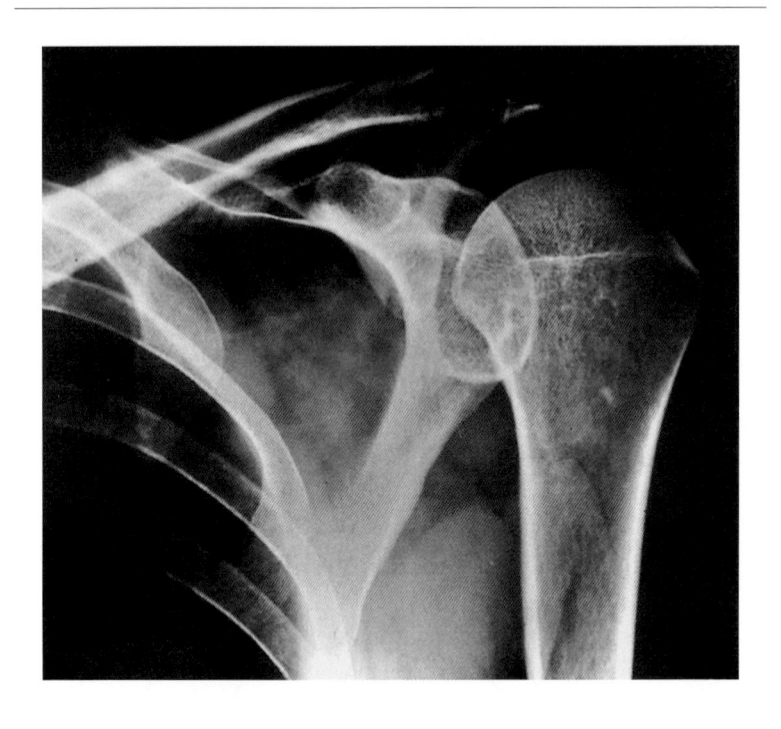

上肢

肩関節　正面（前後）　*103*

1　肩峰　Acromion	10　二頭筋溝　Bicipital groove
2　鎖骨　Clavicle	11　上腕骨小結節　Lesser tubercle of the humerus
3　肩鎖関節　Acromioclavicular joint	12　肩甲骨　Scapula
4　肩甲骨上角　Superior angle of the scapula	13　関節窩　Glenoid fossa
5　肩甲棘　Spine of the scapula	14　関節唇　Glenoid labrum
6　烏口突起　Coracoid process	15　外科頸　Surgical neck
7　上腕骨頭　Humeral head	16　肩甲骨外側縁　Lateral margin of the scapula
8　解剖頸　Anatomical neck	17　肩甲骨内側縁　Medial margin of the scapula
9　上腕骨大結節　Greater tubercle of the humerus	

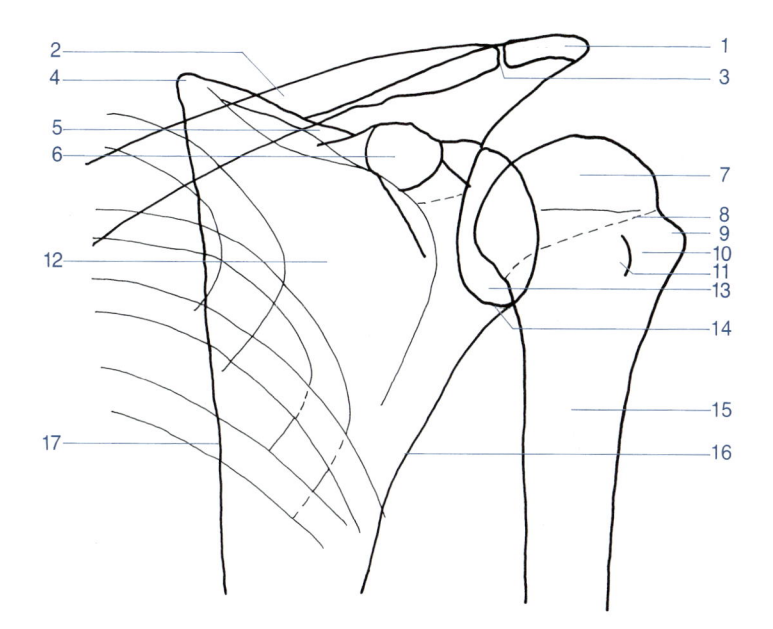

104　上　肢

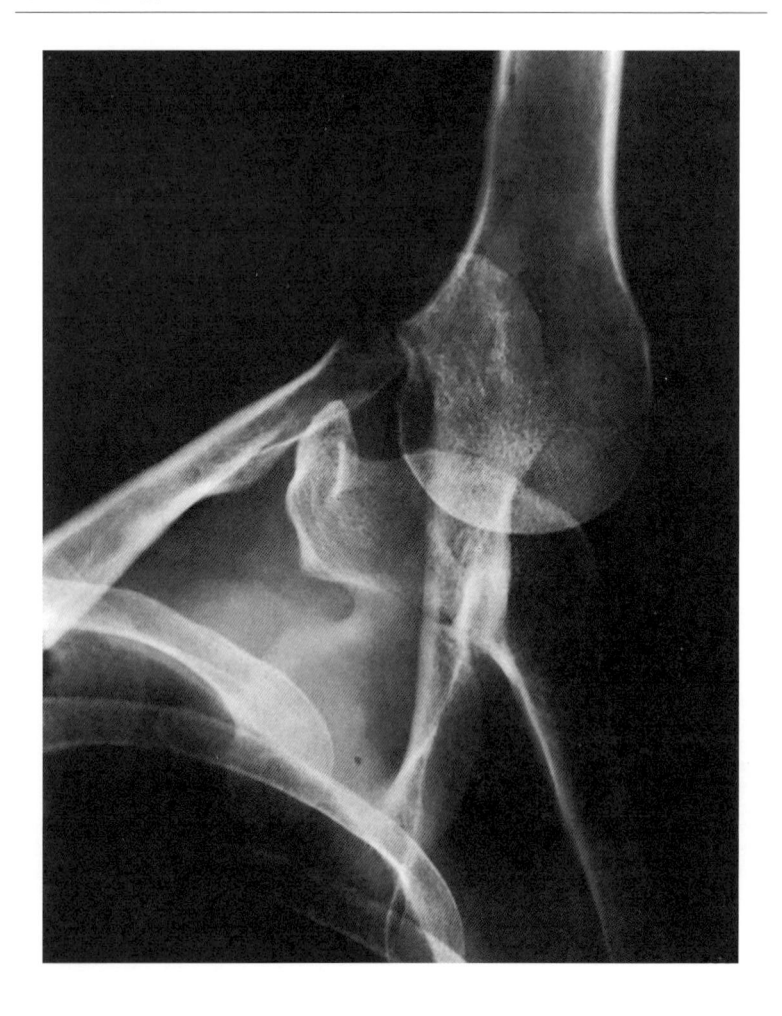

肩関節　外転位（挙上位）正面（前後）　　*105*

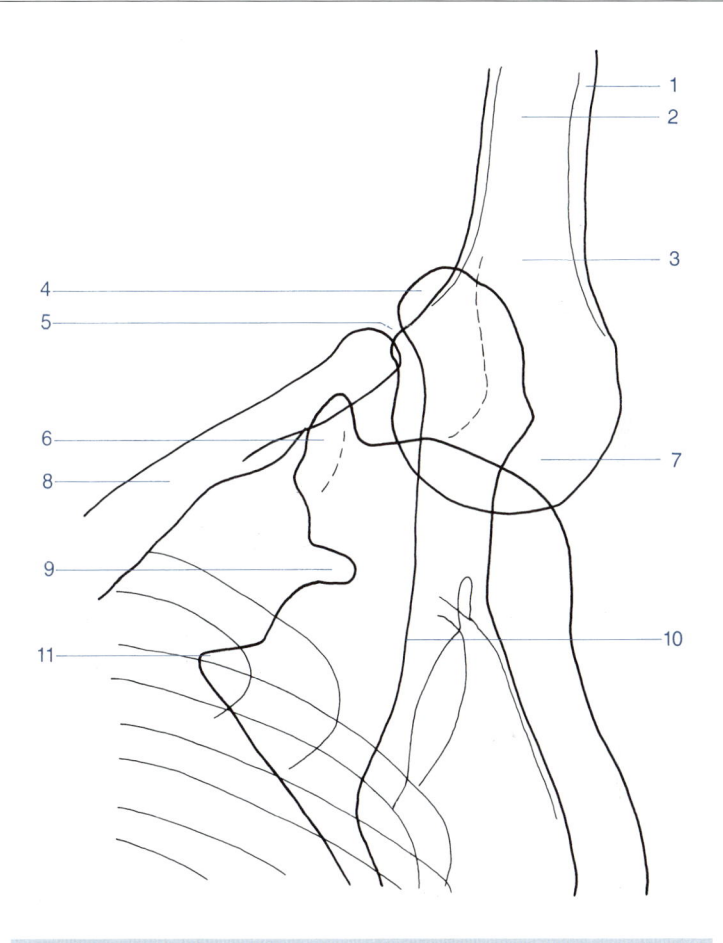

1	骨皮質 Cortex
2	骨幹端 Metaphysis
3	外科頸 Surgical neck
4	肩峰 Acromion
5	肩鎖関節 Acromioclavicular joint
6	烏口突起 Coracoid process
7	上腕骨頭 Humeral head
8	鎖骨 Clavicle
9	肩甲切痕 Suprascapular notch
10	肩甲棘 Spine of the scapula
11	肩甲骨上角 Superior angle of the scapula

106　上　肢

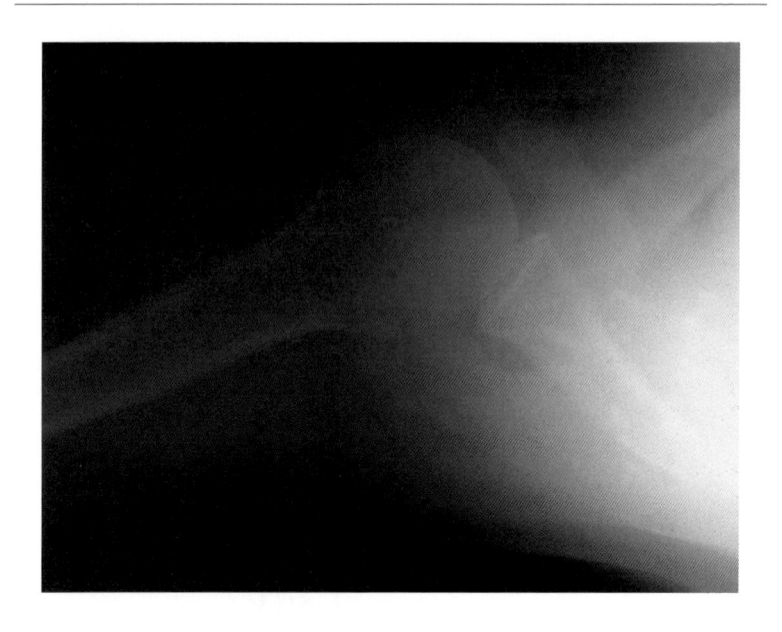

肩関節 軸位 *107*

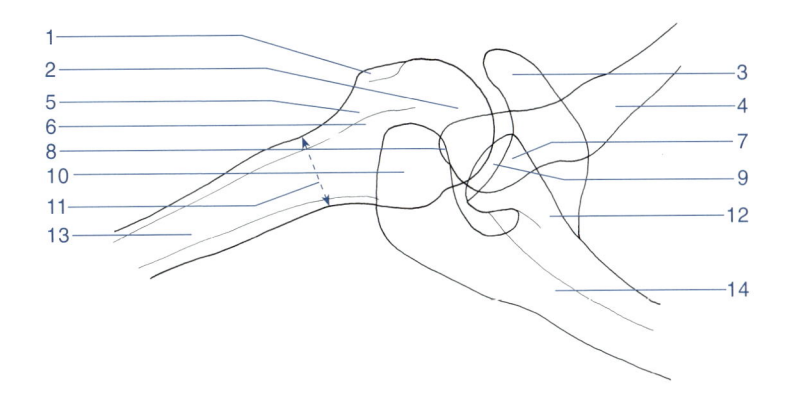

1　上腕骨小結節 Lesser tubercle of the humerus	8　肩鎖関節 Acromioclavicular joint
2　上腕骨頭 Humeral head	9　肩関節(肩甲上腕関節) Glenohumeral joint
3　烏口突起 Coracoid process	10　肩峰 Acromion
4　鎖骨 Clavicle	11　肩甲骨上角 Superior angle of the scapula
5　二頭筋溝 Bicipital groove	12　肩甲頸 Neck of the scapula
6　上腕骨大結節 Greater tubercle of the humerus	13　上腕骨 Humerus
7　関節窩 Glenoid fossa	14　肩甲骨 Scapula

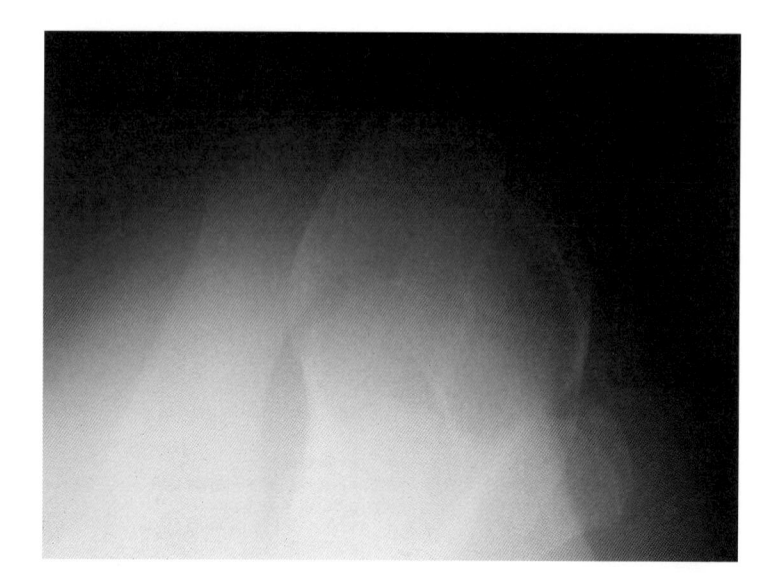

肩関節　接線　**109**

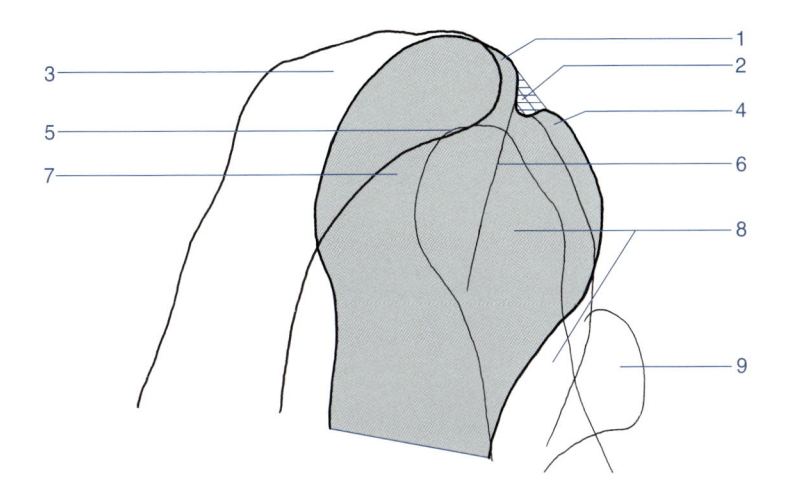

1　上腕骨大結節　Greater tubercle of the humerus
2　二頭筋溝　Bicipital groove
3　肩峰　Acromion
4　上腕骨小結節　Lesser tubercle of the humerus
5　肩鎖関節　Acromioclavicular joint
6　大結節稜　Crest of the greater tubercle
7　上腕骨頭　Humeral head
8　鎖骨　Clavicle
9　烏口突起　Coracoid process

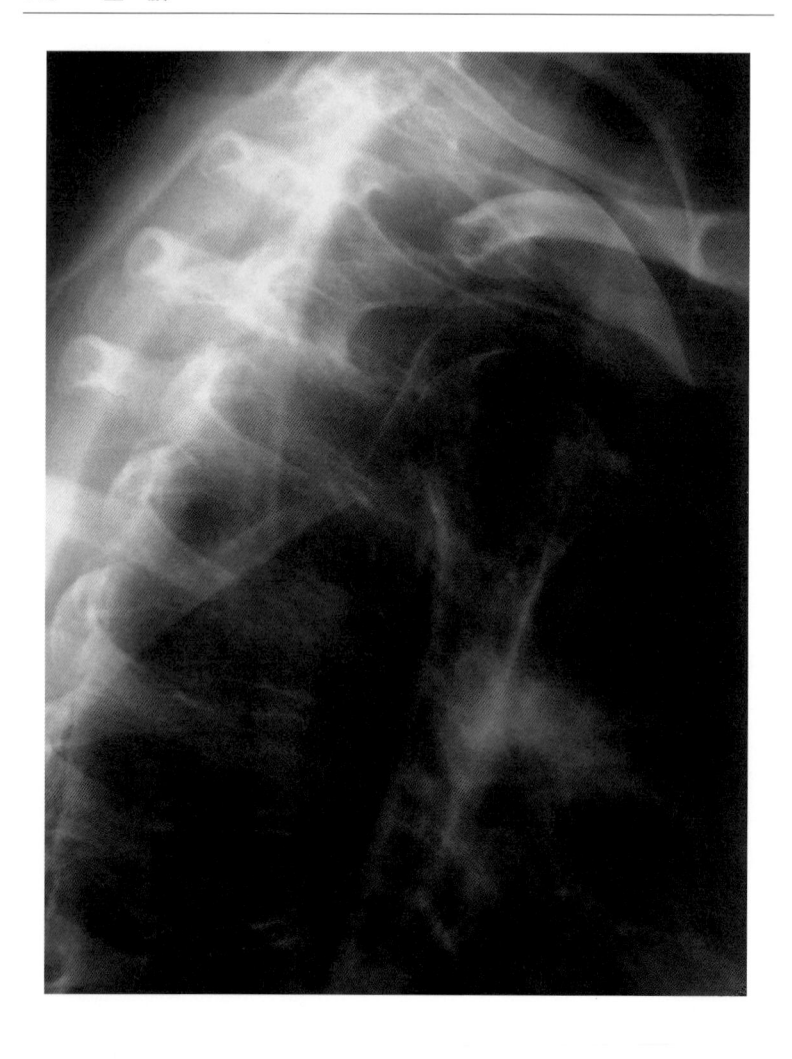

上 肢

肩関節　経胸郭撮影 *111*

1　鎖骨　Clavicle	8　上腕骨小結節　Lesser tubercle of the humerus
2　肩鎖関節　Acromioclavicular joint	9　二頭筋溝　Bicipital groove
3　肩峰　Acromion	10　肩甲骨　Scapula
4　烏口突起　Coracoid process	11　外科頸　Surgical neck
5　上腕骨頭　Humeral head	12　上腕骨　Humerus
6　関節窩　Glenoid fossa	
7　上腕骨大結節　Greater tubercle of the humerus	

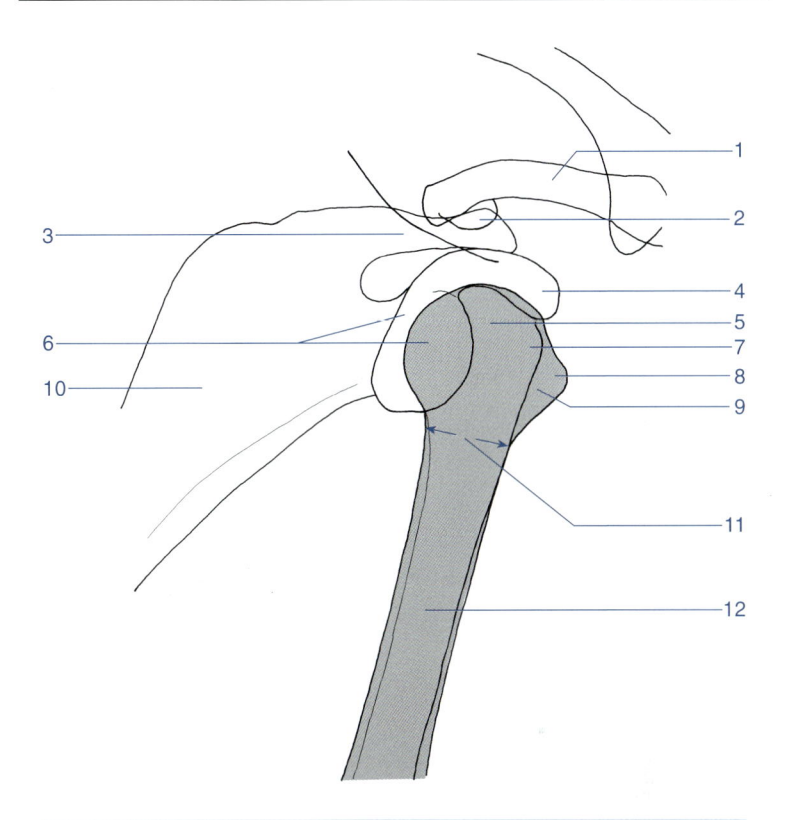

112　上 肢

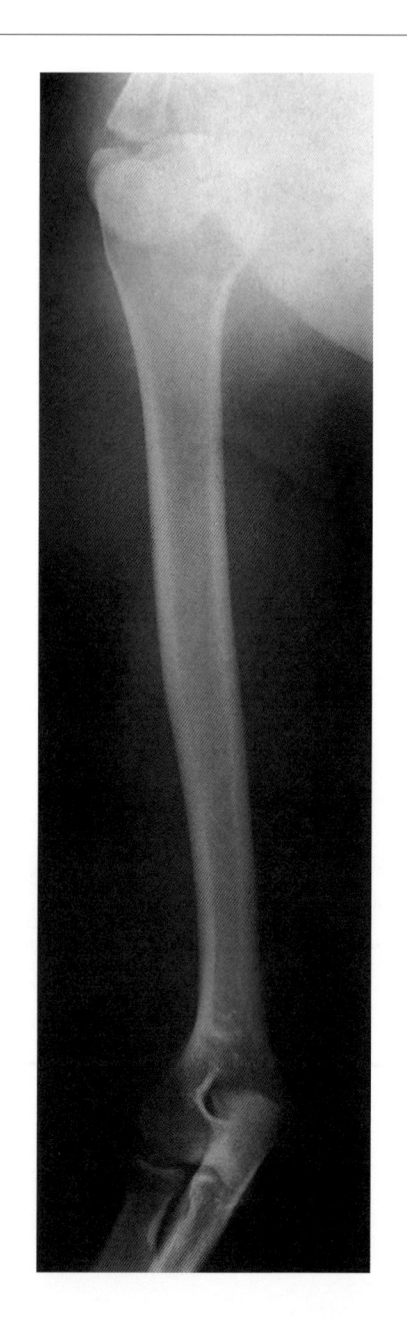

上腕骨 正面(前後)

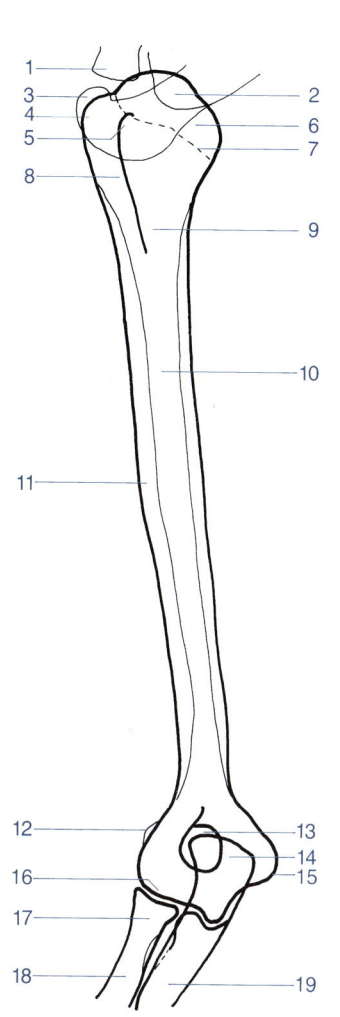

1. 鎖骨 Clavicle
2. 肩甲骨外側角(頸) Lateral angle (neck) of the scapula
3. 肩峰 Acromion
4. 上腕骨大結節 Greater tubercle of the humerus
5. 上腕骨小結節 Lesser tubercle of the humerus
6. 上腕骨頭 Humeral head
7. 解剖頸 Anatomical neck
8. 二頭筋溝 Bicipital groove
9. 外科頸 Surgical neck
10. 上腕骨 Humerus
11. 三角筋粗面 Deltoid tuberosity
12. 外側上顆 Lateral epicondyle
13. 肘頭窩 Olecranon fossa
14. 肘頭 Olecranon
15. 内側上顆 Medial epicondyle
16. 滑車 Trochlea
17. 橈骨頭 Radial head
18. 橈骨 Radius
19. 尺骨 Ulna

114 上　肢

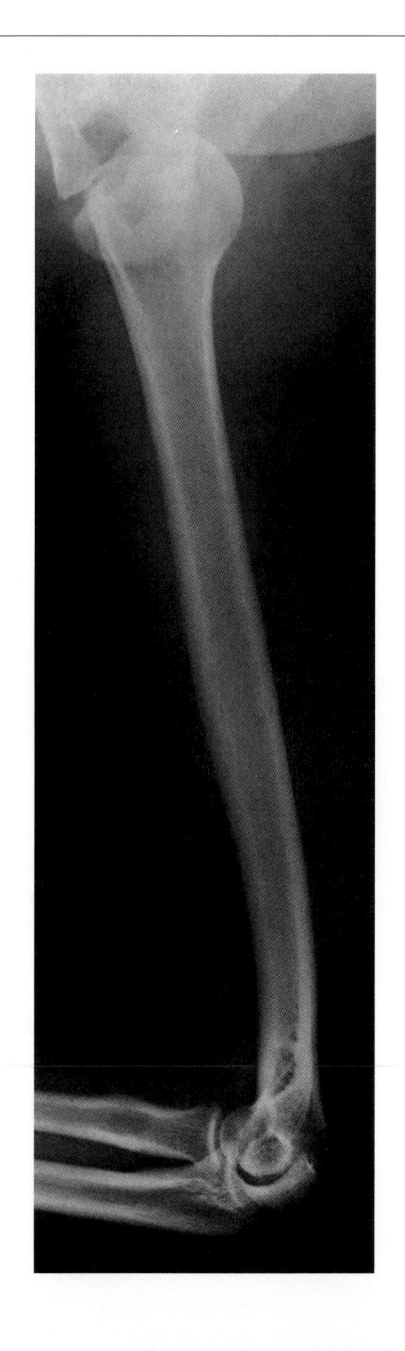

上腕骨　側面　**115**

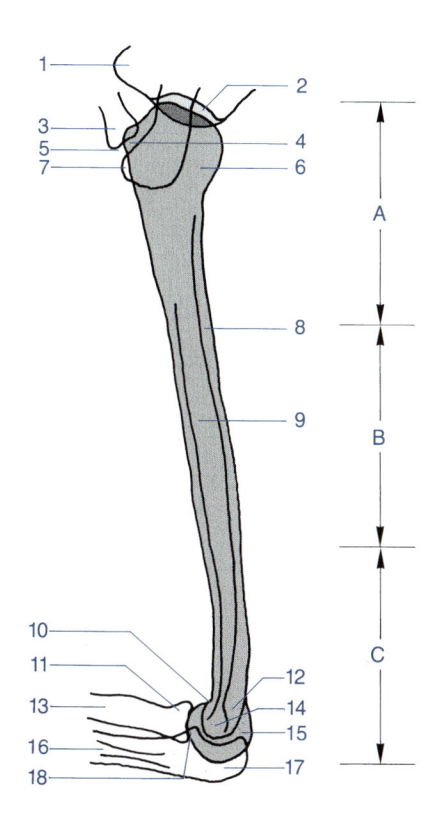

A	上腕骨近位1/3 Proximal third of the humerus	
B	上腕骨中間1/3 Medial third of the humerus	
C	上腕骨遠位1/3 Distal third of the humerus	
1	烏口突起 Coracoid process
2	関節窩 Glenoid fossa
3	鎖骨 Clavicle
4	上腕骨小結節 Lesser tubercle of the humerus
5	肩鎖関節 Acromioclavicular joint
6	上腕骨頭 Humeral head
7	肩峰 Acromion
8	骨皮質 Cortex
9	上腕骨体 Humeral shaft
10	鈎突窩 Coronoid fossa
11	橈骨頭 Radial head
12	肘頭窩 Olecranon fossa
13	橈骨 Radius
14	滑車 Trochlea
15	小頭 Capitellum
16	尺骨 Ulna
17	肘頭 Olecranon
18	鈎状突起 Coronoid process

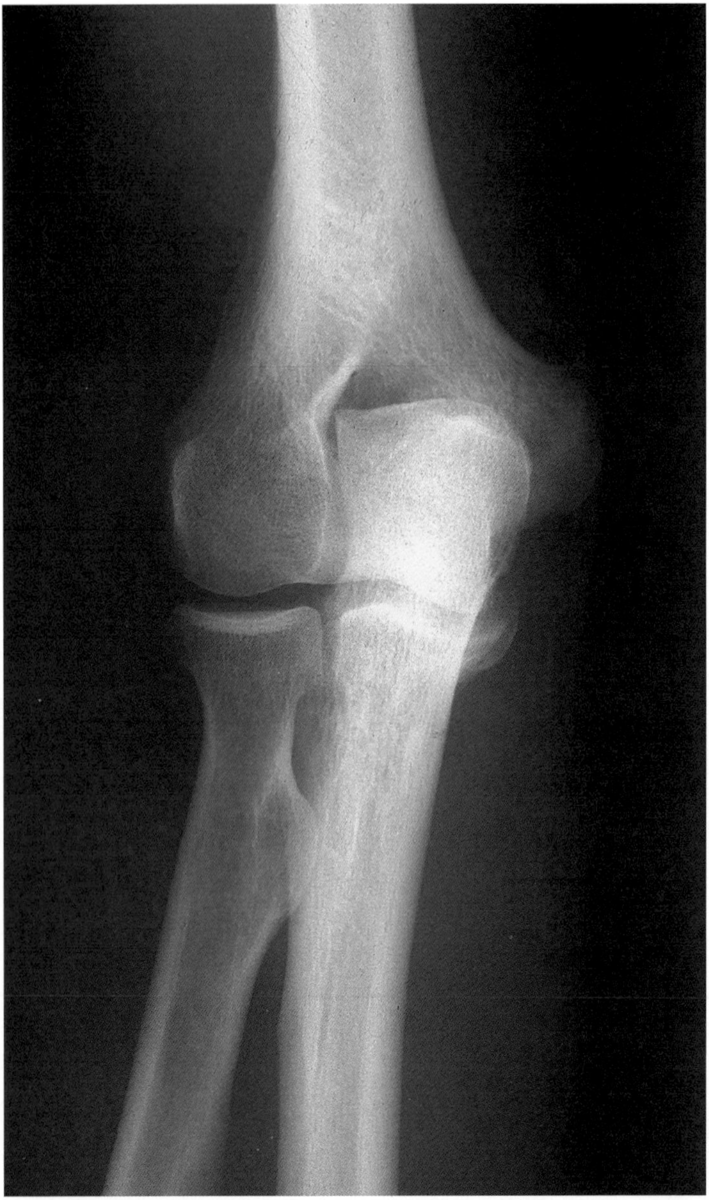

肘関節　正面（前後）　117

1　上腕骨 Humerus	9　小頭 Capitellum
2　肘頭窩 Olecranon fossa	10　滑車 Trochlea
3　上腕骨内側上顆 Medial epicondyle of the humerus	11　腕橈関節 Humeroradial joint
4　上腕骨外側上顆 Lateral epicondyle of the humerus	12　腕尺関節 Humeroulnar joint
5　上腕骨内側上顆尖端 Apex of the medial epicondyle of the humerus	13　鉤状突起 Coronoid process
6　肘頭 Olecranon	14　橈骨頭 Radial head
7　滑車外側縁 Lateral margin of the trochlea	15　上橈尺関節 Proximal radioulnar joint
8　滑車内側縁 Medial margin of the trochlea	16　橈骨頸 Radial neck
	17　橈骨 Radius
	18　尺骨 Ulna

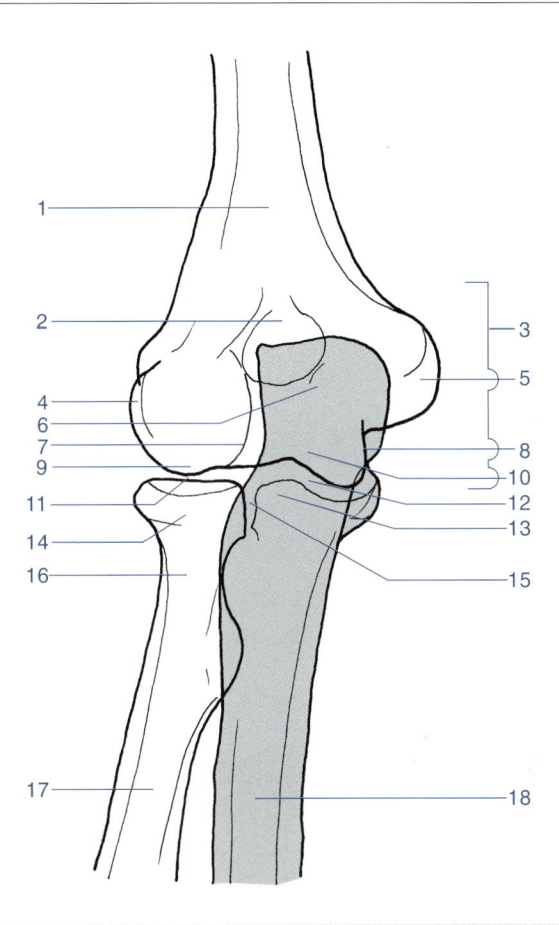

118 上　肢

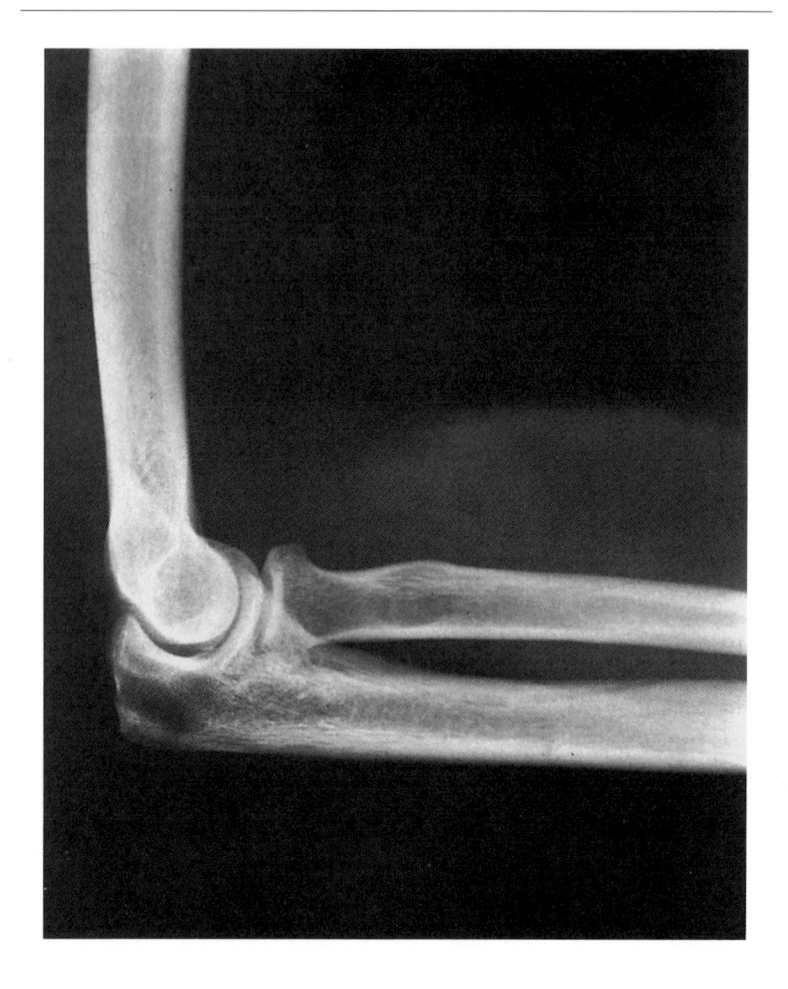

肘関節　側面

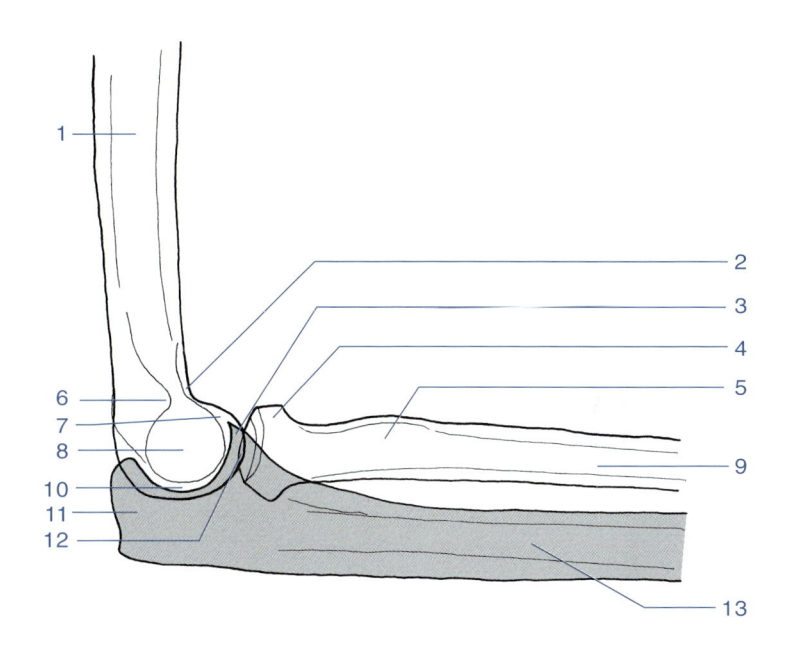

1 上腕骨 Humerus
2 鈎突窩 Coronoid fossa
3 鈎状突起 Coronoid process
4 橈骨頭 Radial head
5 橈骨粗面 Radial tuberosity
6 肘頭窩 Olecranon fossa
7 内側上顆 Medial epicondyle
8 外側上顆 Lateral epicondyle
9 橈骨 Radius
10 腕尺関節 Humeroulnar joint
11 肘頭 Olecranon
12 腕橈関節 Humeroradial joint
13 尺骨 Ulna

120　上　肢

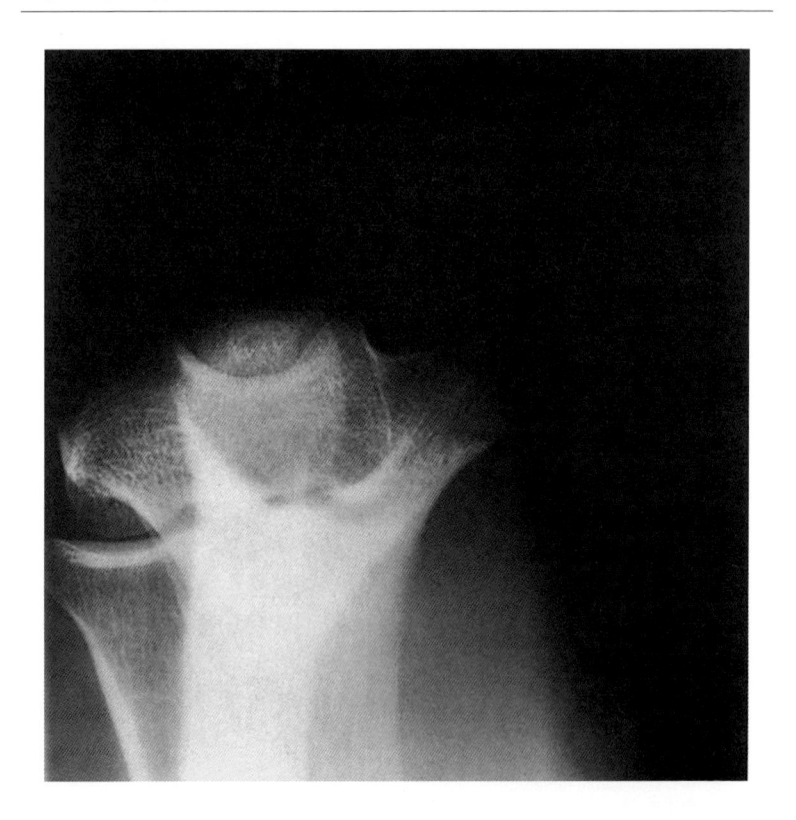

肘関節 軸位

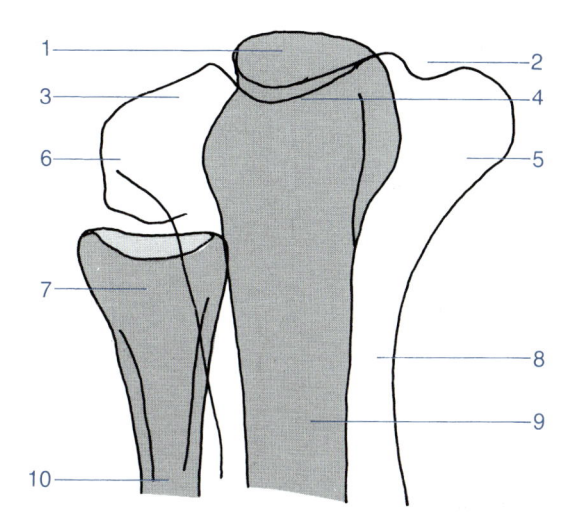

1 肘頭 Olecranon
2 肘部管(尺骨神経溝) Cubital tunnel
3 小頭 Capitellum
4 滑車 Trochlea
5 内側上顆 Medial epicondyle
6 外側上顆 Lateral epicondyle
7 橈骨頭 Radial head
8 上腕骨 Humerus
9 尺骨 Ulna
10 橈骨 Radius

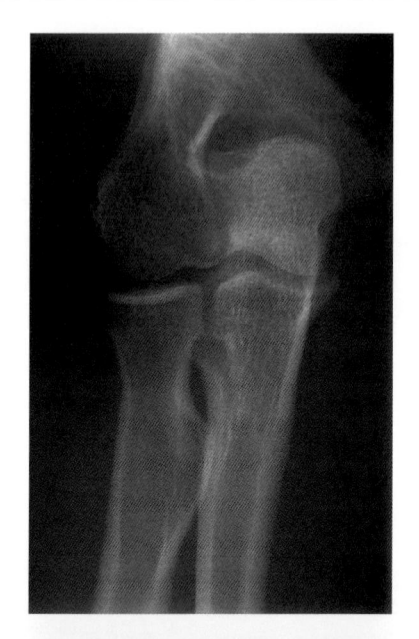

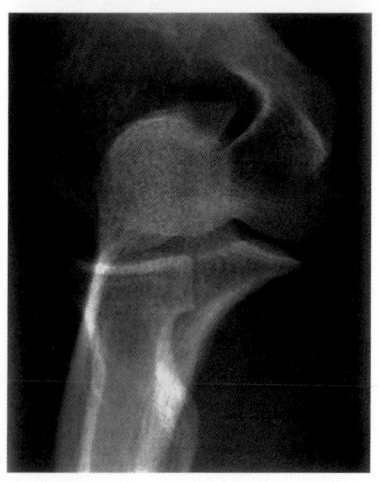

上　肢

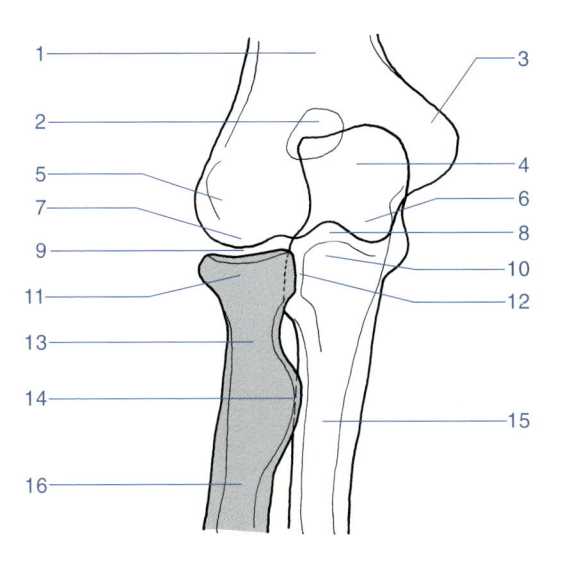

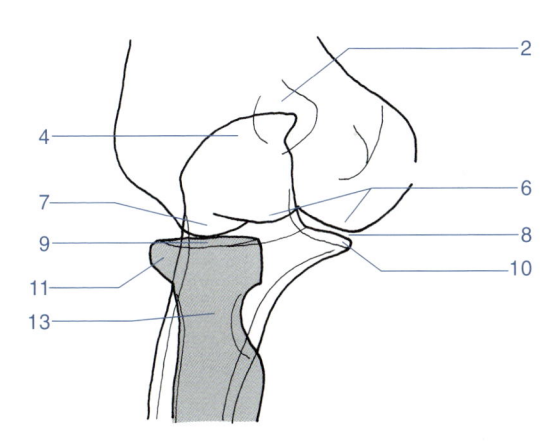

橈骨 斜位

1	上腕骨 Humerus	9	腕橈関節 Humeroradial joint
2	肘頭窩 Olecranon fossa	10	鈎状突起 Coronoid process
3	内側上顆 Medial epicondyle	11	橈骨頭 Radial head
4	肘頭 Olecranon	12	上橈尺関節 Proximal radioulnar joint
5	外側上顆 Lateral epicondyle	13	橈骨頸 Radial neck
6	滑車 Trochlea	14	橈骨粗面 Radial tuberosity
7	小頭 Capitellum	15	尺骨 Ulna
8	腕尺関節 Humeroulnar joint	16	橈骨 Radius

上 肢

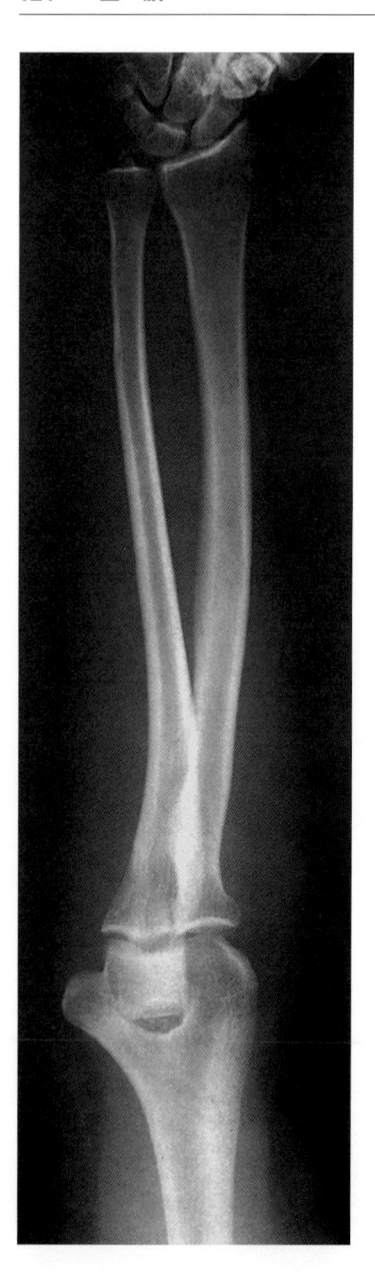

A	手根骨 Carpal bones
B	前腕遠位1/3 Distal third of the forearm
C	前腕中間1/3 Middle third of the forearm
D	前腕近位1/3 Proximal third of the forearm

1. 豆状骨 Pisiform
2. 舟状骨 Scaphoid
3. 三角骨 Triquetrum
4. 月状骨 Lunate

1−4 近位手根列 Proximal carpal row

5. 橈骨茎状突起 Radial styloid process
6. 尺骨茎状突起 Ulnar styloid process
7. 橈骨手根関節 Radiocarpal joint
8. 下橈尺関節 Distal radioulnar joint
9. 橈骨 Radius
10. 骨間膜 Interosseous membrane
11. 尺骨 Ulna
12. 橈骨粗面 Radial tuberosity
13. 上橈尺関節 Proximal radioulnar joint
14. 橈骨頸 Radial neck
15. 鉤状突起 Coronoid process
16. 橈骨頭 Radial head
17. 腕尺関節 Humeroulnar joint
18. 腕橈関節 Humeroradial joint
19. 滑車 Trochlea
20. 小頭 Capitellum
21. 肘頭 Olecranon
22. 上腕骨外側上顆 Lateral epicondyle of the humerus
23. 上腕骨内側上顆 Medial epicondyle of the humerus
24. 肘頭窩 Olecranon fossa
25. 上腕骨 Humerus

前腕骨 正面(前後) 125

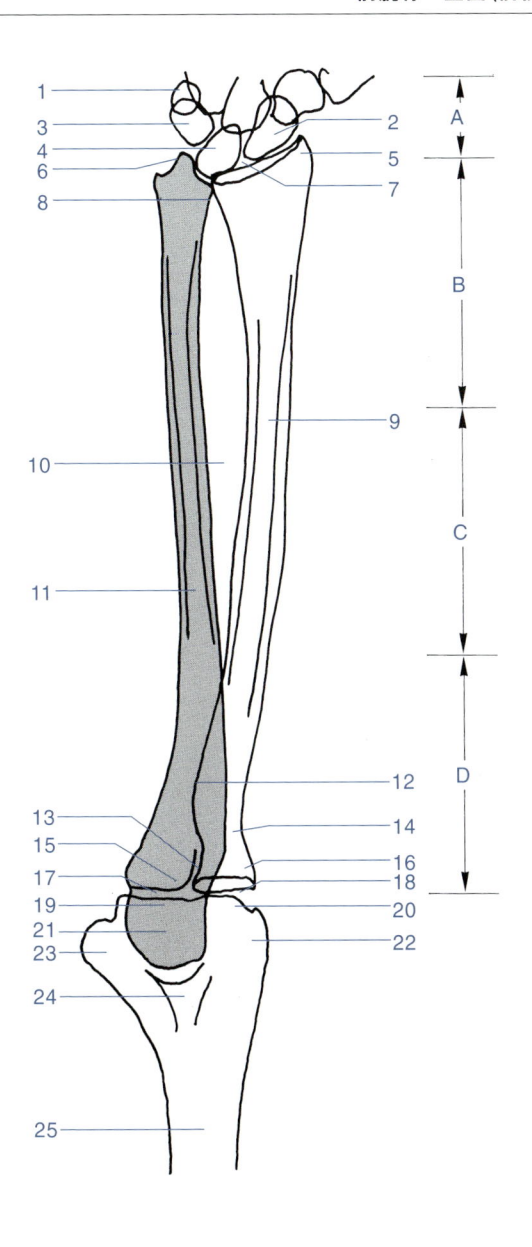

上 肢

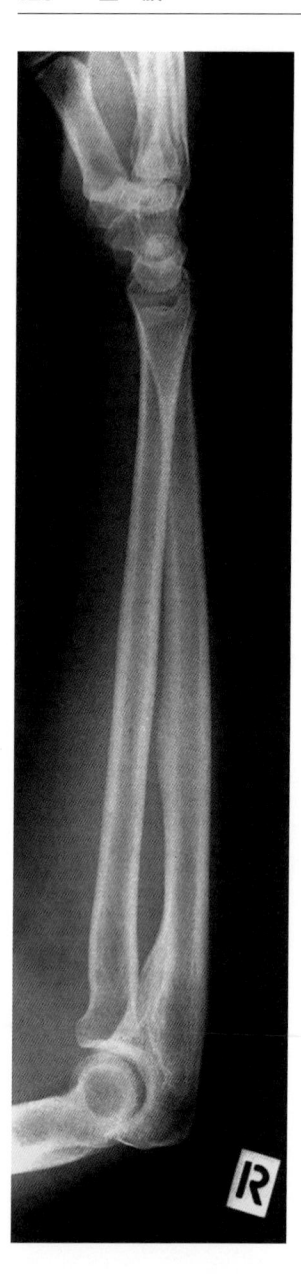

A	手根骨 Carpal bones
B	前腕遠位1/3 Distal third of the forearm
C	前腕中間1/3 Middle third of the forearm
D	前腕近位1/3 Proximal third of the forearm

1	三角骨 Triquetrum
2	舟状骨 Scaphoid
3	豆状骨 Pisiform
4	月状骨 Lunate
1−4	近位手根列 Proximal carpal row
5	橈骨手根関節 Radiocarpal joint
6	尺骨茎状突起 Ulnar styloid process
7	尺骨 Ulna
8	橈骨 Radius
9	骨間膜 Interosseous membrane
10	橈骨頸 Radial neck
11	橈骨頭 Radial head
12	鈎状突起 Coronoid process
13	鈎突窩 Coronoid fossa
14	上腕骨滑車 Trochlea of the humerus
15	上腕骨 Humerus
16	肘頭 Olecranon
17	肘頭窩 Olecranon fossa

前腕骨　側面　127

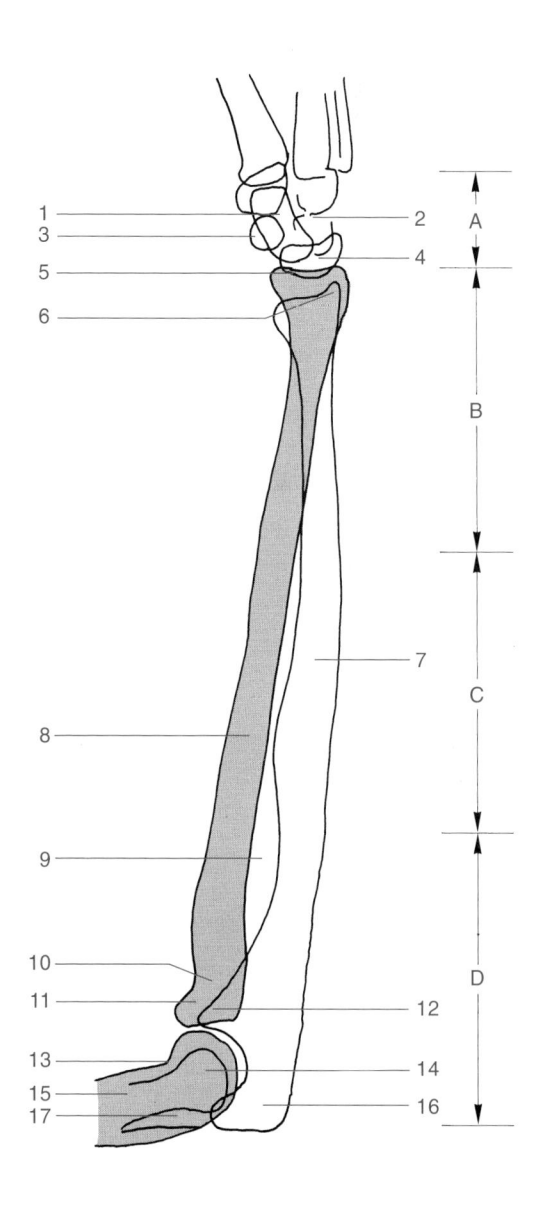

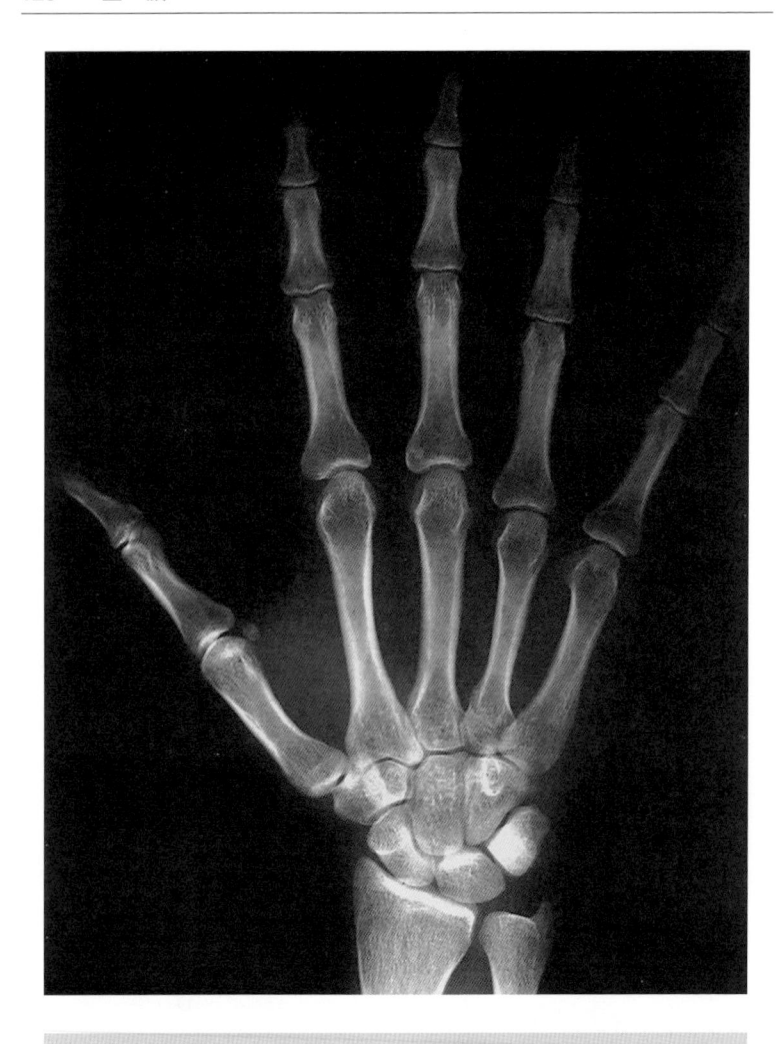

1　末節骨 Distal phalanx(tuft)	7　基節骨 Proximal phalanx
2　末節骨 Distal phalanx	8　中手指節関節(MP関節) Metacarpophalangeal joint
3　遠位指節間関節(DIP関節) Distal interphalangeal joint	9　基節骨底 Base of the proximal phalanx
4　近位指節間関節(PIP関節) Proximal interphalangeal joint	10　中手骨頭 Metacarpal head
5　中節骨 Middle phalanx	11　種子骨 Sesamoid
6　基節骨頭 Head of the proximal phalanx	12　中手骨 Metacarpal
	13　中手骨底 Metacarpal base

手　正面（前後）

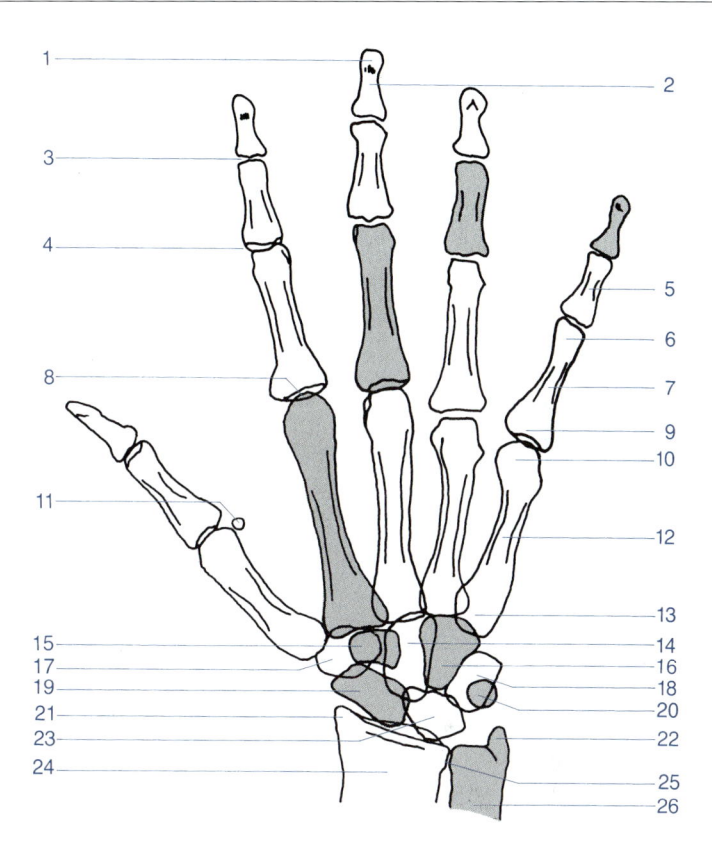

14	有頭骨 Capitate	21	橈骨茎状突起 Radial styloid process
15	小菱形骨 Trapezoid	22	尺骨茎状突起 Ulnar styloid process
16	有鈎骨 Hamate	23	月状骨 Lunate
17	大菱形骨 Trapezium	24	橈骨遠位端 Distal radius
18	三角骨 Triquetrum	25	下橈尺関節 Distal radioulnar joint
19	舟状骨 Scaphoid	26	尺骨遠位端 Distal ulna
20	豆状骨 Pisiform		

130 上　肢

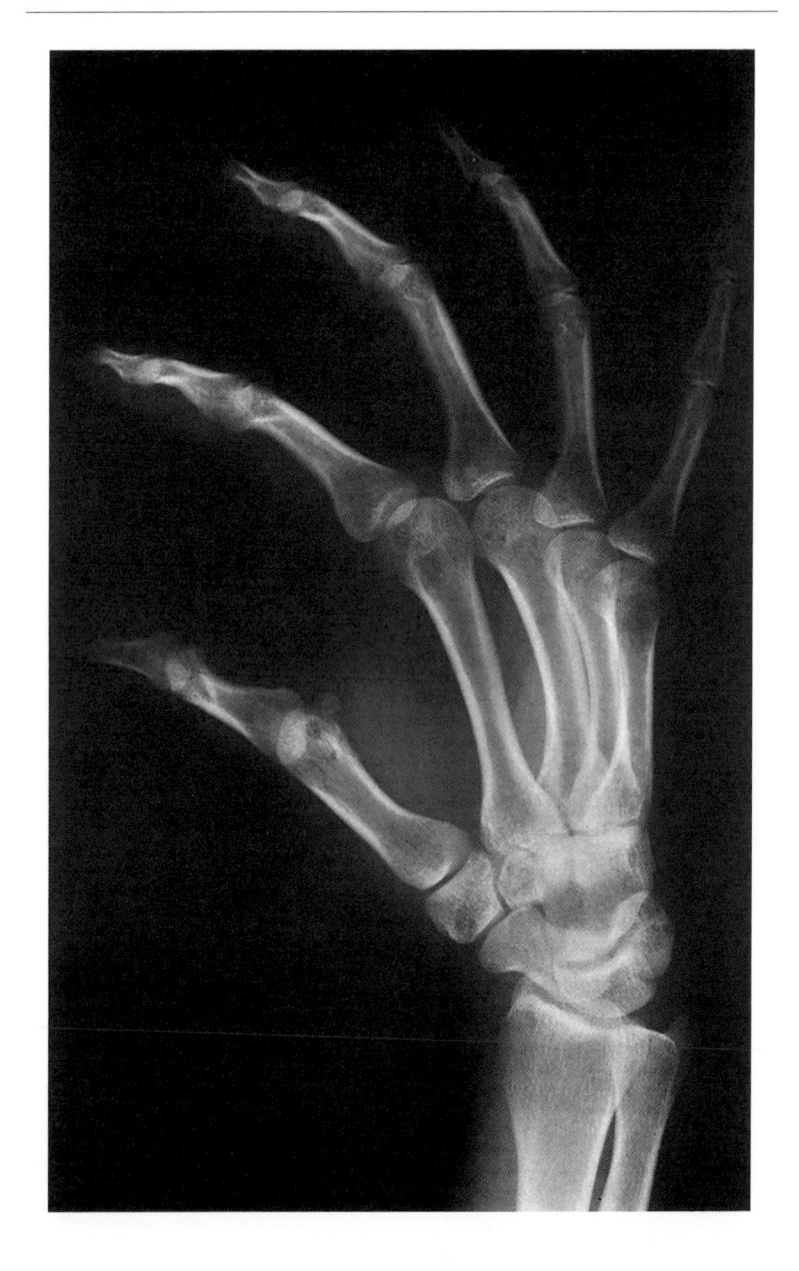

手 斜位

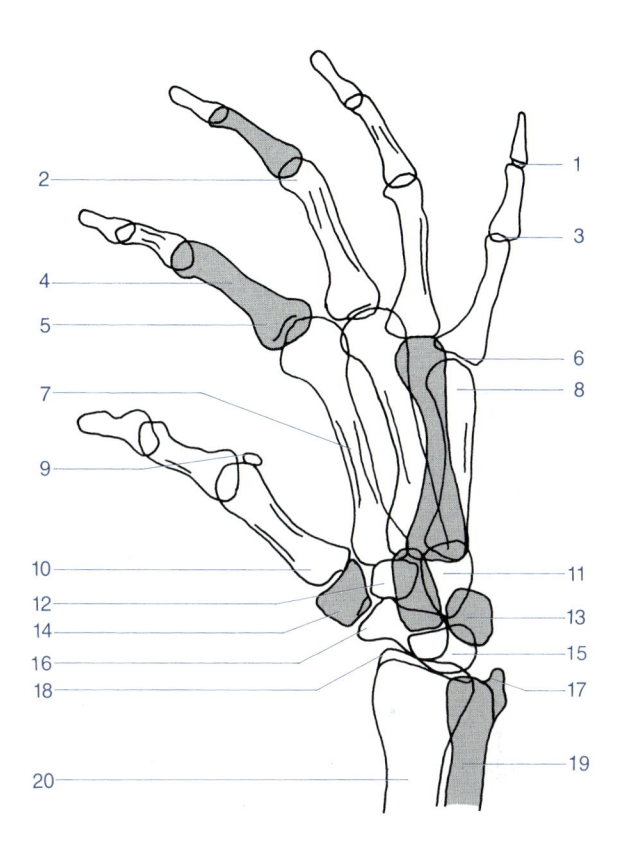

1 遠位指節間関節（DIP関節）Distal interphalangeal joint	10 中手骨底 Metacarpal base
2 基節骨頭 Head of the proximal phalanx	11 有頭骨 Capitate，有鈎骨 Hamate
3 近位指節間関節（PIP関節）Proximal interphalangeal joint	12 小菱形骨 Trapezoid
4 基節骨 Proximal phalanx	13 三角骨 Triquetrum
5 基節骨底 Base of the proximal phalanx	14 大菱形骨 Trapezium
6 中手指節関節（MP関節）Metacarpophalangeal joint	15 月状骨 Lunate
7 中手骨 Metacarpal	16 舟状骨 Scaphoid
8 中手骨頭 Metacarpal head	17 尺骨茎状突起 Ulnar styloid process
9 種子骨 Sesamoid	18 橈骨茎状突起 Radial styloid process
	19 尺骨遠位端 Distal ulna
	20 橈骨遠位端 Distal radius

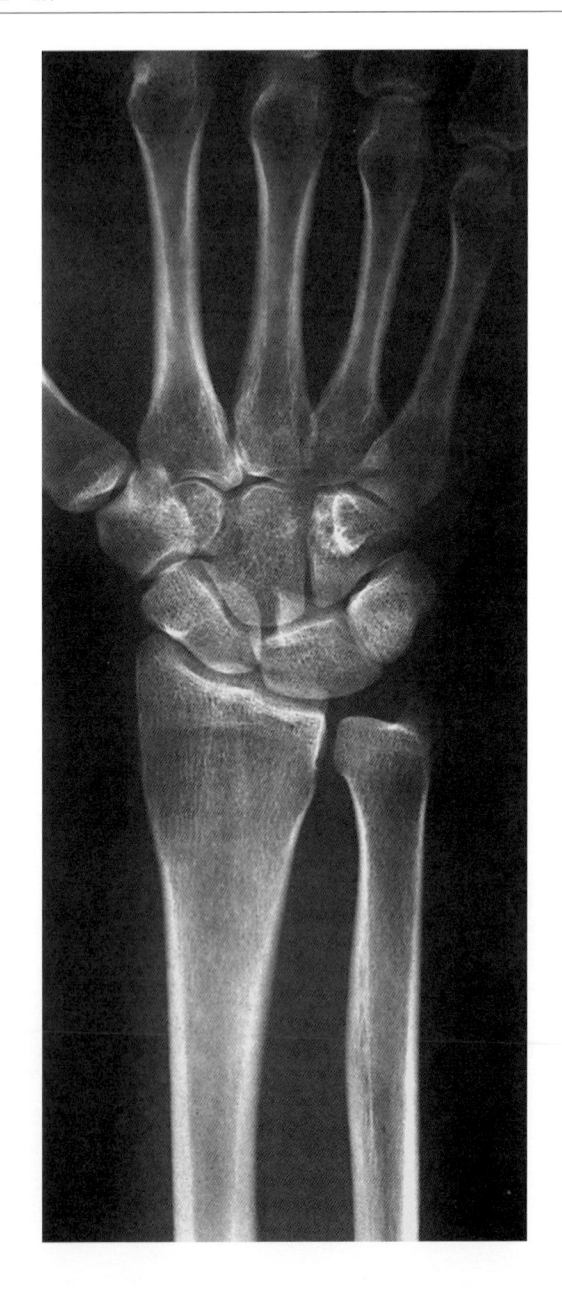

上 肢

手関節　正面(前後)

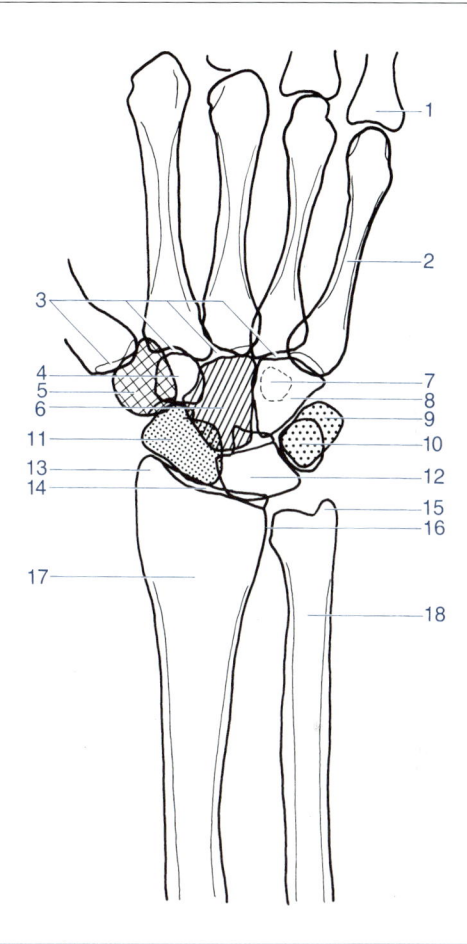

1	基節骨 Proximal phalanx
2	第5中手骨 Fifth metacarpal
3	手根中手関節(CM関節) Carpometacarpal joint
4	小菱形骨 Trapezoid
5	大菱形骨 Trapezium
6	有頭骨 Capitate
7	有鈎骨鈎 Hook of the Hamate
8	有鈎骨 Hamate
9	三角骨 Triquetrum
10	豆状骨 Pisiform
11	舟状骨 Scaphoid
12	月状骨 Lunate
13	橈骨茎状突起 Radial styloid process
14	橈骨手根関節 Radiocarpal joint
15	尺骨茎状突起 Ulnar styloid process
16	下橈尺関節 Distal radioulnar joint
17	橈骨 Radius
18	尺骨 Ulna

134 上 肢

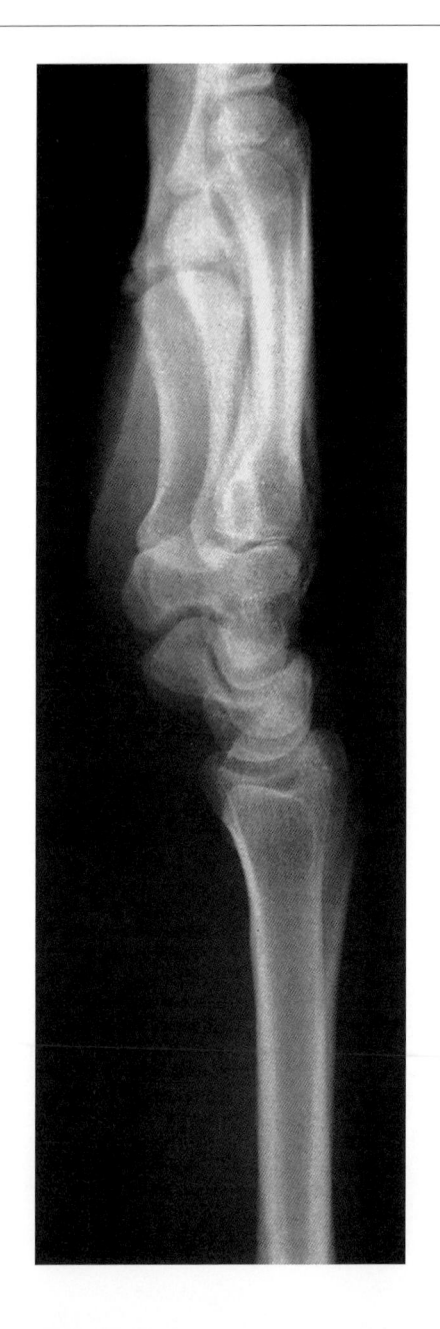

手関節　側面　　*135*

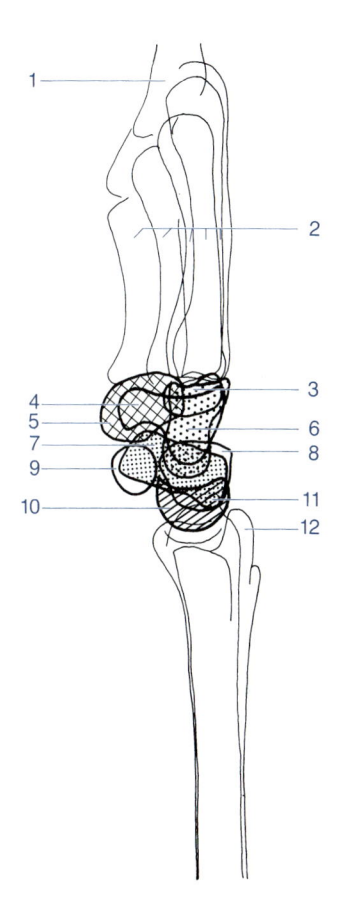

1	基節骨 Proximal phalanx	7	舟状骨 Scaphoid
2	中手骨 Metacarpals	8	三角骨 Triquetrum
3	小菱形骨 Trapezoid	9	豆状骨 Pisiform
4	有鈎骨鈎 Hook of the Hamate	10	月状骨 Lunate
5	大菱形骨 Trapezium	11	橈骨茎状突起 Radial styloid process
6	有頭骨 Capitate	12	尺骨茎状突起 Ulnar styloid process

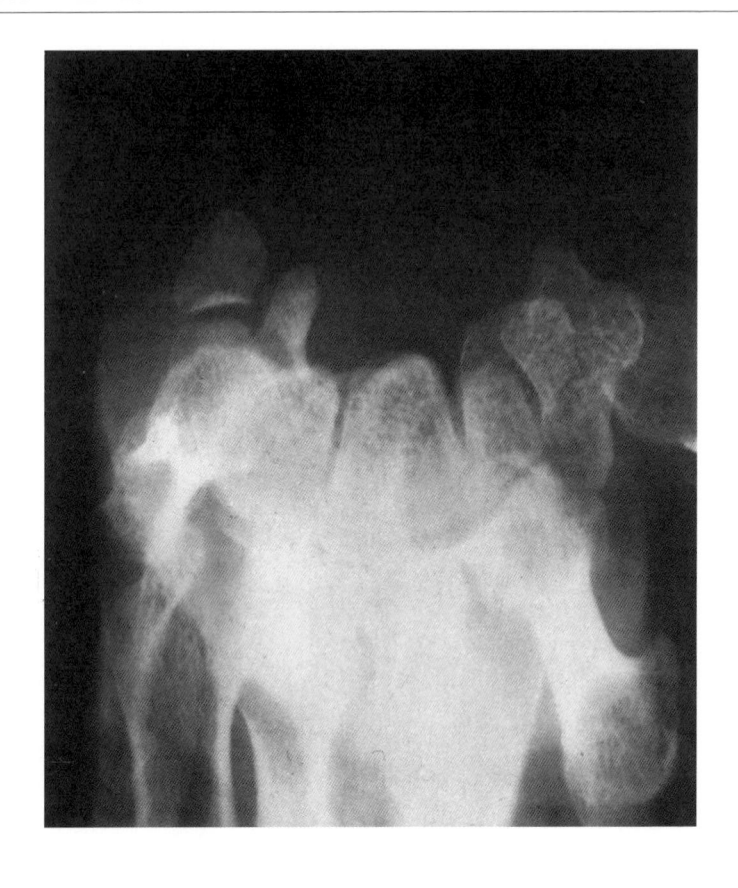

上　肢

手根管撮影   **137**

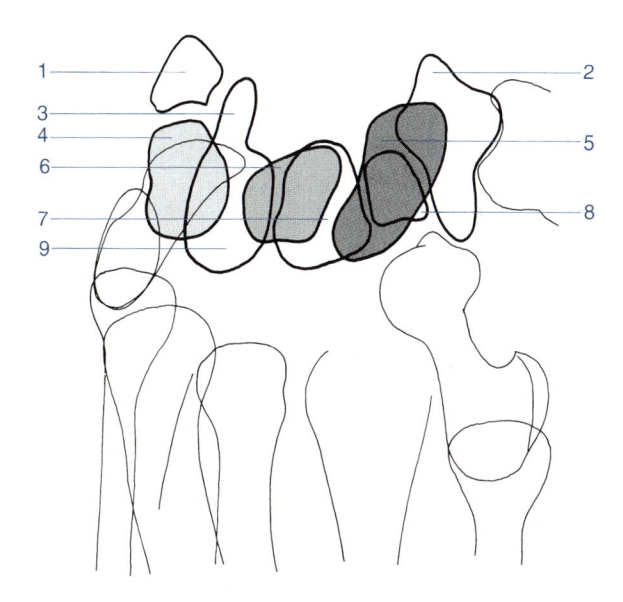

1 豆状骨 Pisiform
2 大菱形骨 Trapezium
3 有鈎骨鈎 Hook of the Hamate
4 三角骨 Triquetrum
5 舟状骨 Scaphoid
6 月状骨 Lunate
7 有頭骨 Capitate
8 小菱形骨 Trapezoid
9 有鈎骨 Hamate

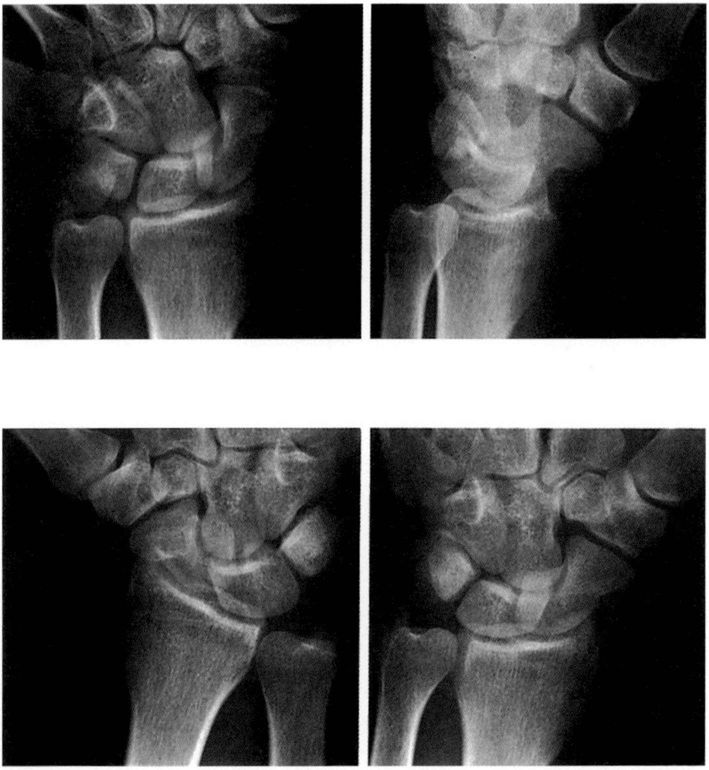

舟状骨撮影 139

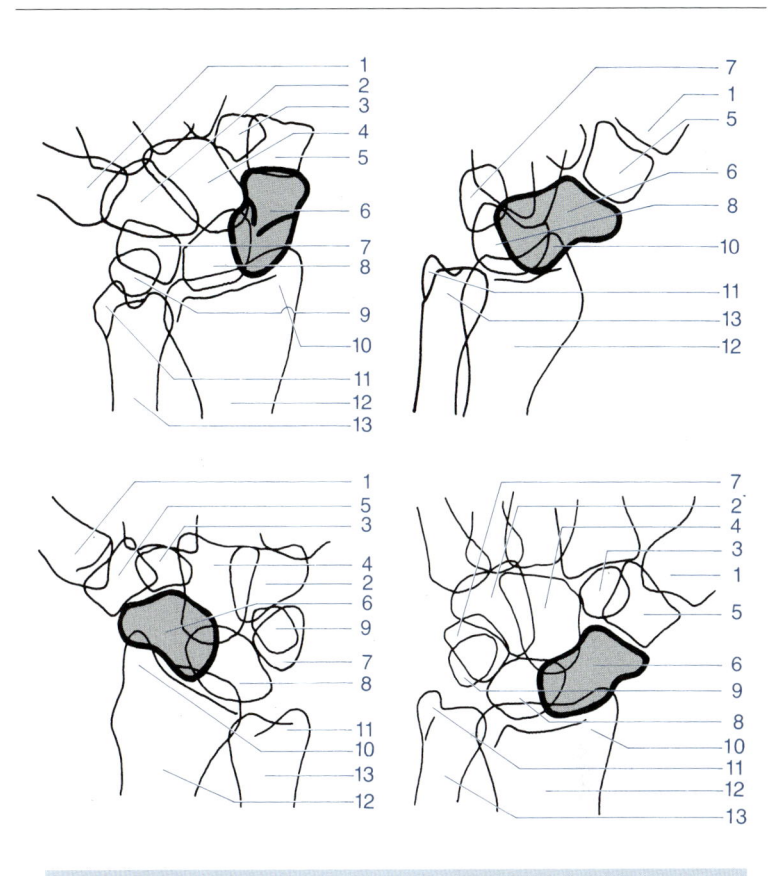

1	中手骨 Metacarpal
2	有鈎骨 Hamate
3	小菱形骨 Trapezoid
4	有頭骨 Capitate
5	大菱形骨 Trapezium
6	舟状骨 Scaphoid
7	三角骨 Triquetrum
8	月状骨 Lunate
9	豆状骨 Pisiform
10	橈骨茎状突起 Radial styloid process
11	尺骨茎状突起 Ulnar styloid process
12	橈骨 Radius
13	尺骨 Ulna

140 上　肢

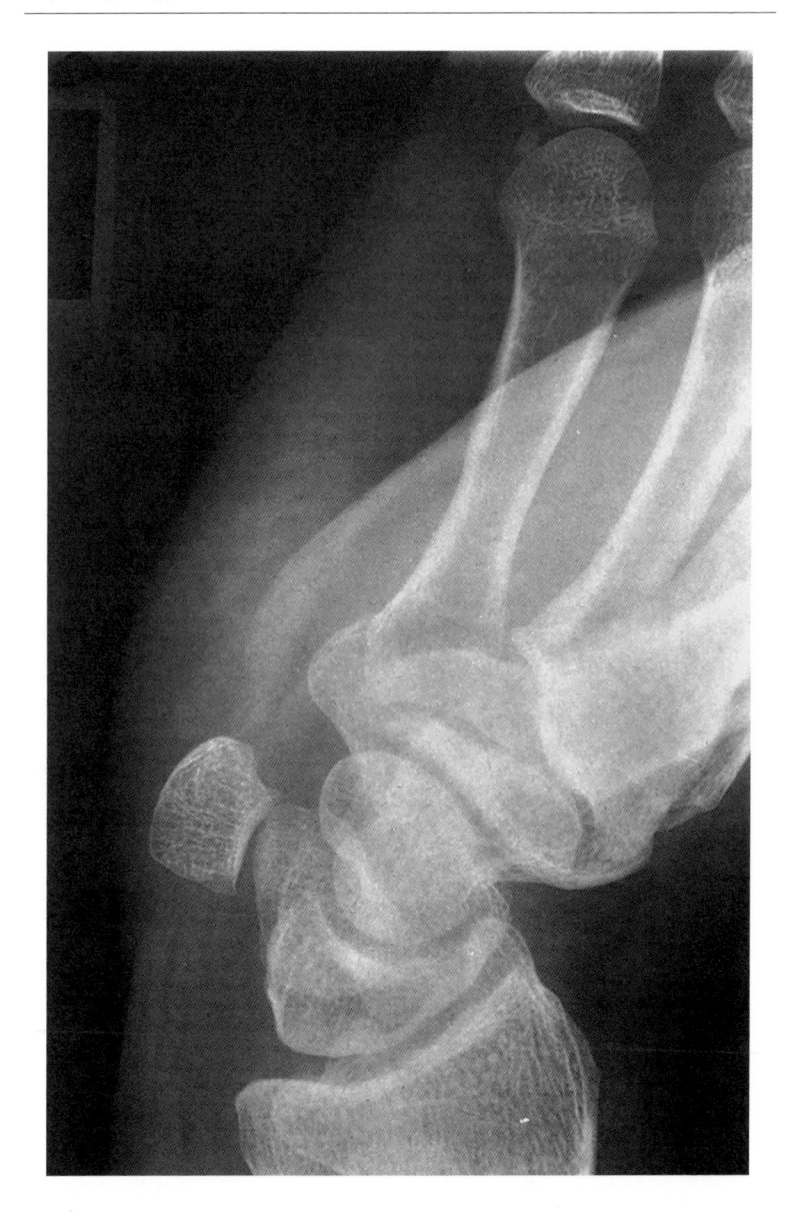

豆状骨　特殊撮影

1　中手骨 Metacarpals	7　三角骨 Triquetrum
2　有鈎骨 Hamate	8　有頭骨 Capitate
3　小菱形骨 Trapezoid	9　月状骨 Lunate
4　舟状骨 Scaphoid	10　橈骨 Radius
5　豆状骨 Pisiform	11　尺骨茎状突起 Ulnar styloid process
6　大菱形骨 Trapezium	

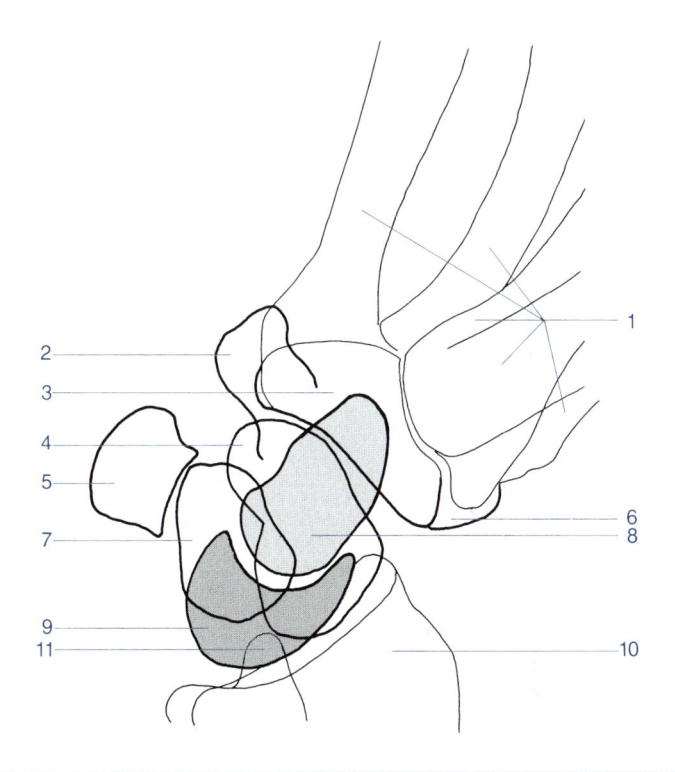

142　上　肢

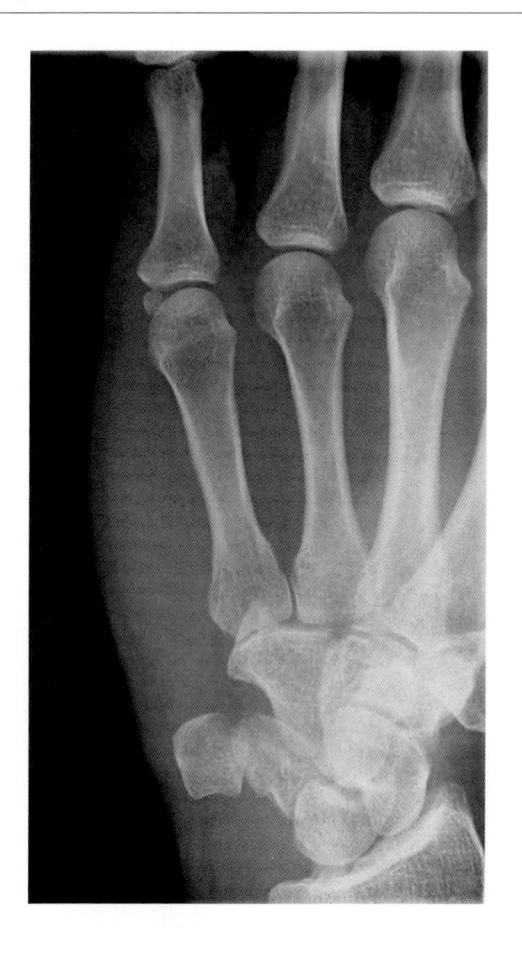

中手骨　斜位

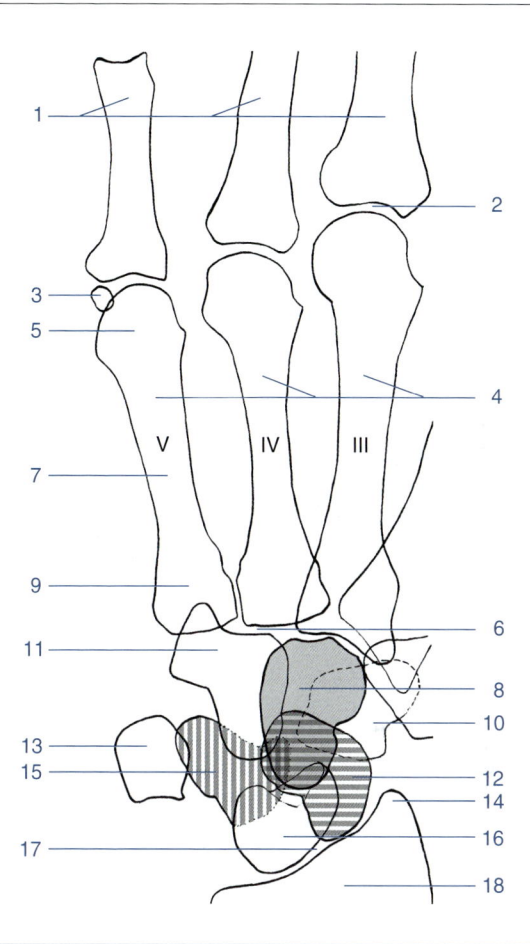

1	基節骨　Proximal phalanges
2	中手指節関節（MP関節）Metacarpophalangeal joint
3	種子骨　Sesamoid
4	第3〜第5中手骨　Third through fifth metacarpals
5	第5中手骨頭　Fifth metacarpal head
6	手根中手関節（CM関節）Carpometacarpal joint
7	第5中手骨体　Fifth metacarpal shaft
8	有頭骨　Capitate
9	第5中手骨底　Fifth metacarpal base
10	大菱形骨　Trapezium，小菱形骨　Trapezoid　重なっている
11	有鈎骨　Hamate
12	舟状骨　Scaphoid
13	豆状骨　Pisiform
14	橈骨茎状突起　Radial styloid process
15	三角骨　Triquetrum
16	月状骨　Lunate
17	橈骨手根関節　Radiocarpal joint
18	橈骨　Radius

144 上　肢

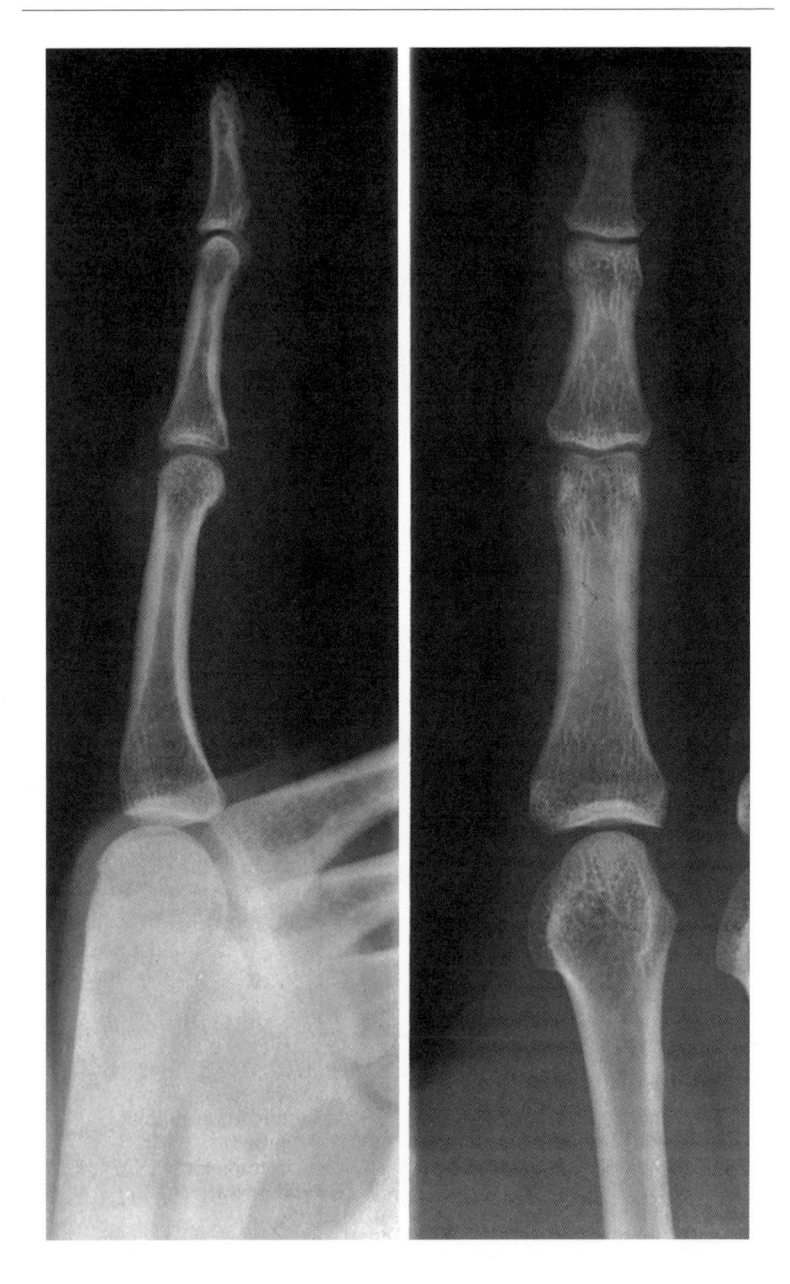

手指 2方向　**145**

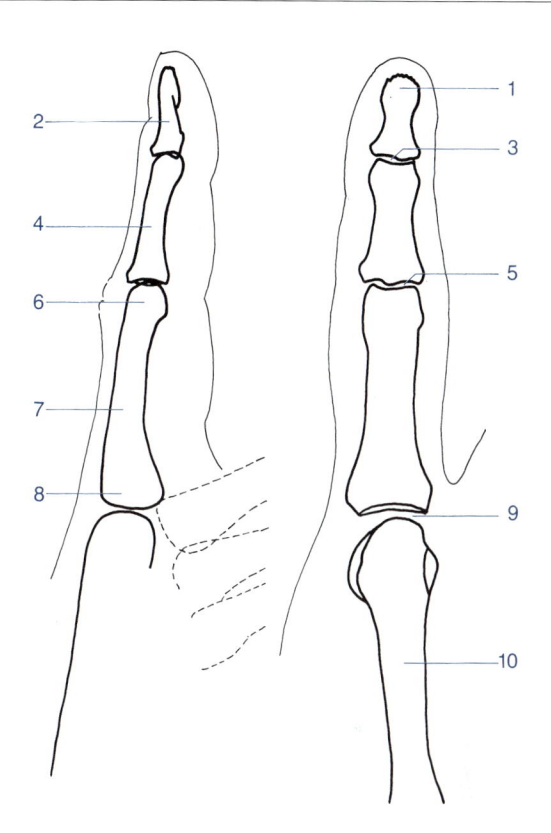

1　末節骨（指腹）Distal phalanx（tuft）	6　基節骨頭 Head of the proximal phalanx
2　末節骨 Distal phalanx	7　基節骨 Proximal phalanx
3　遠位指節間関節（DIP関節）Distal interphalangeal joint	8　基節骨底 Base of the proximal phalanx
4　中節骨 Middle phalanx	9　中手指節関節（MP関節）Metacarpophalangeal joint
5　近位指節間関節（PIP関節）Proximal interphalangeal joint	10　中手骨 Metacarpal

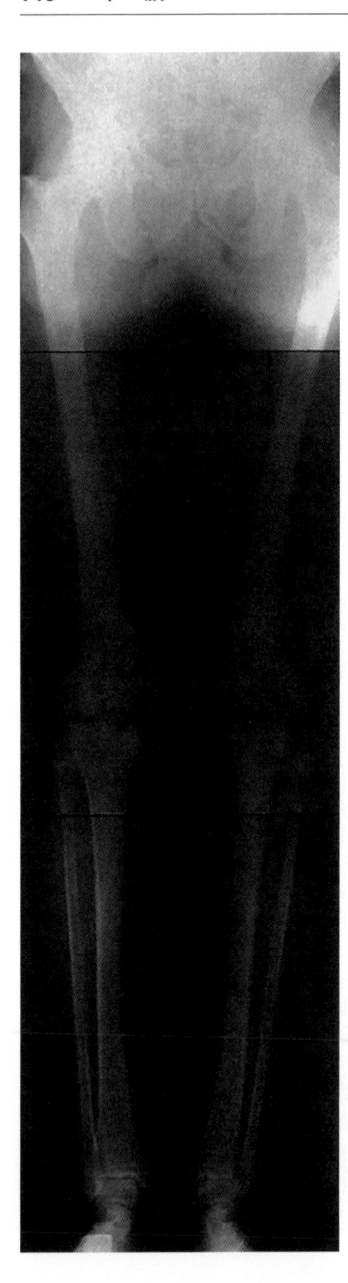

A	大腿骨遠位1/3 Distal third of the femur
B	大腿骨中間1/3 Middle third of the femur
C	大腿骨近位1/3 Proximal third of the femur
D	下腿遠位1/3 Proximal third of the lower leg
E	下腿中間1/3 Middle third of the lower leg
F	下腿遠位1/3 Distal third of the lower leg
1	股関節腔 Joint space of the hip
2	恥骨 Pubis
3	大腿骨頭 Femoral head
4	大転子 Greater trochanter
5	閉鎖孔 Obturator foramen
6	坐骨 Ischium
7	坐骨結節 Ischial tuberosity
8	大腿骨 Femur
9	膝蓋骨 Patella
10	大腿骨内側顆および外側顆 Medial and lateral femoral condyles
11	膝関節腔 Joint space of the knee
12	顆間隆起 Intercondylar eminence
13	脛骨内側顆および外側顆 Medial and lateral tibial condyles
14	脛骨 Tibia
15	腓骨 Fibula
16	内果 Medial malleolus
17	外果 Lateral malleolus
18	距骨滑車 Trochlea of the talus
19	足関節 Ankle joint

全下肢荷重撮影　正面(前後)　　*147*

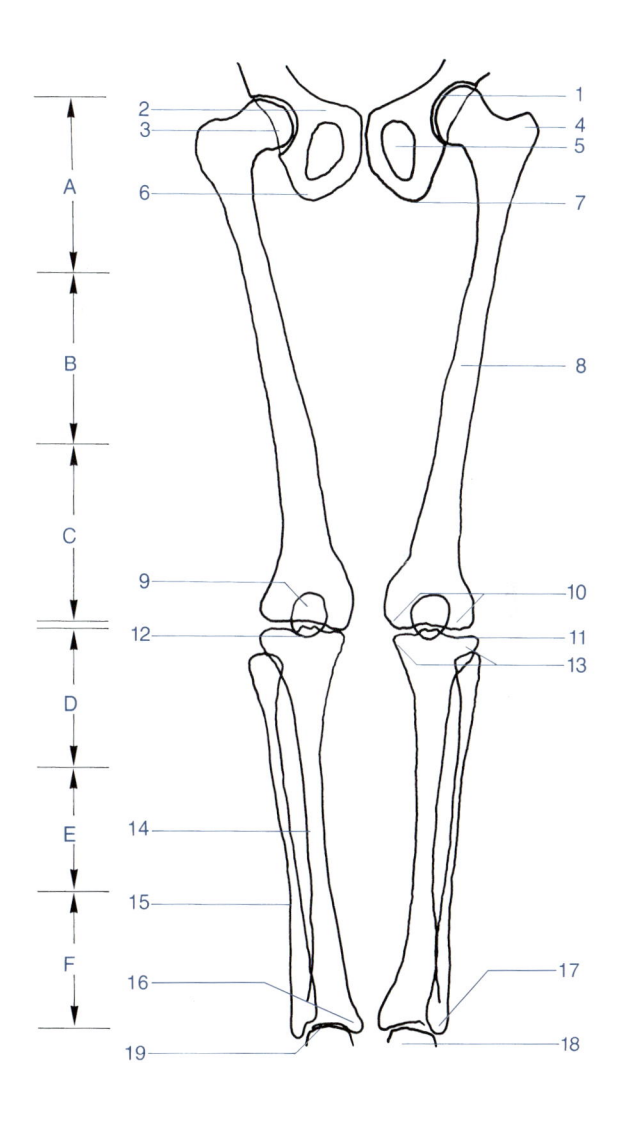

148　下　肢

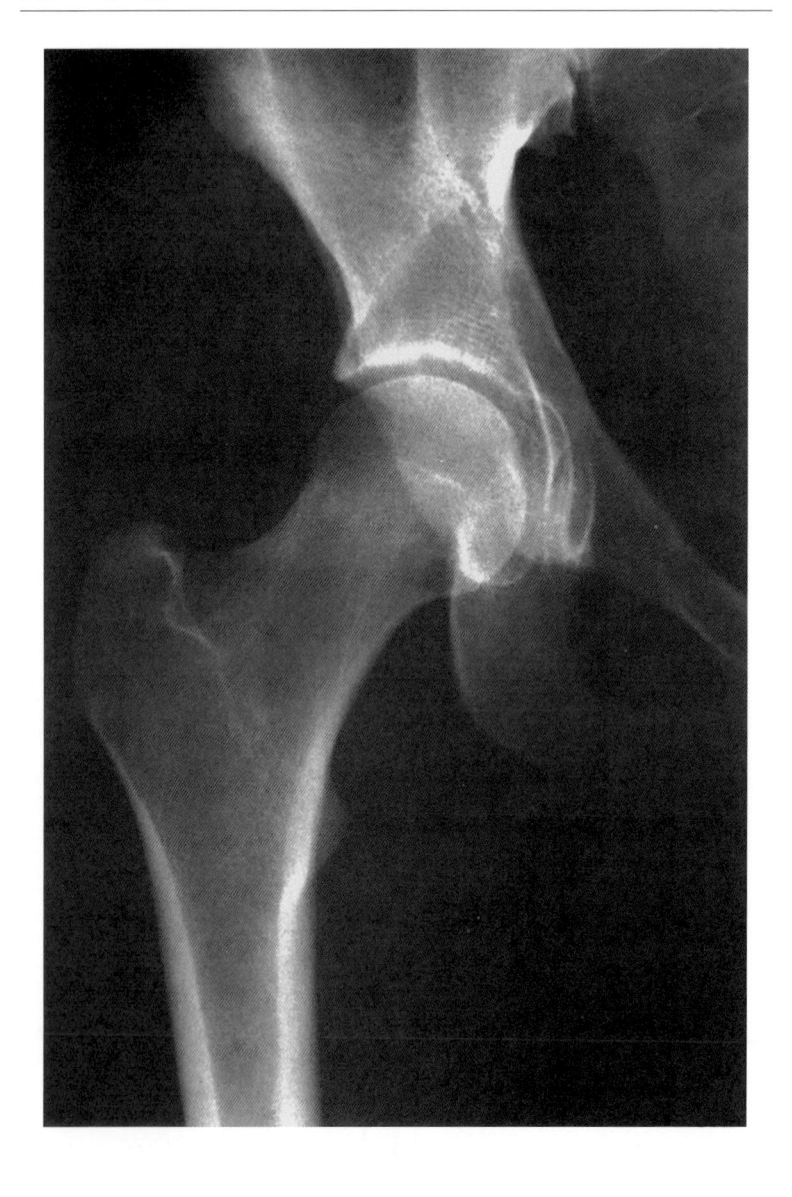

股関節　正面（前後） 149

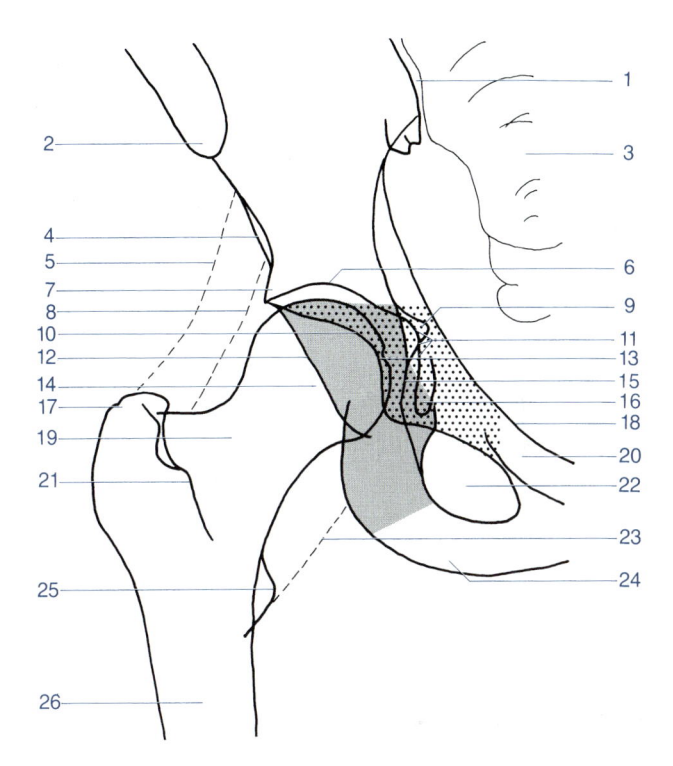

1	仙腸関節 Sacroiliac joint
2	上前腸骨棘 Anterior superior iliac spine
3	仙骨 Sacrum
4	下前腸骨棘 Anterior inferior iliac spine
5	殿筋間の脂肪線 Intergluteal fat stripe
6	臼蓋 Roof of the acetabulum
7	寛骨臼蓋 Acetabular convexity（臼蓋嘴 Promontory）
8	小殿筋内側の脂肪線 Fat stripe medial to the gluteus minimus
9	坐骨棘 Spine of the ischium
10	寛骨臼前縁 Anterior acetabular rim
11	臼底 Floor of the acetabulum
12	寛骨臼後縁 Posterior acetabular rim
13	大腿骨頭窩 Fovea of the femoral head
14	大腿骨頭 Femoral head
15	腸骨坐骨線 Ilioischial line
16	Köhler の涙痕 Köhler's teardrop figure
17	大転子 Greater trochanter
18	分界線 Terminal line
19	大腿骨頸 Femoral neck
20	恥骨上枝 Superior pubic ramus
21	転子間稜 Intertrochanteric crest
22	閉鎖孔 Obturator foramen
23	腸腰筋内側の脂肪線 Fat stripe medial to the iliopsoas
24	坐骨結節 Ischial tuberosity
25	小転子 Lesser trochanter
26	大腿骨 Femur

坐骨 Ischium (**後柱** Posterior column)
恥骨 Pubis (**前柱** Anterior column)

150　下　肢

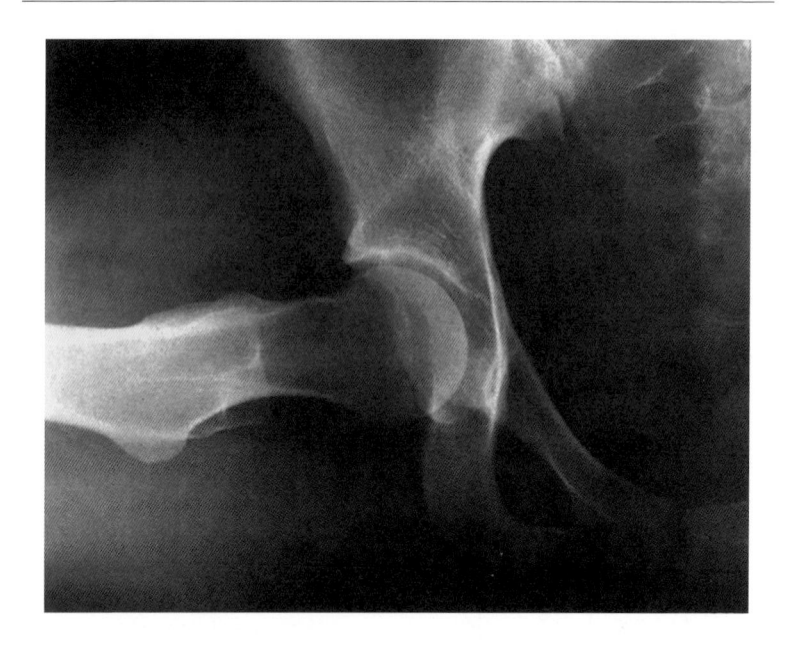

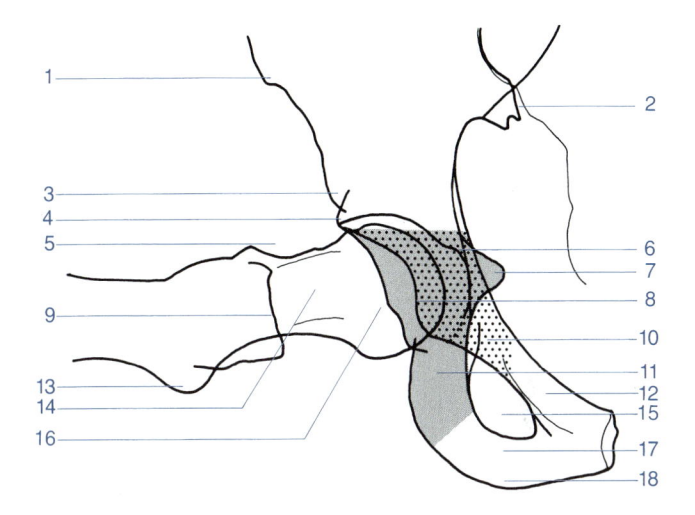

股関節 Lauenstein法

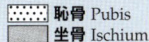

1 上前腸骨棘 Anterior superior iliac spine
2 仙腸関節 Sacroiliac joint
3 下前腸骨棘 Anterior inferior iliac spine
4 寛骨臼上縁 Superior acetabular rim
5 寛骨臼後縁 Posterior acetabular rim
6 臼底 Floor of the acetabulum
7 坐骨棘 Spine of the ischium
8 寛骨臼前縁 Anterior acetabular rim
9 大転子 Greater trochanter
10 恥骨 Pubis（前柱 Anterior column）
11 坐骨 Ischium（後柱 Posterior column）
12 恥骨上枝 Superior pubic ramus
13 小転子 Lesser trochanter
14 大腿骨頸 Femoral neck
15 閉鎖孔 Obturator foramen
16 大腿骨頭 Femoral head
17 恥骨下枝 Inferior pubic ramus
18 坐骨結節 Ischial tuberosity

恥骨 Pubis
坐骨 Ischium

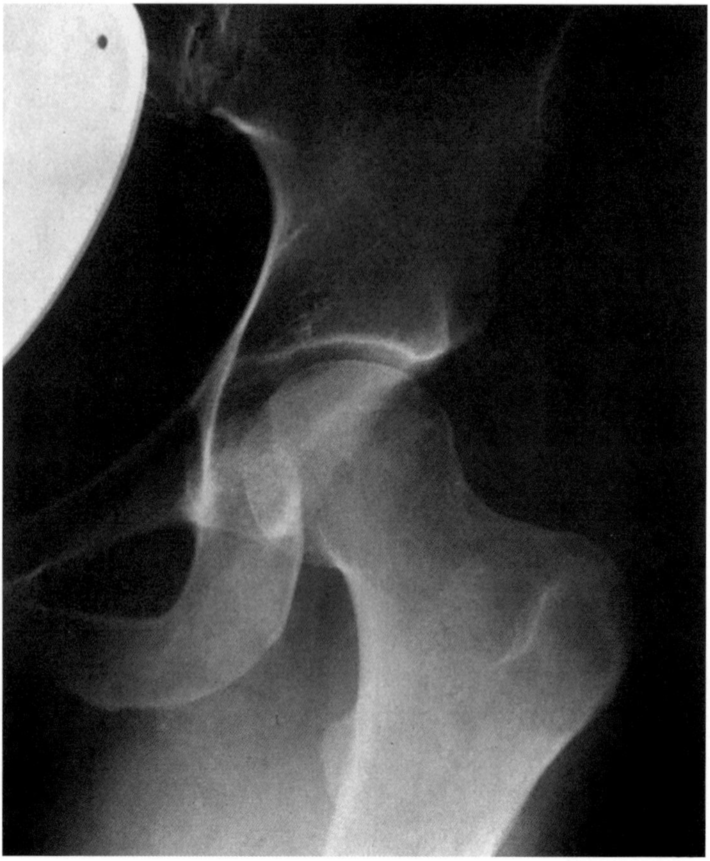

股関節　接線（Schneider I 法）　**153**

1　仙腸関節 Sacroiliac joint	10　恥骨 Pubis（前柱 Anterior column）
2　腸骨 Ilium	11　寛骨臼後縁 Posterior acetabular rim
3　上前腸骨棘 Anterior superior iliac spine	12　坐骨 Ischium
4　下前腸骨棘 Anterior inferior iliac spine	13　大腿骨頸 Femoral neck
5　臼蓋 Roof of the acetabulum	14　閉鎖孔 Obturator foramen
6　寛骨臼上縁 Superior acetabular rim	15　大転子 Greater trochanter
7　坐骨棘 Spine of the ischium	16　坐骨結節 Ischial tuberosity
8　大腿骨頭の関節面前部 Anterior articular surface of the femoral head	17　転子間稜 Intertrochanteric crest
9　寛骨臼前縁 Anterior acetabular rim	18　小転子 Lesser trochanter

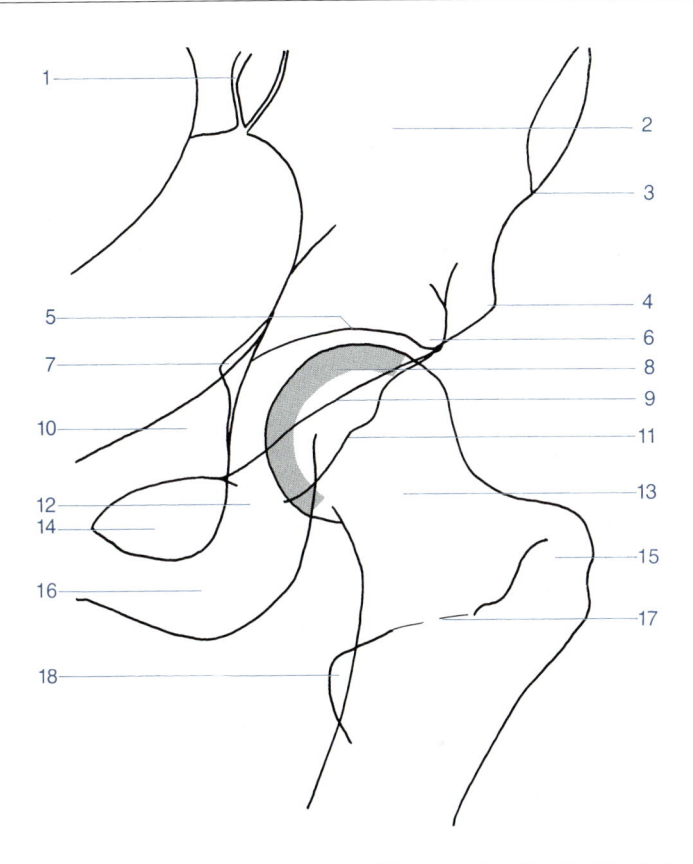

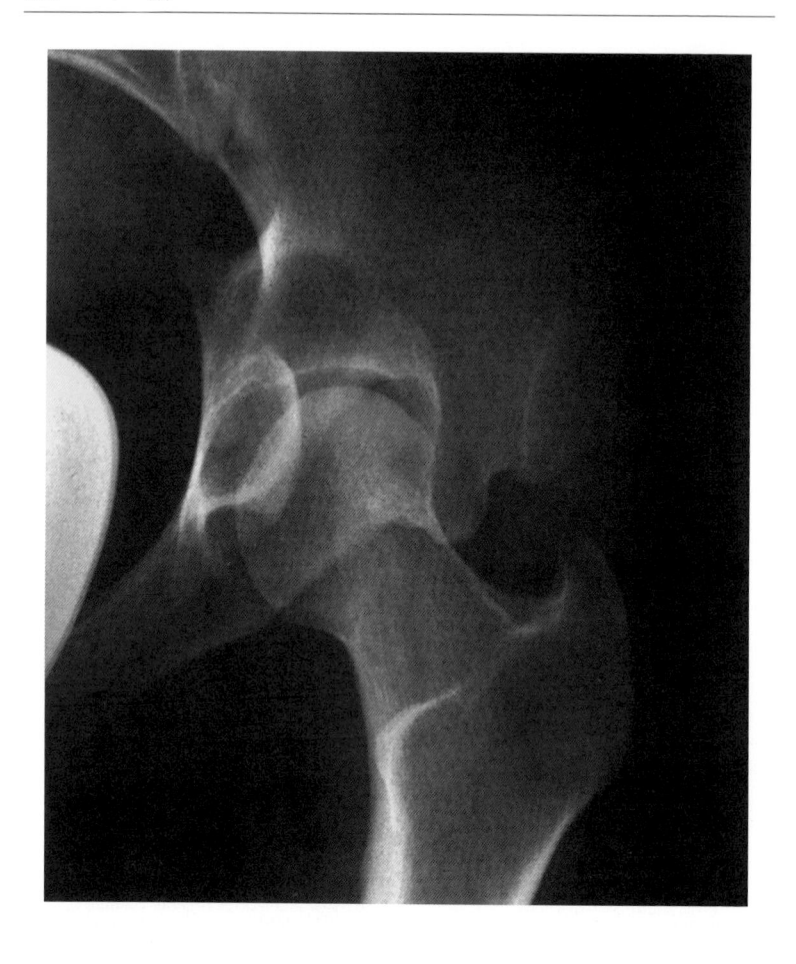

下 肢

股関節　接線（Schneider Ⅱ 法）　**155**

1　仙腸関節 Sacroiliac joint	8　寛骨臼前縁 Anterior acetabular rim
2　腸骨 Ilium	9　大転子 Greater trochanter
3　坐骨棘 Spine of the ischium	10　大腿骨頸 Femoral neck
4　臼蓋 Roof of the acetabulum	11　坐骨 Ischium
5　大腿骨頭の関節面後部 Posterior articular surface of the femoral head	12　恥骨 Pubis
6　上前腸骨棘 Anterior superior iliac spine	13　転子間稜 Intertrochanteric crest
7　臼底 Floor of the acetabulum	14　小転子 Lesser trochanter

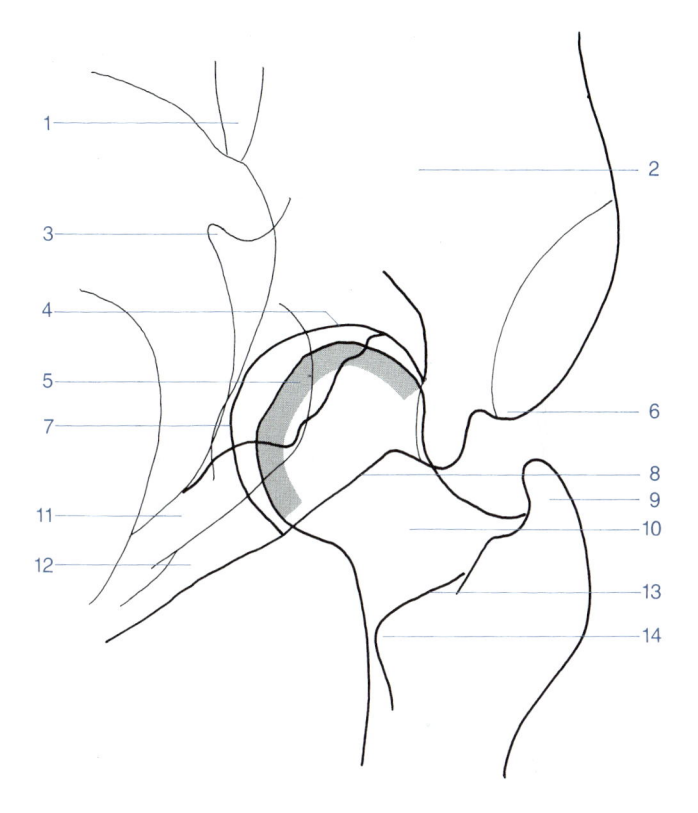

156 下 肢

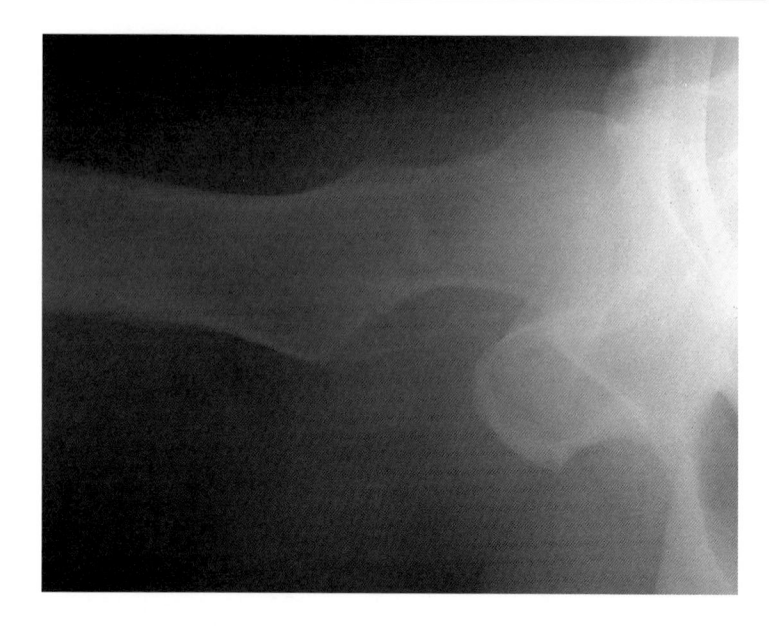

股関節　軸位

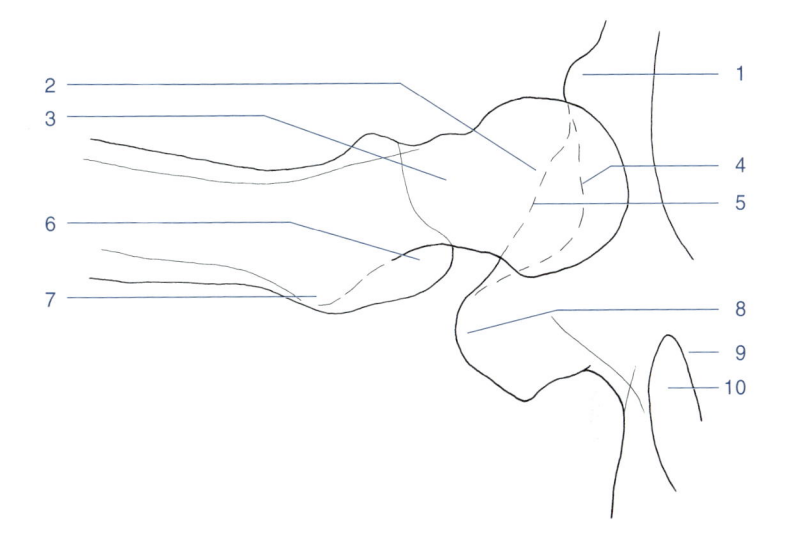

1 下前腸骨棘 Anterior inferior iliac spine
2 大腿骨頭 Femoral head
3 大腿骨頸 Femoral neck
4 寛骨臼前縁 Anterior acetabular rim
5 寛骨臼後縁 Posterior acetabular rim
6 大転子 Greater trochanter
7 小転子 Lesser trochanter
8 坐骨結節 Ischial tuberosity
9 恥骨 Pubis
10 閉鎖孔 Obturator foramen

158　下　肢

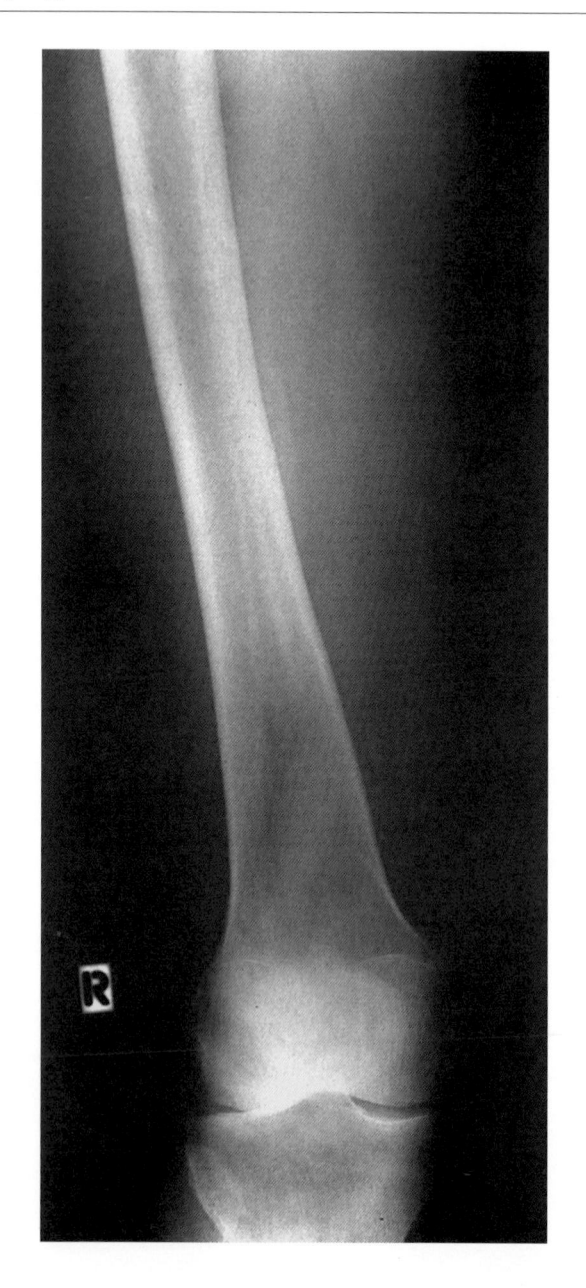

大腿骨　正面（前後） 159

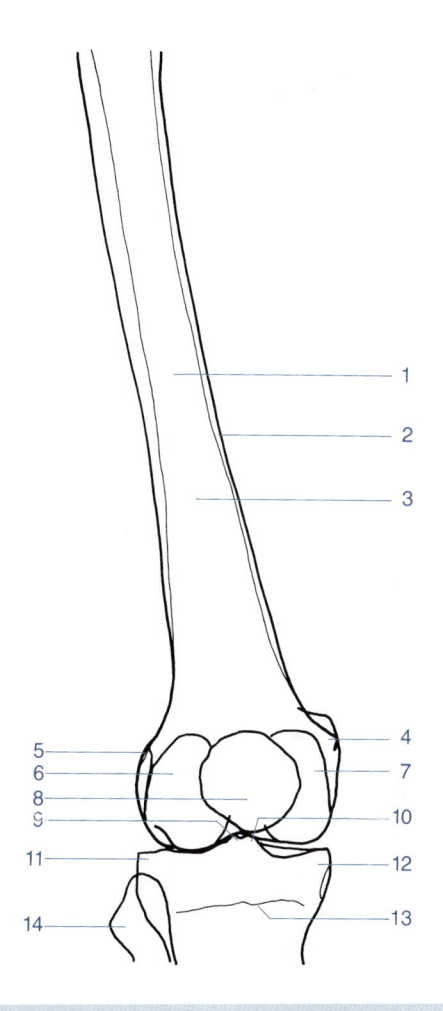

1 大腿骨体　Femoral shaft
2 骨皮質　Cortex
3 骨髄腔　Medullary canal
4 大腿骨内側上顆　Medial femoral epicondyle
5 大腿骨外側上顆　Lateral femoral epicondyle
6 大腿骨外側顆　Lateral femoral condyle
7 大腿骨内側顆　Medial femoral condyle
8 膝蓋骨　Patella
9 外側顆間結節　Lateral intercondylar tubercle
10 内側顆間結節　Medial intercondylar tubercle
11 脛骨外側顆　Lateral tibial condyle
12 脛骨内側顆　Medial tibial condyle
13 成長板　Growth plate
14 腓骨頭　Fibular head

160　下 肢

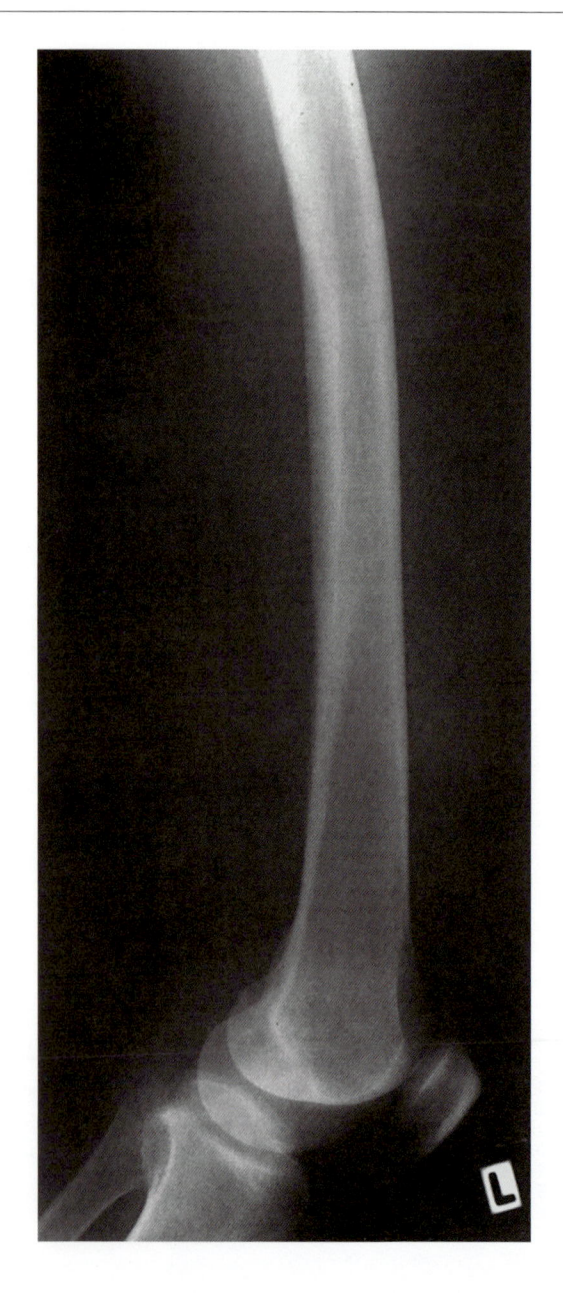

大腿骨 側面

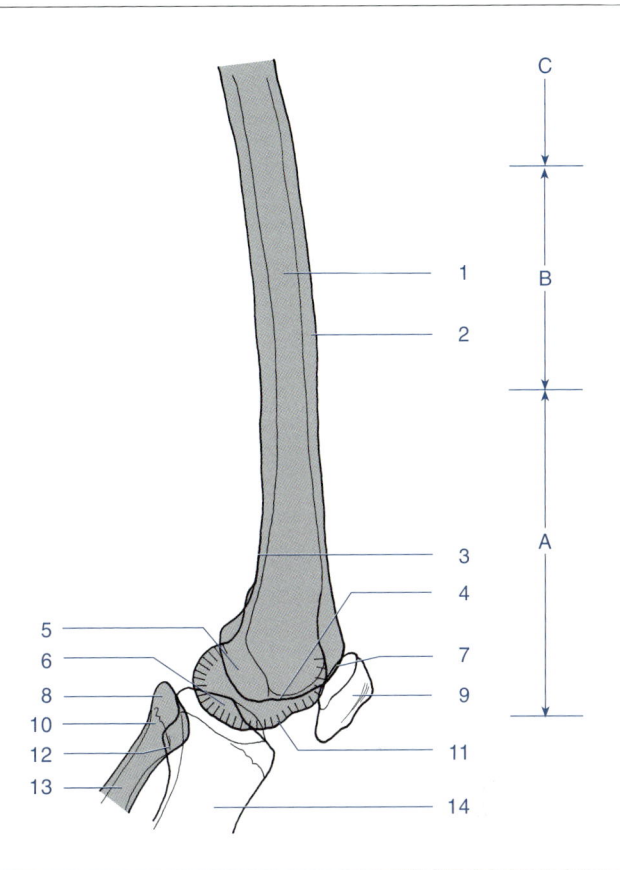

A	大腿骨遠位1/3	Distal third of the femur
B	大腿骨中間1/3	Middle third of the femur
C	大腿骨近位1/3	Proximal third of the femur

1. 大腿骨 Femur
2. 骨皮質 Cortex
3. 膝窩 Popliteal fossa
4. 大腿骨外側顆 Lateral femoral condyle
5. 顆間窩 Intercondylar fossa
6. 顆間隆起 Intercondylar eminence
7. 膝蓋大腿関節 Patellofemoral joint
8. 腓骨頭の尖端 Apex of the fibular head
9. 膝蓋骨 Patella
10. 腓骨頭 Fibular head
11. 大腿骨内側顆 Medial femoral condyle
    a 対側の大腿骨外側顆(4)は腓骨(13)と関節を形成する
    b 膝蓋骨(9)と大腿骨の関節面は，どのような体位で撮影された場合でも，外側面の方が内側面よりも長く描出される．
12. 脛腓関節 Tibiofibular joint
13. 腓骨 Fibula
14. 脛骨 Tibia

162　下　肢

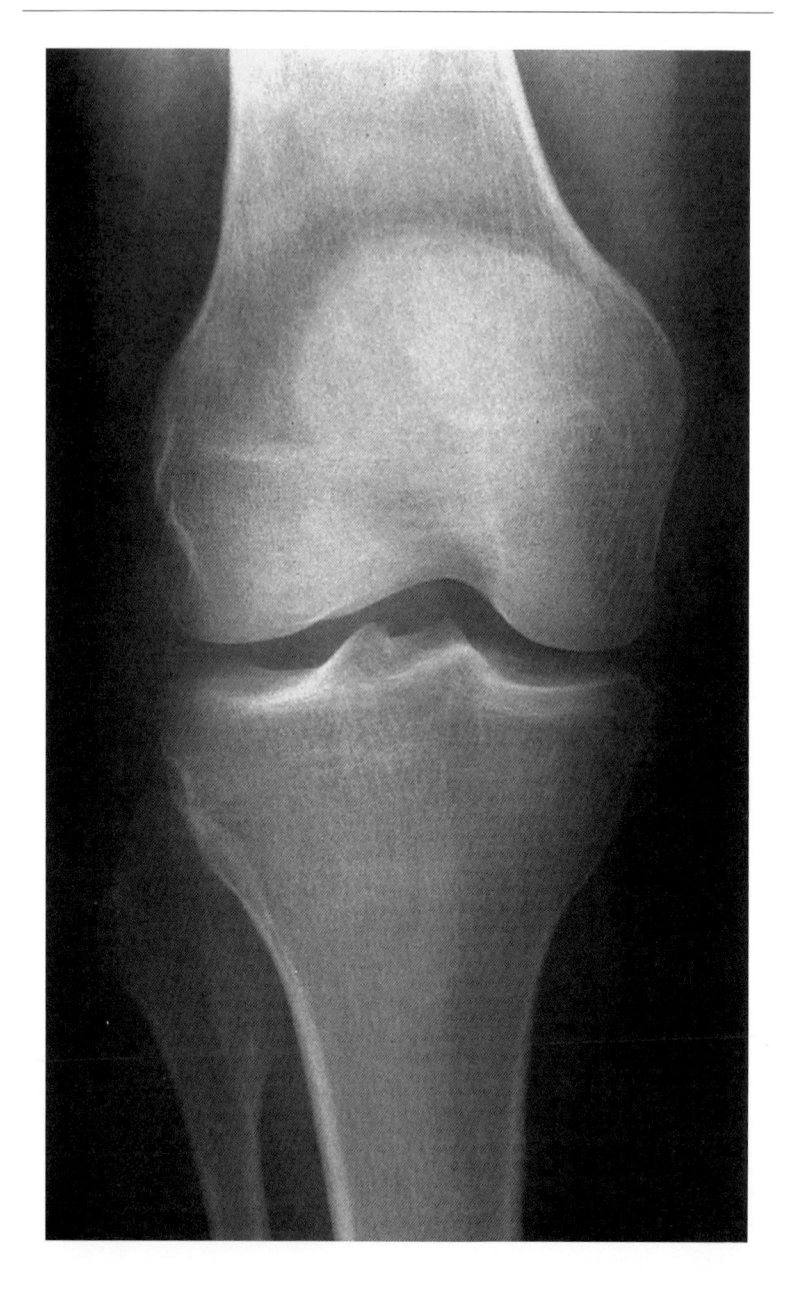

膝関節　正面（前後）　　*163*

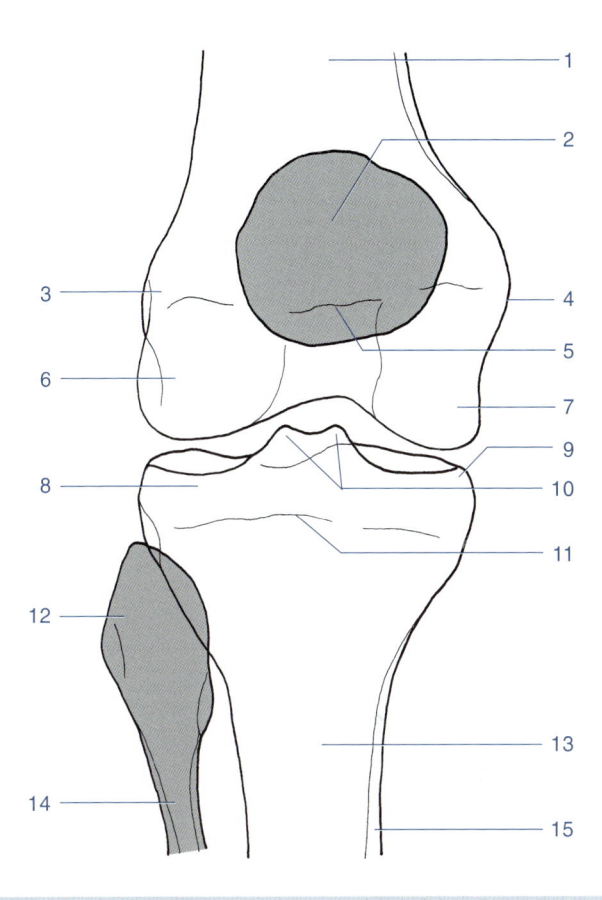

1 大腿骨 Femur
2 膝蓋骨 Patella
3 大腿骨外側上顆 Lateral femoral epicondyle
4 大腿骨内側上顆 Medial femoral epicondyle
5 成長板 Growth plate
6 大腿骨外側顆 Lateral femoral condyle
7 大腿骨内側顆 Medial femoral condyle
8 脛骨外側顆 Lateral tibial condyle
9 脛骨内側顆 Medial tibial condyle
10 内側および外側顆間結節 Medial and lateral intercondylar tubercles
11 骨端板 Epiphyseal plate
12 腓骨頭 Fibular head
13 脛骨 Tibia
14 腓骨 Fibula
15 骨皮質 Cortex

164　下　肢

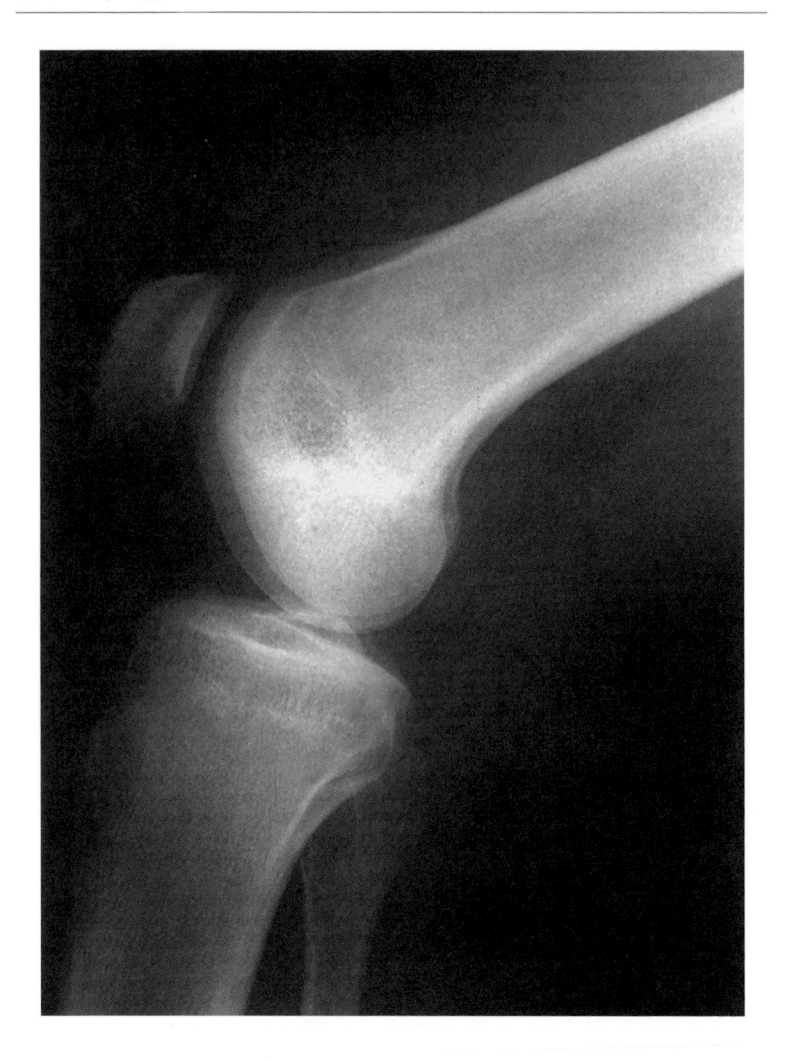

膝関節　側面

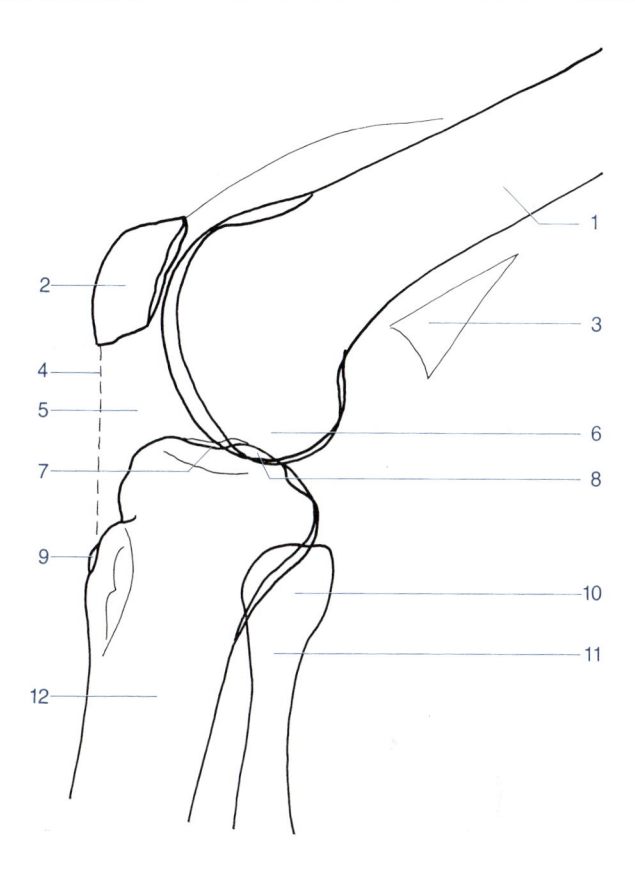

1　大腿骨　Femur	7　脛骨高原　Tibial plateau
2　膝蓋骨　Patella	8　顆間隆起　Intercondylar eminence
3　膝後方の脂肪　Posterior fat	9　脛骨粗面　Tibial tuberosity
4　膝蓋靱帯　Patellar ligament	10　腓骨頭　Fibular head
5　膝蓋下脂肪体　Infrapatellar fat pad	11　腓骨頸　Fibular neck
6　大腿骨外側顆　Lateral femoral condyle	12　脛骨　Tibia

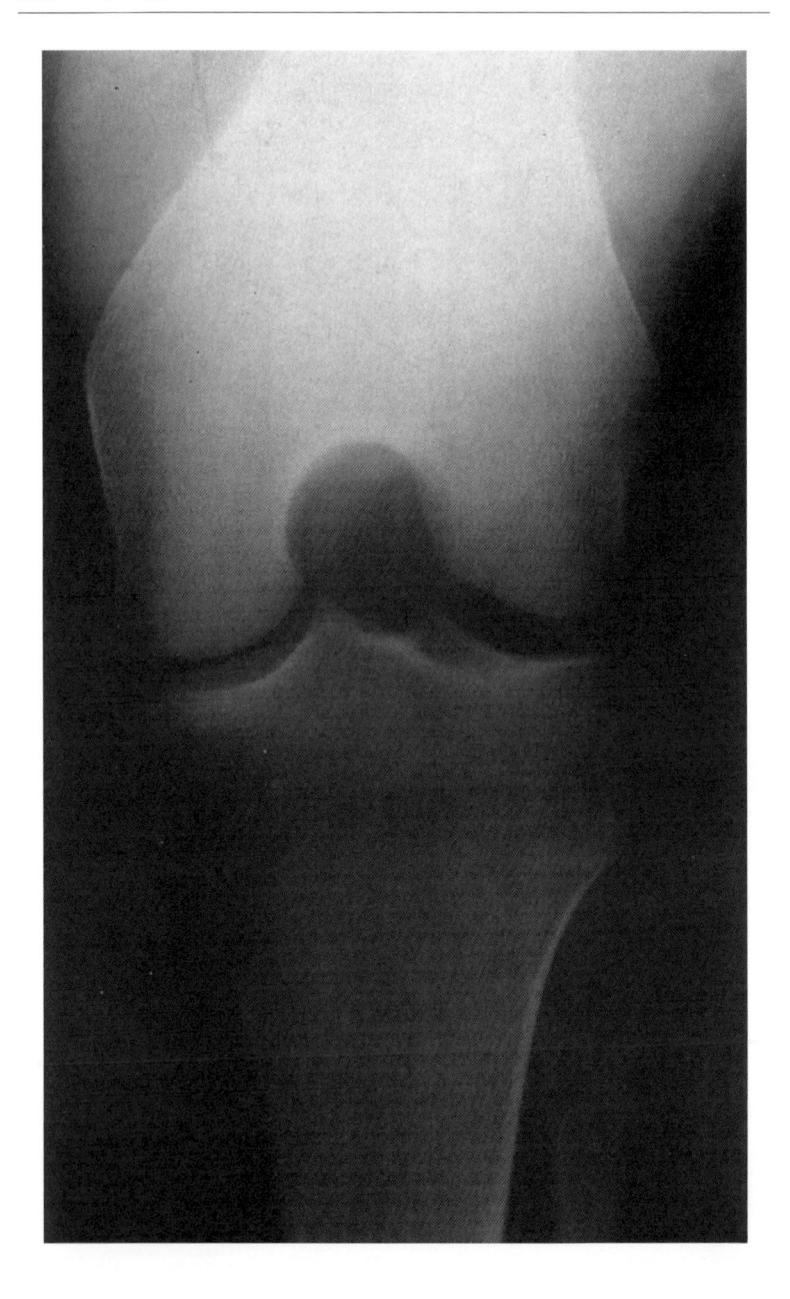

下 肢

膝関節　顆間窩撮影（Frik法）

1　大腿骨　Femur	10　外側脛骨高原　Lateral tibial plateau
2　膝蓋骨　Patella	11　内側脛骨高原　Medial tibial plateau
3　大腿骨内側上顆　Medial femoral epicondyle	12　脛骨粗面　Tibial tuberosity
4　大腿骨外側上顆　Lateral femoral epicondyle	13　成長板　Growth plate
5　顆間窩　Intercondylar fossa	14　腓骨頭　Fibular head
6　大腿骨外側顆　Lateral femoral condyle	15　腓骨頸　Fibular neck
7　大腿骨内側顆　Medial femoral condyle	16　脛骨　Tibia
8　外側顆間結節　Lateral intercondylar tubercle	17　骨間膜　Interosseous membrane
9　内側顆間結節　Medial intercondylar tubercle	

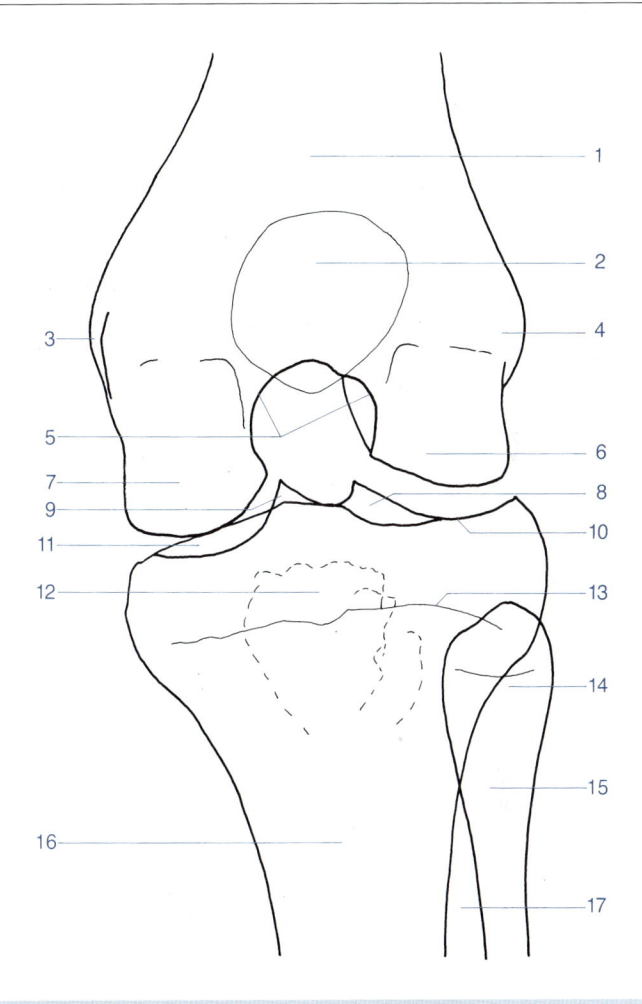

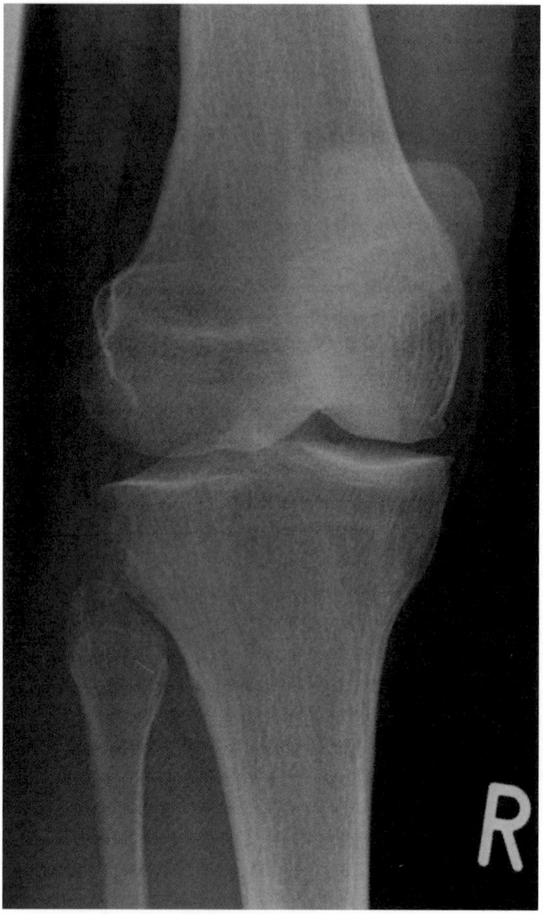
R

膝関節 45°内旋位　**169**

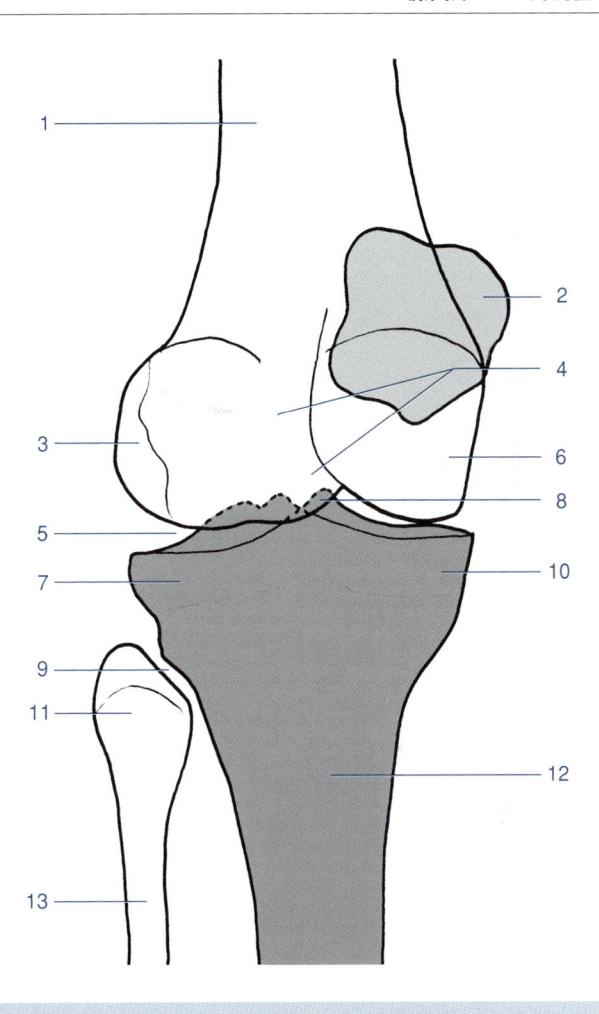

1　大腿骨体 Femoral shaft	8　顆間隆起 Intercondylar eminence
2　膝蓋骨内側縁 Medial margin of the patella	9　脛腓関節 Tibiofibular joint
3　大腿骨外側顆 Lateral femoral condyle	10　脛骨内側顆 Medial tibial condyle
4　顆間窩 Intercondylar fossa	11　腓骨頭 Fibular head
5　膝関節 Knee (関節腔 Joint space)	12　脛骨体 Tibial shaft
6　大腿骨内側顆 Medial femoral condyle	13　腓骨体 Fibular shaft
7　脛骨外側顆 Lateral tibial condyle	

170　下　肢

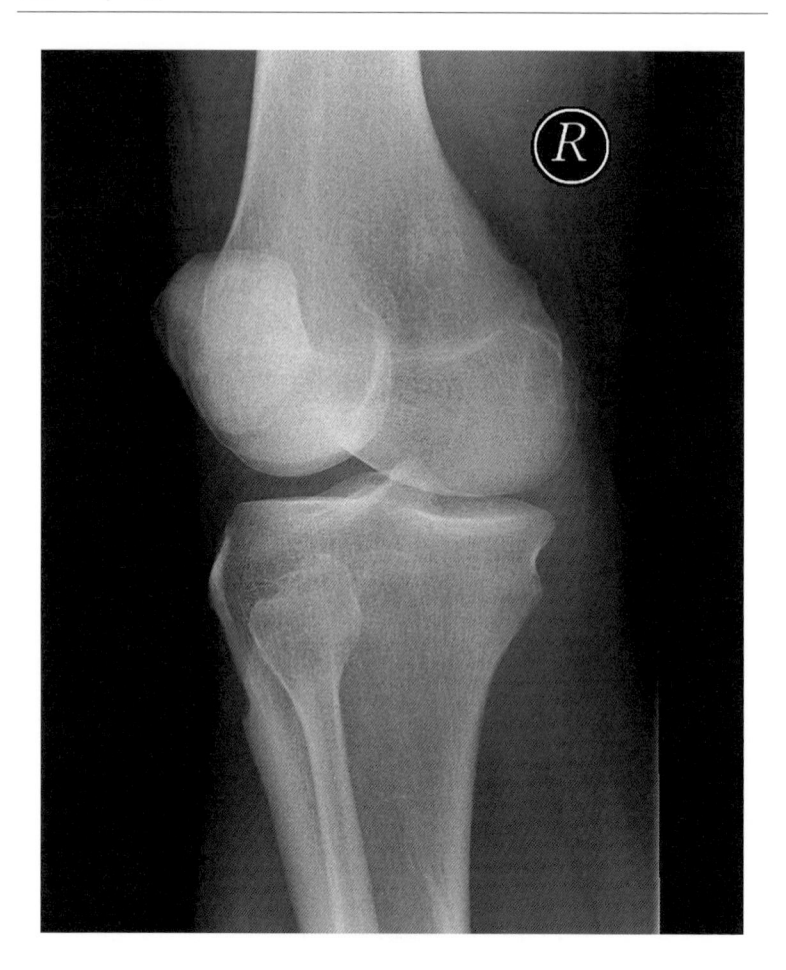

膝関節 45°外旋位 *171*

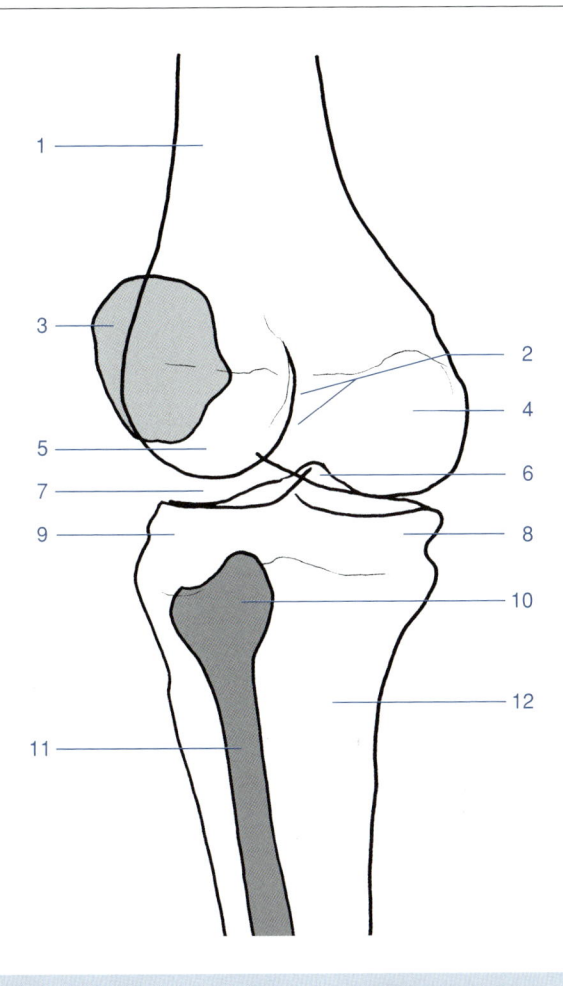

1	大腿骨体 Femoral shaft
2	顆間窩 Intercondylar fossa
3	膝蓋骨外側縁 Lateral margin of the patella
4	大腿骨内側顆 Medial femoral condyle
5	大腿骨外側顆 Lateral femoral condyle
6	顆間隆起 Intercondylar eminence
7	膝関節 Knee (関節腔 Joint space)
8	脛骨内側顆 Medial tibial condyle
9	脛骨外側顆 Lateral tibial condyle
10	腓骨頭 Fibular head
11	腓骨体 Fibular shaft
12	脛骨体 Tibial shaft

172　下 肢

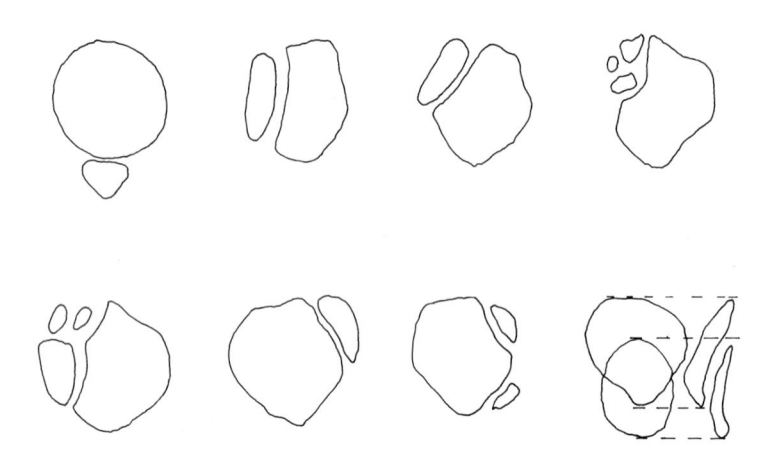

よくみられる分裂膝蓋骨の形態（Schaerによる）

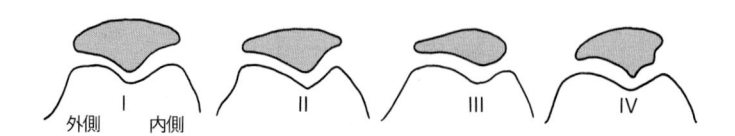

Wibergによる膝蓋骨の形態の分類（右膝）

外側　内側

膝蓋骨 軸位(30°, 60°, 90°屈曲位) 173

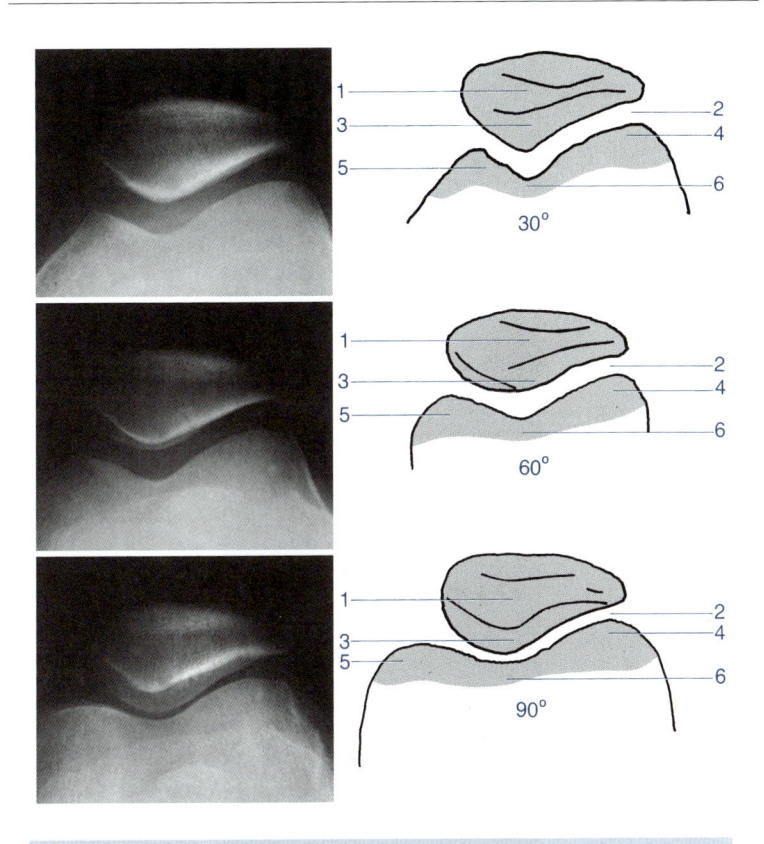

- 1 膝蓋骨 Patella
- 2 膝蓋大腿関節 Patellofemoral joint
- 3 関節面 Articular surface
- 4 大腿骨外側顆 Lateral femoral condyle
  一般的にこちらのほうが大きい
- 5 大腿骨内側顆 Medial femoral condyle
- 6 顆間窩 Intercondylar fossa

174 下 肢

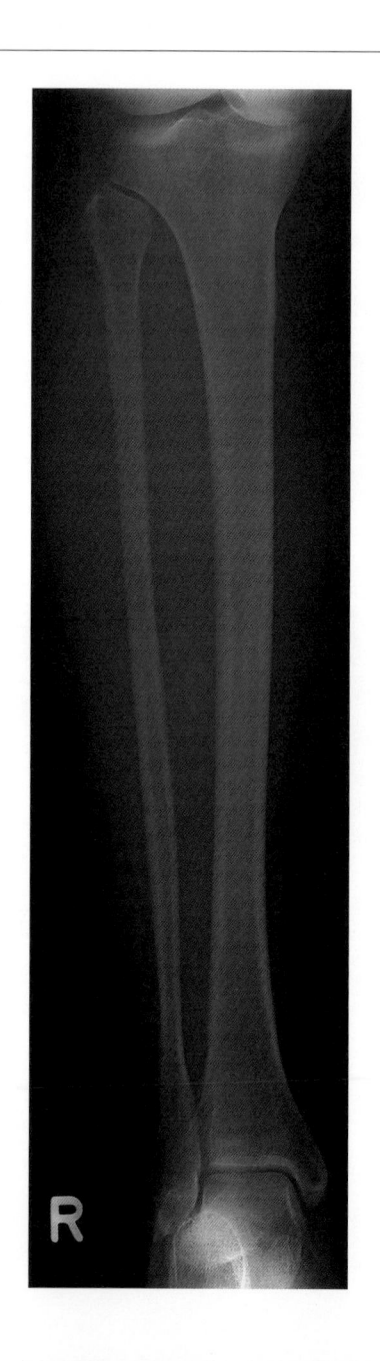

下腿骨 正面(前後)

1 大腿骨内側顆 Medial femoral condyle	9 骨間膜 Interosseous membrane
2 大腿骨外側顆 Lateral femoral condyle	10 腓骨 Fibula
3 内側および外側顆間結節 Medial and lateral intercondylar tubercles	11 脛骨 Tibia
4 脛骨内側顆 Medial tibial condyle	12 骨皮質 Cortex
5 脛骨外側顆 Lateral tibial condyle	13 骨髄腔 Medullary canal
6 脛骨粗面 Tibial tuberosity	14 成長板 Growth plate
7 腓骨頭 Fibular head	15 外果 Lateral malleolus
8 腓骨頸 Fibular neck	16 内果 Medial malleolus
	17 距骨 Talus

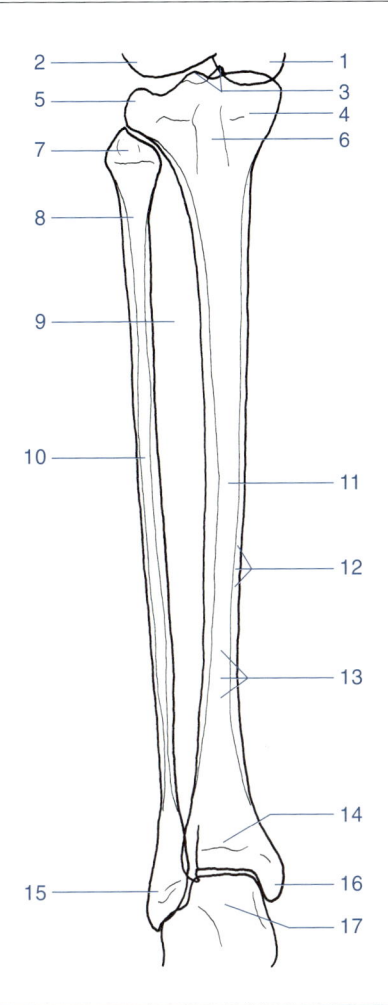

176　下 肢

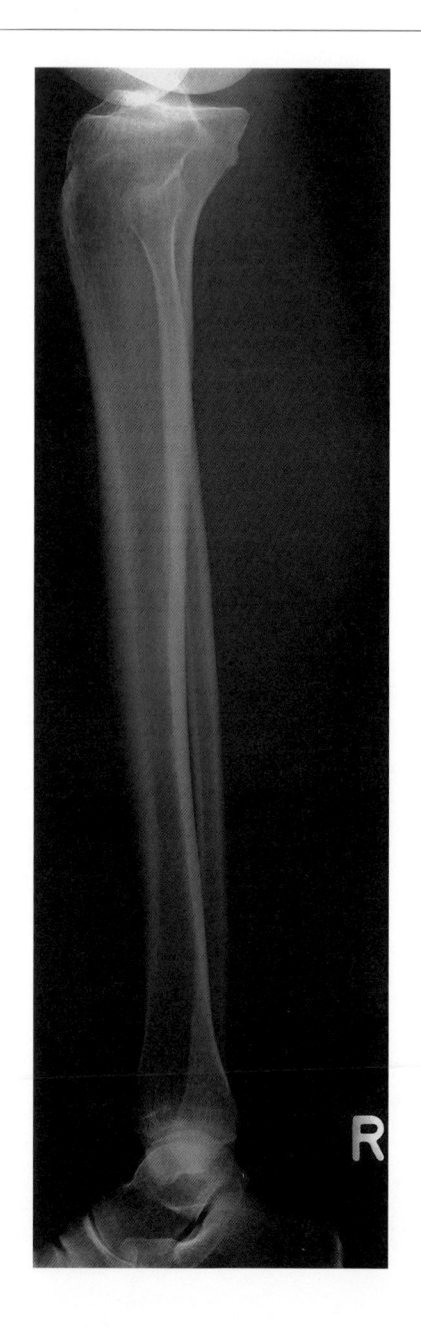

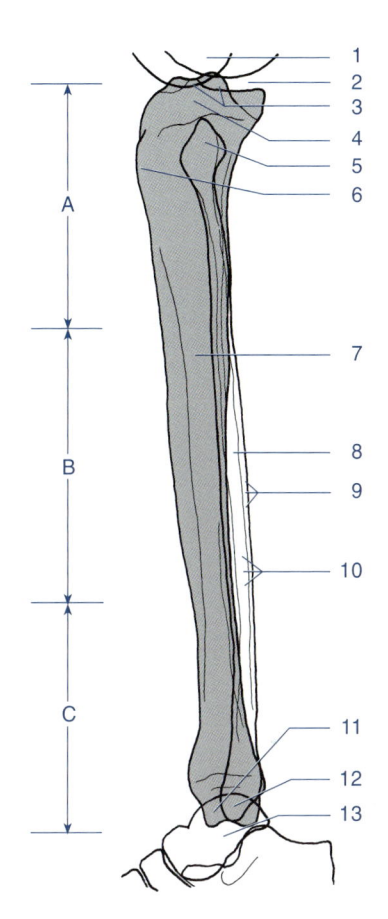

下腿骨 側面 177

A	下腿近位1/3 Proximal third of the lower leg
B	下腿中間1/3 Middle third of the lower leg
C	下腿遠位1/3 Distal third of the lower leg
1	大腿骨内側顆および外側顆 Medial and lateral femoral condyles
2	膝関節 Knee joint
3	顆間隆起 Intercondylar eminence
4	脛骨内側顆および外側顆 Medial and lateral tibial condyles
5	腓骨頭 Fibular head
6	脛骨粗面 Tibial tuberosity （小児では近位脛骨突起 Proximal tibial apophysis）
7	脛骨 Tibia
8	腓骨 Fibula
9	骨皮質 Cortex
10	骨髄腔 Medullary canal
11	内果 Medial malleolus
12	外果 Lateral malleolus
13	距骨 Talus

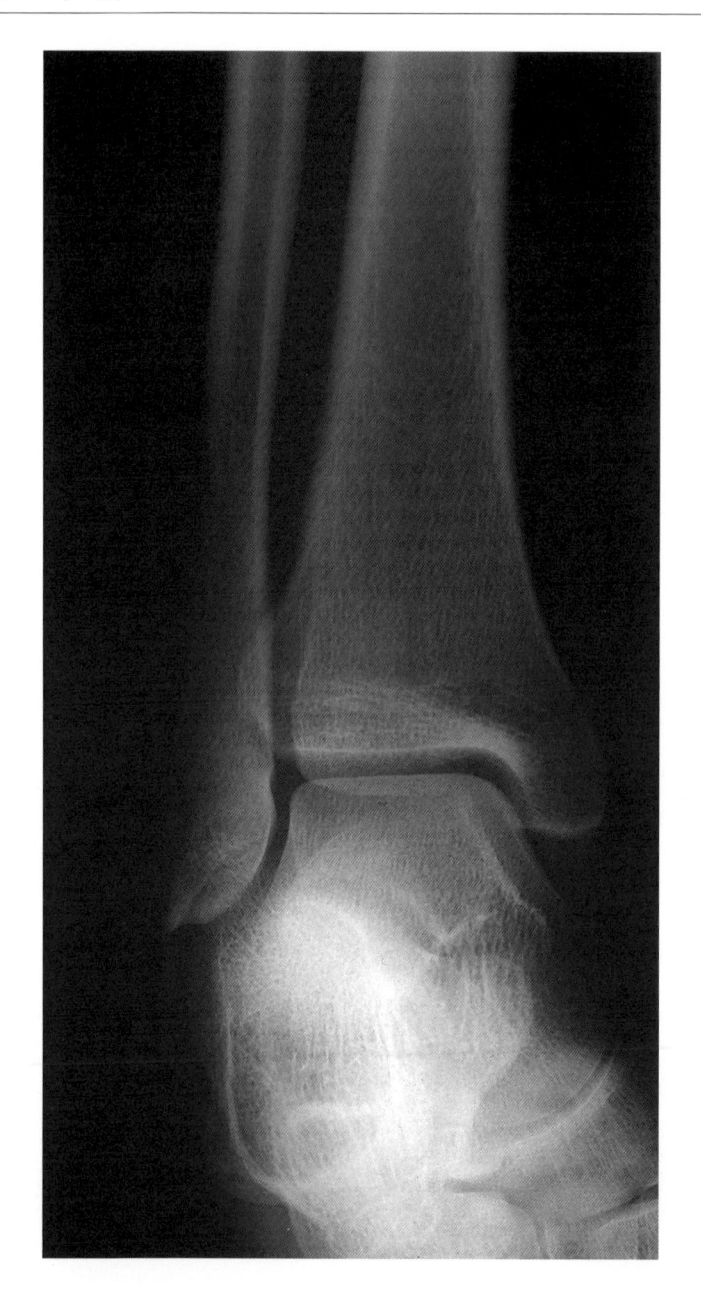

下 肢

足関節　正面（前後）

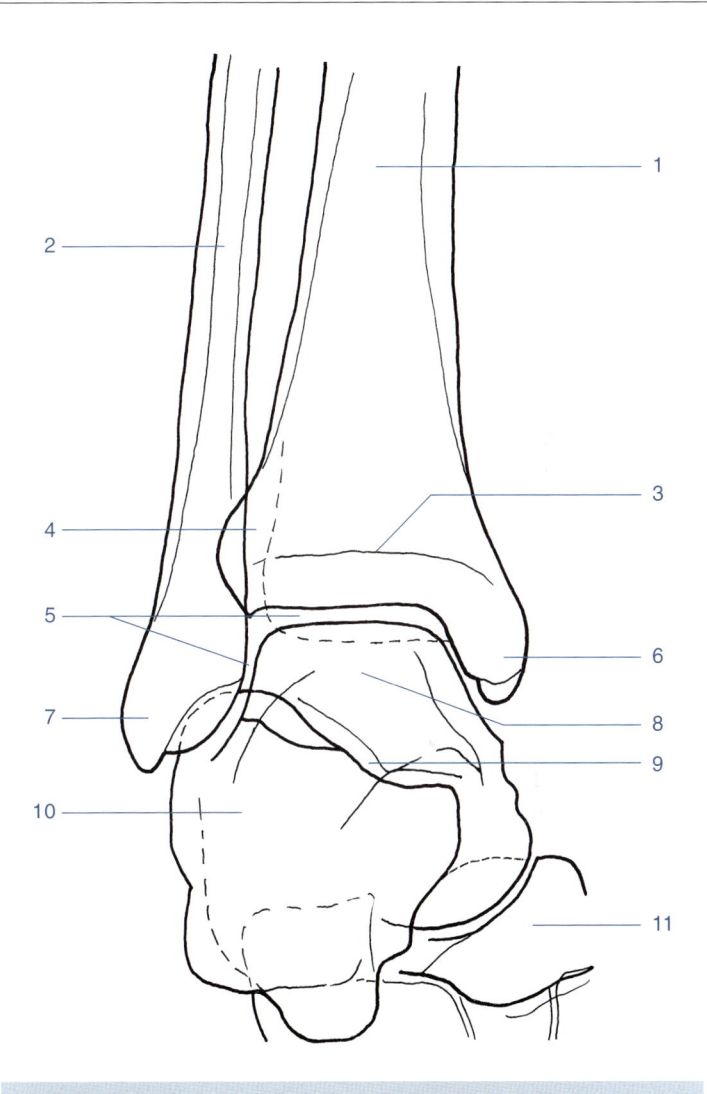

1　脛骨　Tibia	7　外果　Lateral malleolus
2　腓骨　Fibula	8　距骨滑車　Trochlea of the talus
3　成長板　Growth plate	9　距骨下関節　Subtalar joint
4　腓骨　Fibular notch	10　踵骨　Calcaneus
5　足関節　Ankle joint	11　舟状骨　Navicular
6　内果　Medial malleolus	

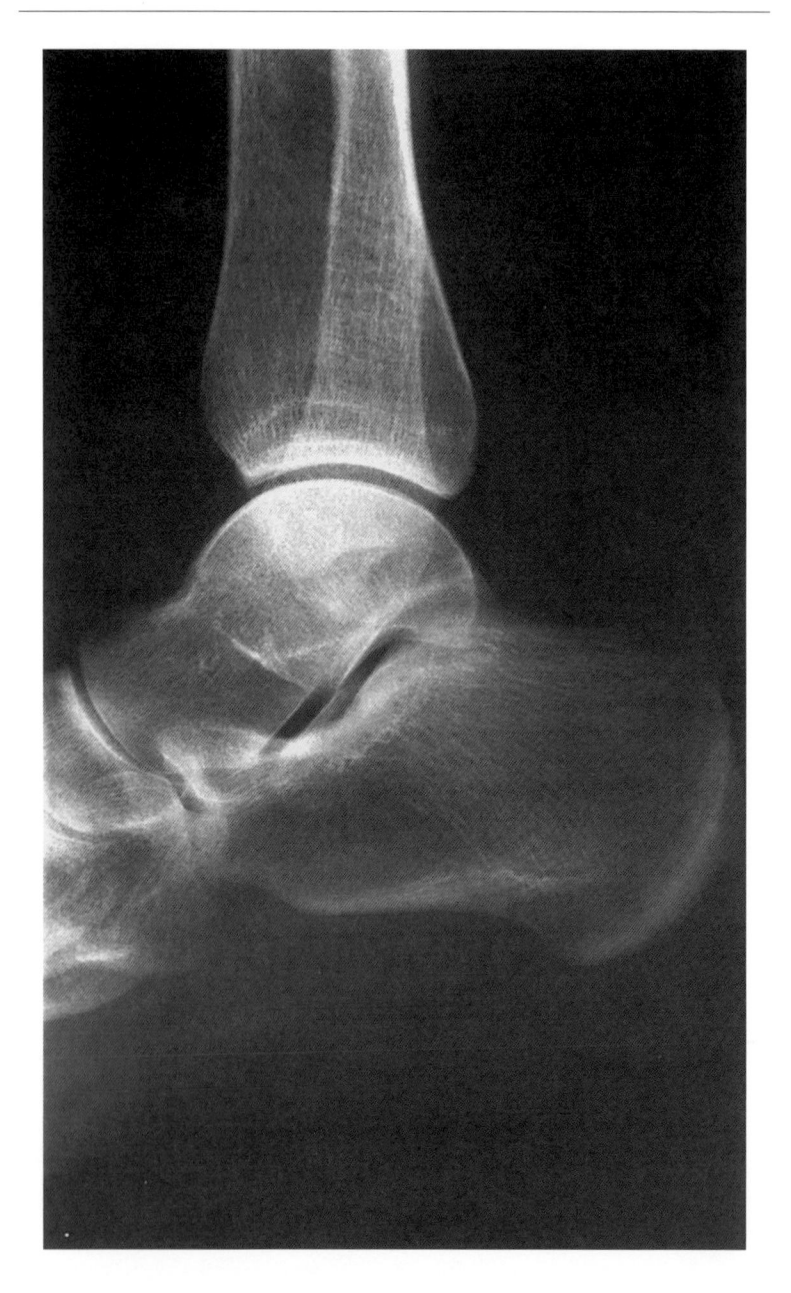

下 肢

足関節 側面

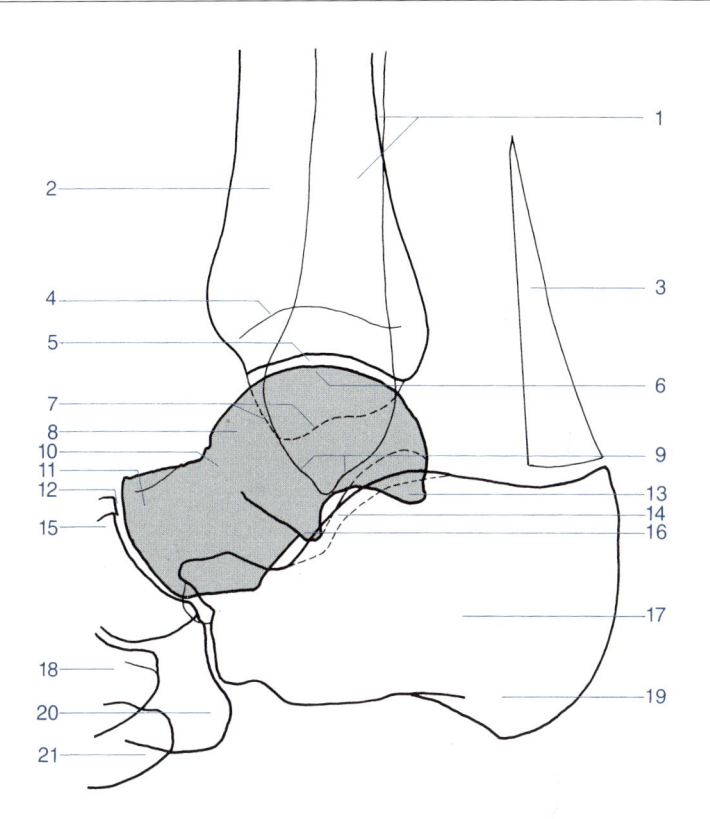

1 腓骨 Fibula	12 距舟関節 Talonavicular joint
2 脛骨 Tibia	13 距骨後突起 Posterior process of the talus
3 アキレス腱 Achilles tendon	14 足根洞 Tarsal sinus
4 成長板 Growth plate	15 舟状骨 Navicular
5 足関節 Ankle joint	16 距骨外側突起 Lateral process of the talus
6 距骨滑車 Trochlea of the talus	17 踵骨 Calcaneus
7 内果 Medial malleolus	18 内側楔状骨 Medial cuneiform
8 距骨 Talus	19 踵骨隆起 Tuberosity of the calcaneus
9 外果 Lateral malleolus	20 立方骨 Cuboid
10 距骨頸 Neck of the talus	21 第5中足骨底 Base of the fifth metatarsal
11 距骨頭 Head of the talus	

182　下 肢

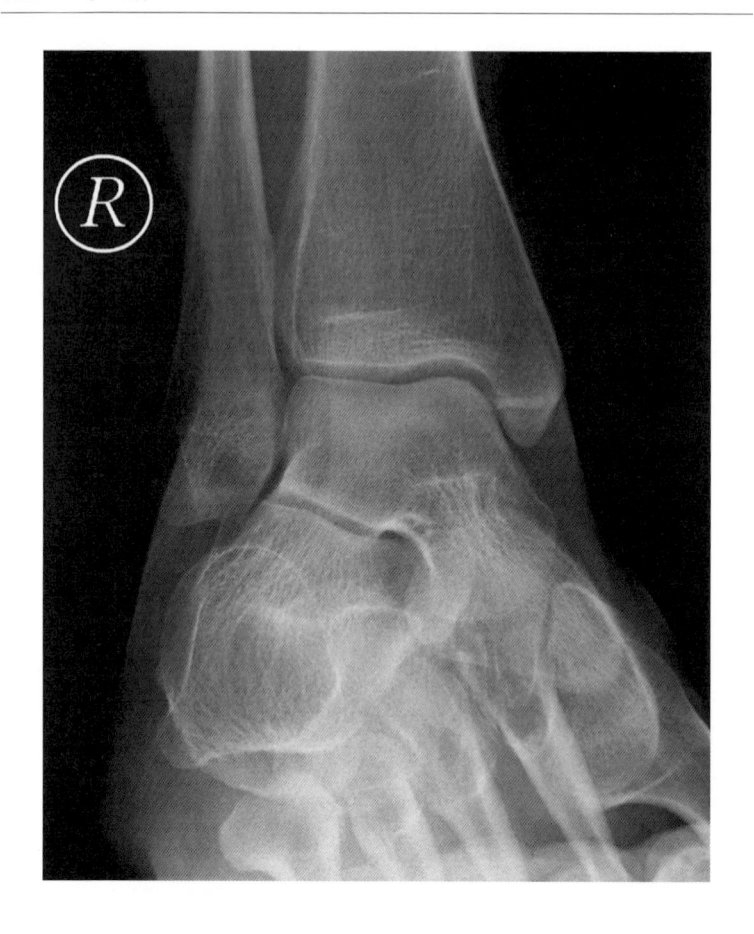

足関節　斜位1　　183

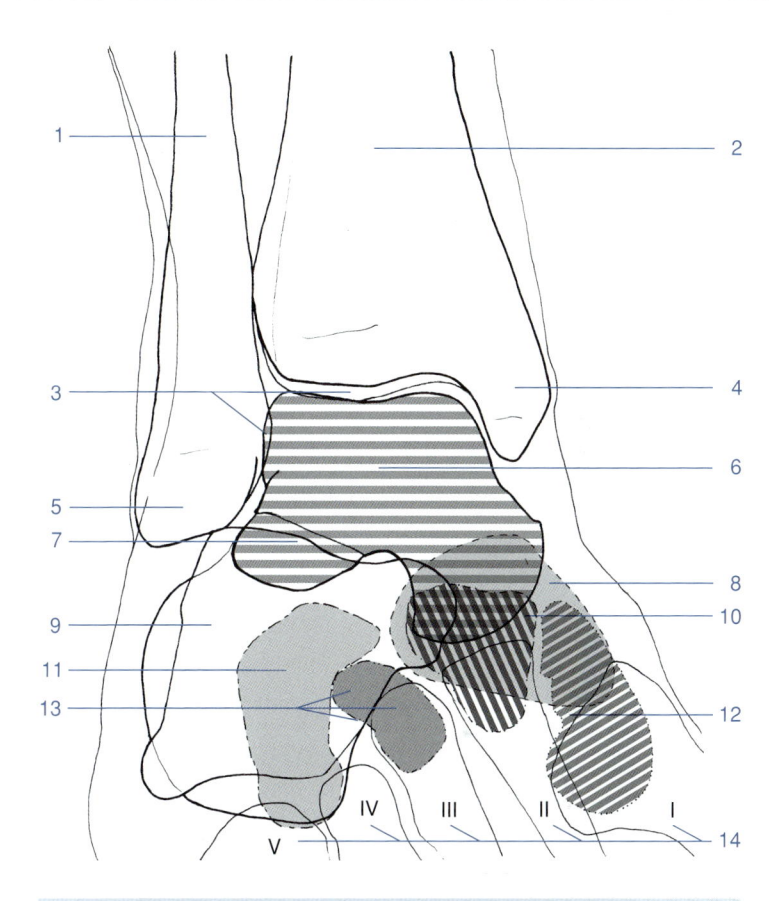

1　腓骨 Fibula	8　舟状骨 Navicular
2　脛骨 Tibia	9　踵骨 Calcaneus
3　足関節腔 Ankle joint space	10　中間楔状骨 Intermediate cuneiform
（距腿関節 Talocrural joint）	11　立方骨 Cuboid
4　内果 Medial malleolus	12　内側楔状骨 Medial cuneiform
5　外果 Lateral malleolus	13　外側楔状骨 Lateral cuneiform
6　距骨 Talus	14　中足骨 Metatarsals
7　距踵関節 Talocalcaneal joint	
（距骨下関節 Subtalar joint の後方部分）	

184 下　肢

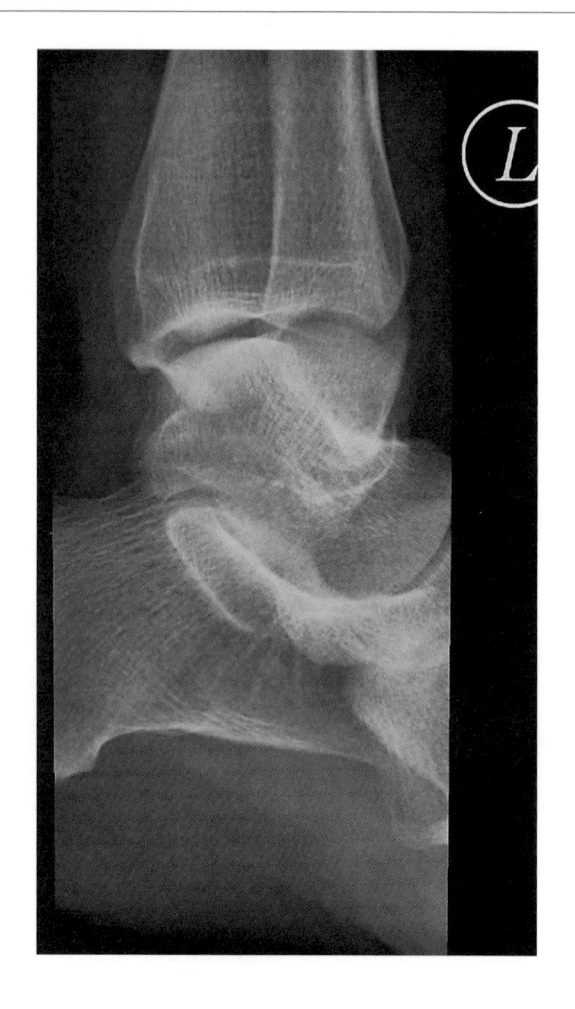

足関節 斜位2　　185

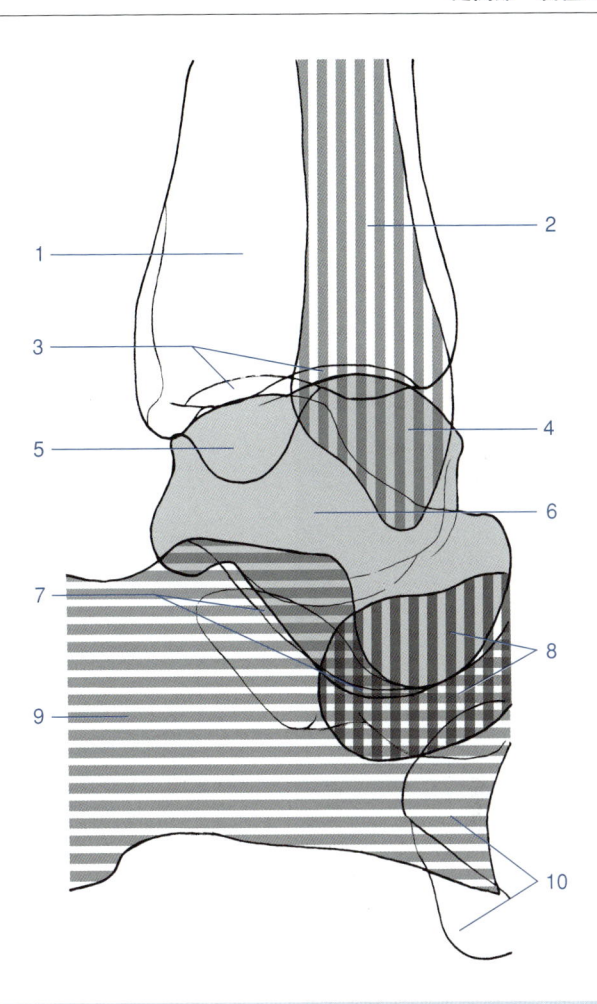

1 脛骨 Tibia
2 腓骨 Fibula
3 足関節腔 Ankle joint space
　（距腿関節 Talocrural joint）
4 外果 Lateral malleolus
5 内果 Medial malleolus
6 距骨 Talus
7 距踵関節 Talocalcaneal joint
　（距骨下関節 Subtalar joint の後方部分）
8 舟状骨 Navicular
9 踵骨 Calcaneus
10 立方骨 Cuboid

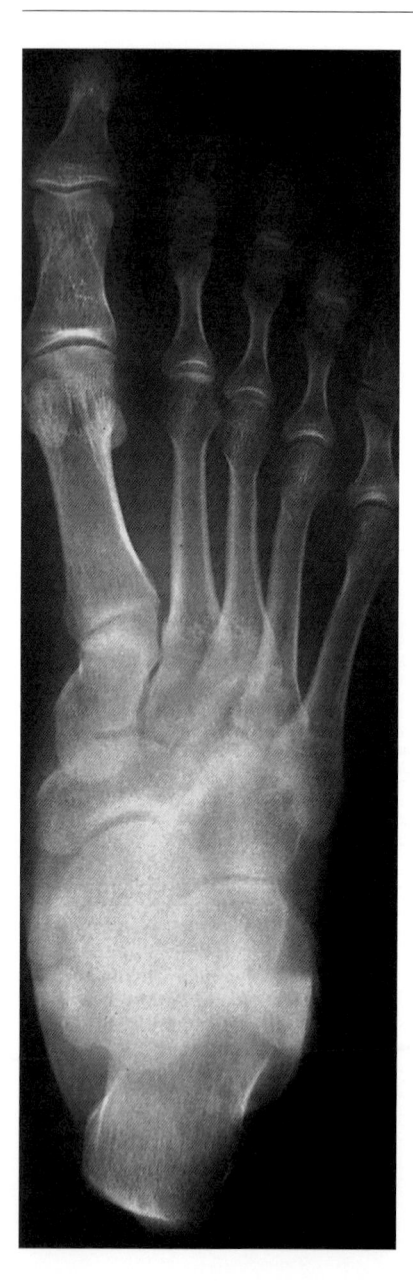

1 末節骨 Distal phalanx（tuft）
2 末節骨 Distal phalanx of the great toe
3 母指指節間関節（IP関節）Interphalangeal joint of the great toe
4 遠位指節間関節（DIP関節）Distal interphalangeal joint
5 近位指節間関節（PIP関節）Proximal interphalangeal joint
6 末節骨 Distal phalanx
7 中節骨 Middle phalanx
8 基節骨頭 Head of the proximal phalanx
9 基節骨 Proximal phalanx
10 種子骨 Sesamoid
11 指節骨底 Base of the phalanx
12 中足指節関節（MP関節）Metatarsophalangeal joint
13 中足骨 Metatarsal
14 中足骨頭 Metatarsal head
15 内側楔状骨 Medial cuneiform
16 中間楔状骨 Intermediate cuneiform
17 外側楔状骨 Lateral cuneiform
18 第5中足骨底 Base of the fifth metatarsal
19 舟状骨 Navicular
20 距骨頭 Head of the talus
21 立方骨 Cuboid
22 内果 Medial malleolus
23 外果 Lateral malleolus
24 踵骨 Calcaneus
25 足根中足関節 Tarsometatarsal joints（Lisfranc関節）
26 横足根関節 Transverse tarsal joint（Chopart関節）

足　正面（前後）　187

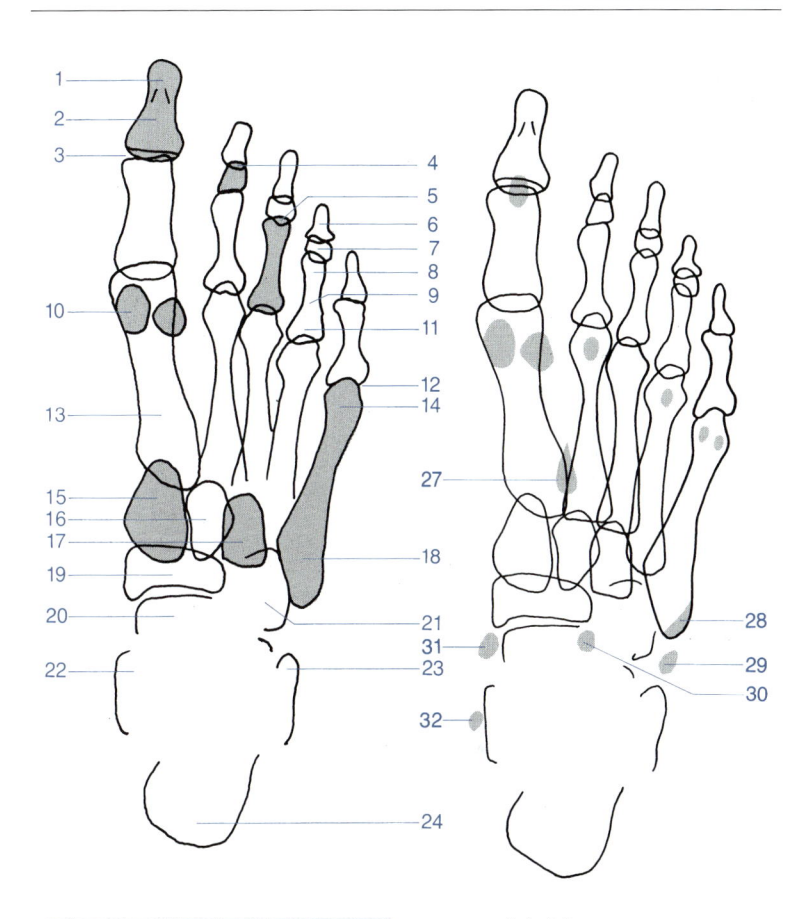

足によくみられる種子骨と副骨（過剰骨）

27　中足骨間骨　Os intermetatarseum
28　ヴェサリウス骨　Os vesalianum
29　腓骨筋骨　Os peroneum
30　第2立方骨　Secondary cuboid
31　外脛骨　Os tibiale externum
32　上距骨　Os supratalare

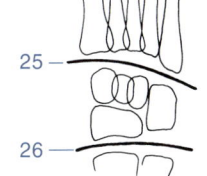

188　下　肢

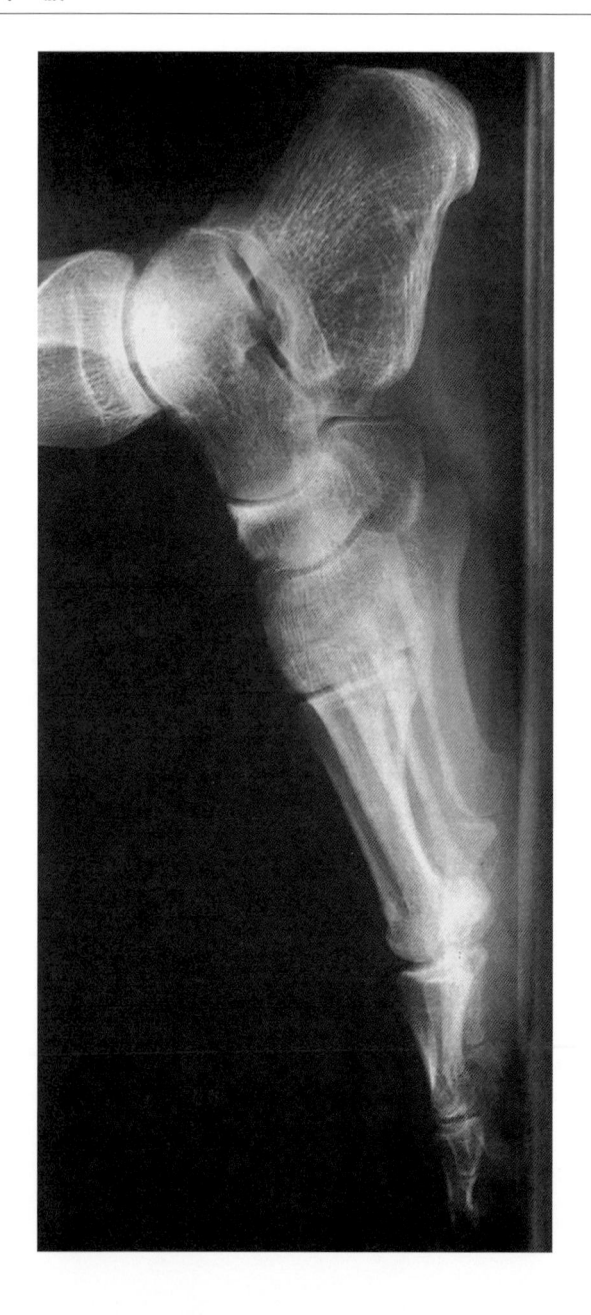

足　側面

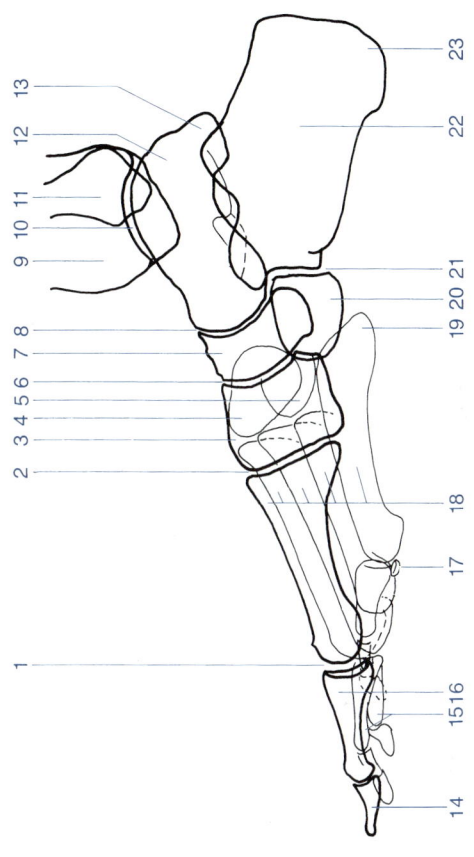

1 中足指節関節 (MP関節) Metatarsophalangeal joint
2 足根中足関節 Tarsometatarsal joint
3 内側楔状骨 Medial cuneiform
4 中間楔状骨 Intermediate cuneiform
5 外側楔状骨 Lateral cuneiform
6 楔舟関節 Cuneonavicular joint
7 舟状骨 Navicular
8 距踵舟関節 Talocalcaneonavicular joint
9 脛骨 Tibia
10 足関節 Ankle joint
11 腓骨 Fibula
12 距骨 Talus
13 距骨後突起 Posterior process of the talus
14 末節骨 Distal phalanx
15 中節骨 Middle phalanx
16 基節骨 Proximal phalanx
17 種子骨 Sesamoid
18 中足骨 Metatarsal
19 第5中足骨底 Base of fifth metatarsal
20 立方骨 Cuboid
21 踵立方関節 Calcaneocuboid joint
22 踵骨 Calcaneus
23 踵骨隆起 Tuberosity of the calcaneus

190　下　肢

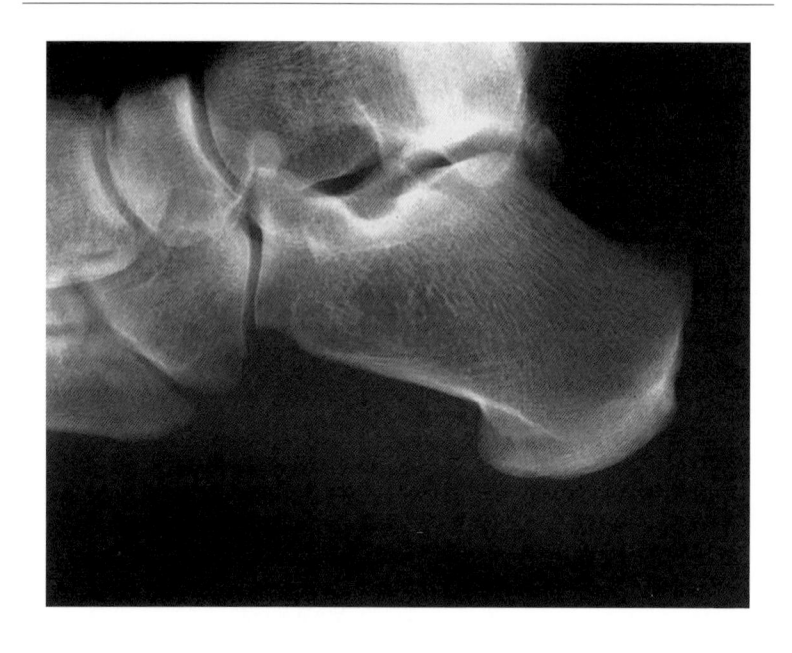

踵骨 側面 **191**

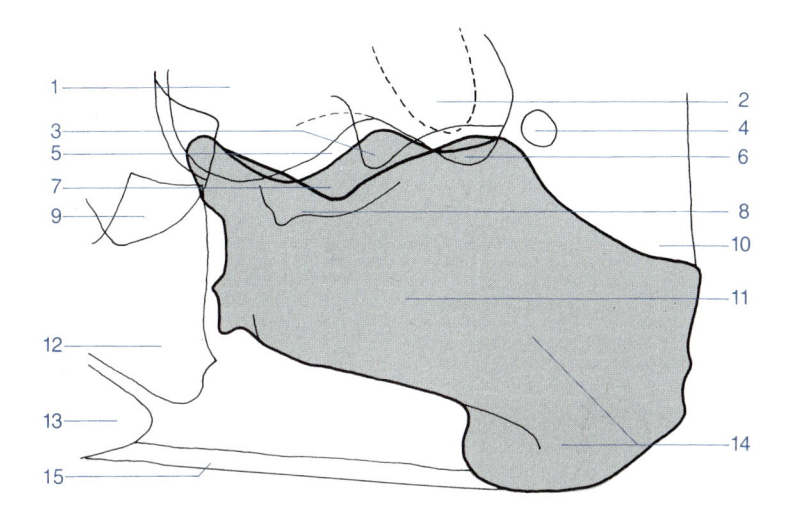

1 距骨 Talus
2 外果 Lateral malleolus
3 距骨外側突起 Lateral process of the talus
4 三角骨 Os trigonum*
5 距骨下関節 Subtalar joint
6 距骨後突起 Posterior process of the talus
7 足根洞 Tarsal sinus
8 載距突起 Sustentaculum tali
9 舟状骨 Navicular
10 アキレス腱 Achilles tendon
11 踵骨 Calcaneus
12 立方骨 Cuboid
13 第5中足骨底 Base of fifth metatarsal
14 踵骨隆起 Tuberosity of the calcaneus
15 足底腱膜 Plantar aponeurosis

*訳注
ときに距骨後突起が独立骨としてみられるもの．
距骨の骨折と間違われることがあるので注意

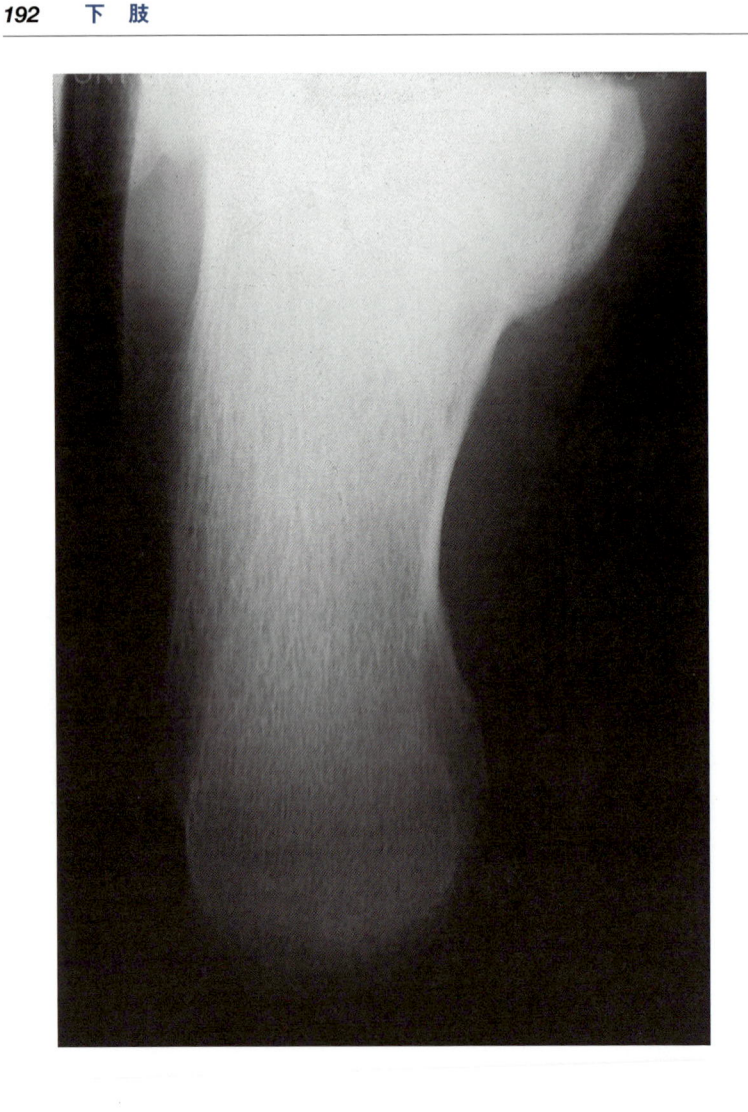

下肢

踵骨　接線　193

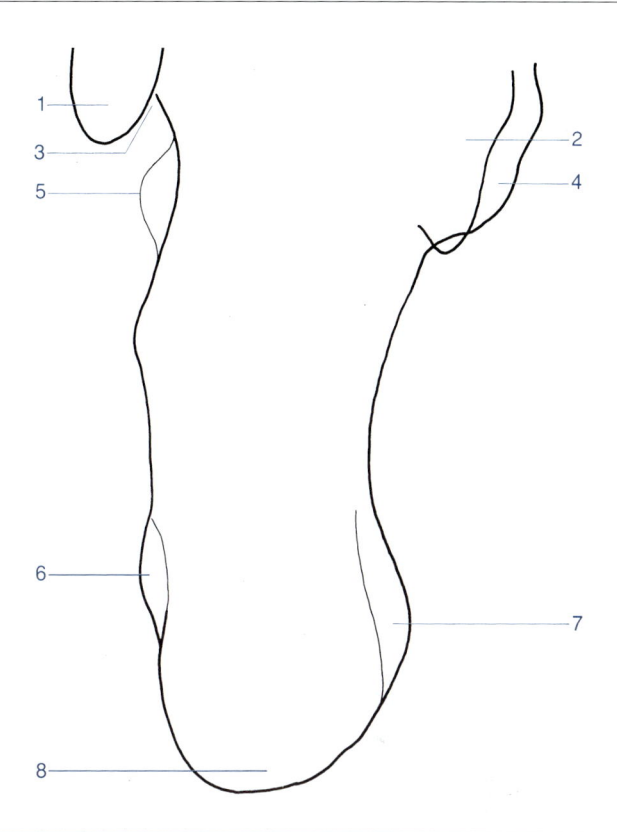

1 外果 Lateral malleolus
2 距骨 Talus
3 長腓骨筋腱溝 Groove for the peroneus longus tendon
4 載距突起 Sustentaculum tali
5 腓骨筋滑車 Peroneal trochlea
6 踵骨隆起外側突起 Lateral process of the tuberosity of the calcaneus
7 踵骨隆起内側突起 Medial process of the tuberosity of the calcaneus
8 踵骨隆起 Tuberosity of the calcaneus

194　下　肢

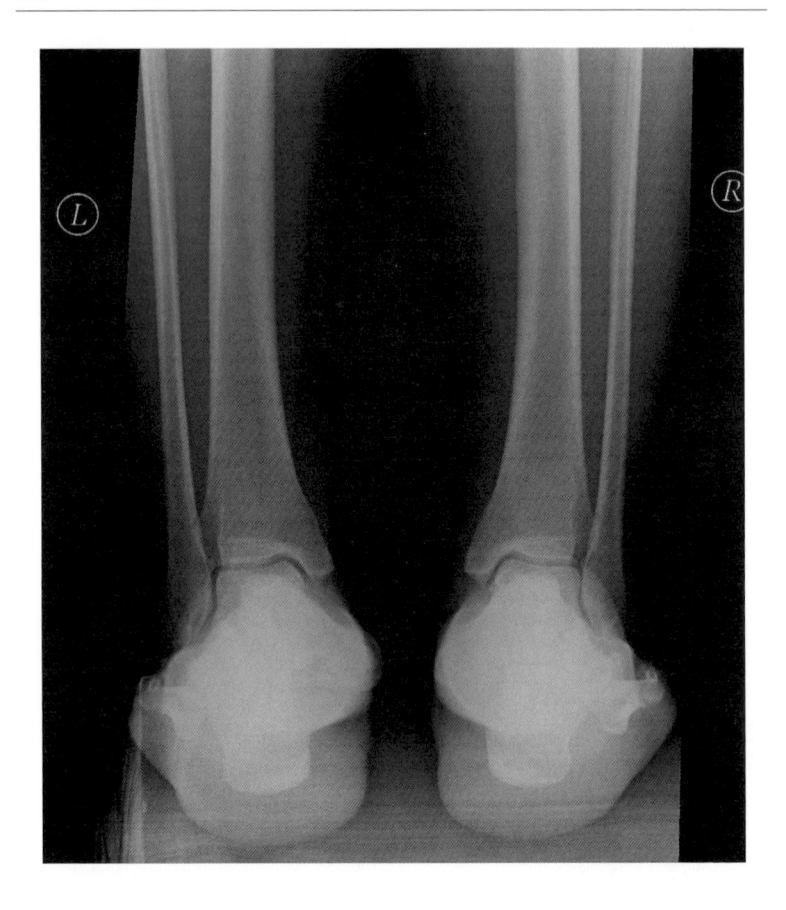

足 立位負荷正面(前後)

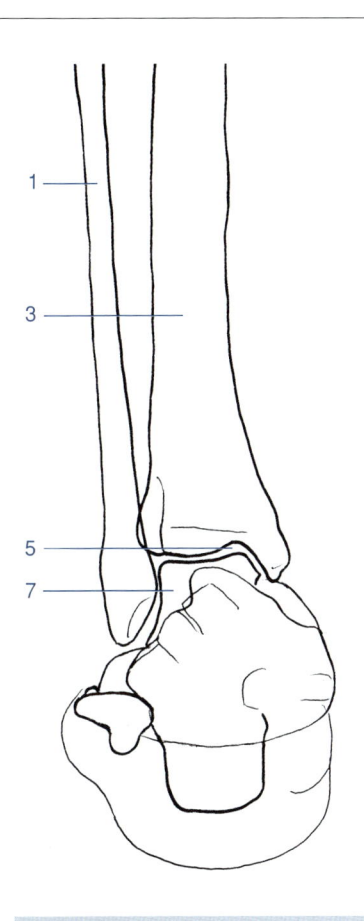

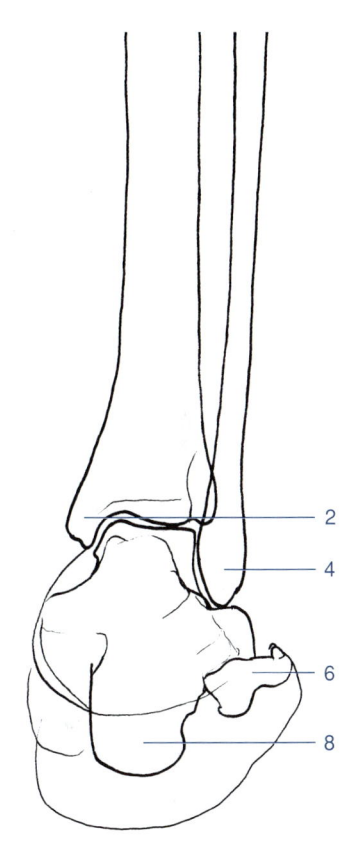

1 腓骨 Fibula
2 内果 Medial malleolus
3 脛骨 Tibia
4 外果 Lateral malleolus
5 足関節腔 Ankle joint space
 (距腿関節 Talocrural joint)
6 第5中足骨 Fifth metatarsal
7 距骨 Talus
8 踵骨 Calcaneus

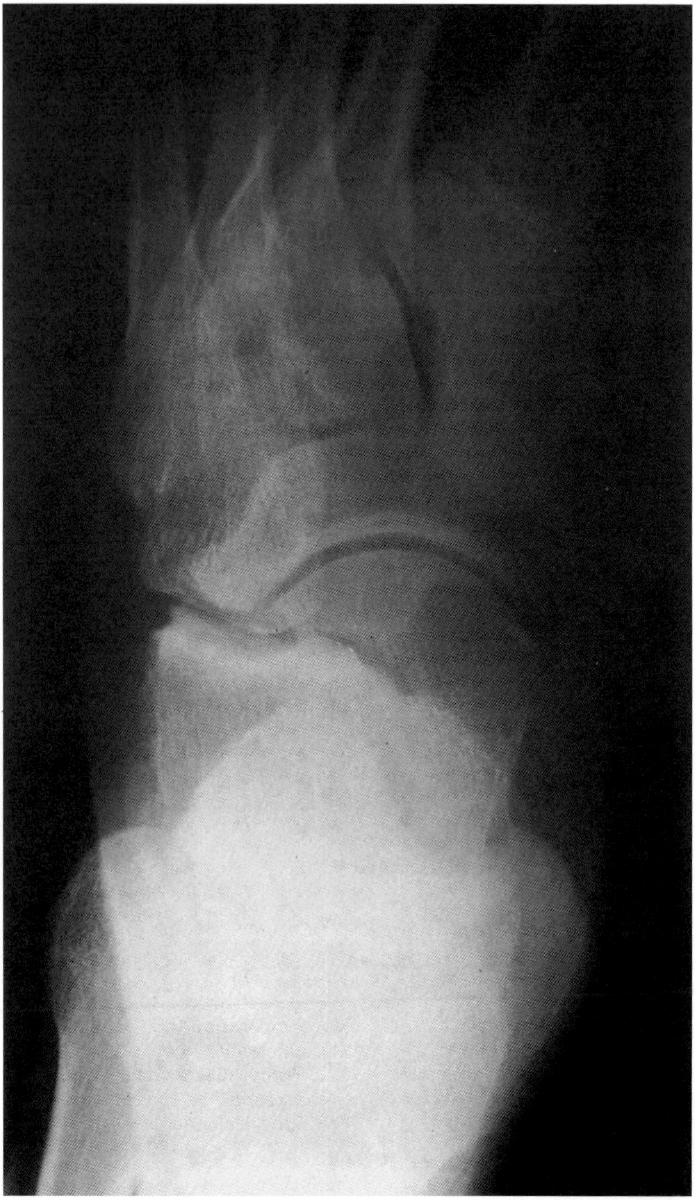

中足部　正面（前後）

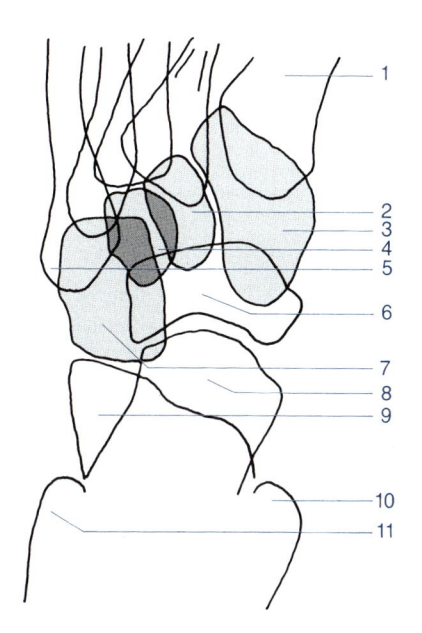

1　中足骨 Metatarsal	7　立方骨 Cuboid
2　中間楔状骨 Intermediate cuneiform	8　距骨頭 Head of the talus
3　内側楔状骨 Medial cuneiform	9　踵骨 Calcaneus
4　外側楔状骨 Lateral cuneiform	10　内果 Medial malleolus
5　第5中足骨底 Base of fifth metatarsal	11　外果 Lateral malleolus
6　舟状骨 Navicular	

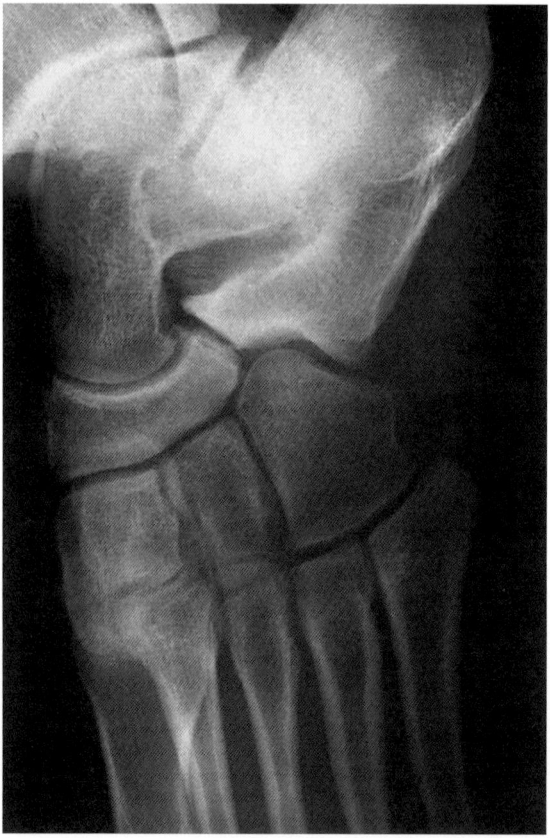

中足部 斜位

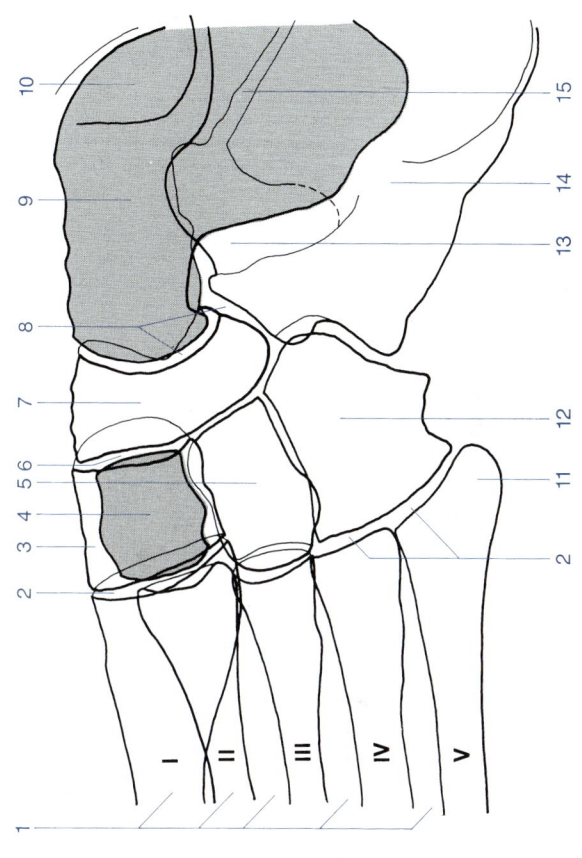

1 中足骨 Metatarsals
2 足根中足関節 Tarsometatarsal joint
3 内側楔状骨 Medial cuneiform
4 中間楔状骨 Intermediate cuneiform
5 外側楔状骨 Lateral cuneiform
6 楔舟関節 Cuneonavicular joint
7 舟状骨 Navicular
8 距踵舟関節 Talocalcaneonavicular joint
9 距骨 Talus
10 内果/外果 Malleolus
11 第5中足骨底 Base of fifth metatarsal
12 立方骨 Cuboid
13 足根洞 Tarsal sinus
14 踵骨 Calcaneus
15 距骨下関節 Subtalar joint
（および距踵舟関節 Talocalcaneonavicular joint）

200　下　肢

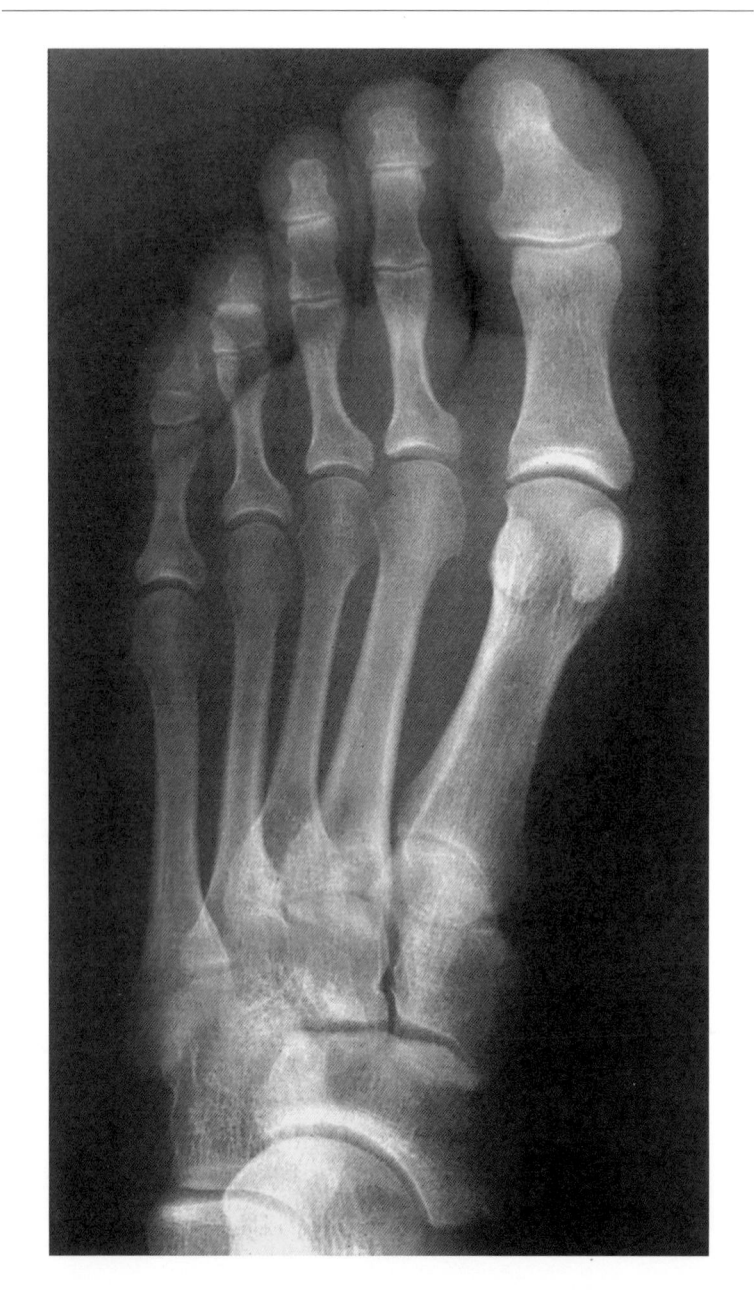

前足部　正面（前後）　**201**

1　末節骨 Distal phalanx	9　内側楔状骨 Medial cuneiform
2　中節骨 Middle phalanx	10　中間楔状骨 Intermediate cuneiform
3　基節骨 Proximal phalanx	11　外側楔状骨 Lateral cuneiform
4　遠位指節間関節（DIP関節）Distal interphalangeal joint	12　足根間関節 Intertarsal joint
5　近位指節間関節（PIP関節）Proximal interphalangeal joint	13　足根中足関節 Tarsometatarsal joint
6　中足指節関節（MP関節）Metatarso phalangeal joint	14　第5中足骨底 Base of fifth metatarsal
7　種子骨 Sesamoids	15　立方骨 Cuboid
8　中足骨 Metatarsals	16　舟状骨 Navicular
	17　距踵舟関節 Talocalcaneonavicular joint
	18　踵立方関節 Calcaneocuboid joint

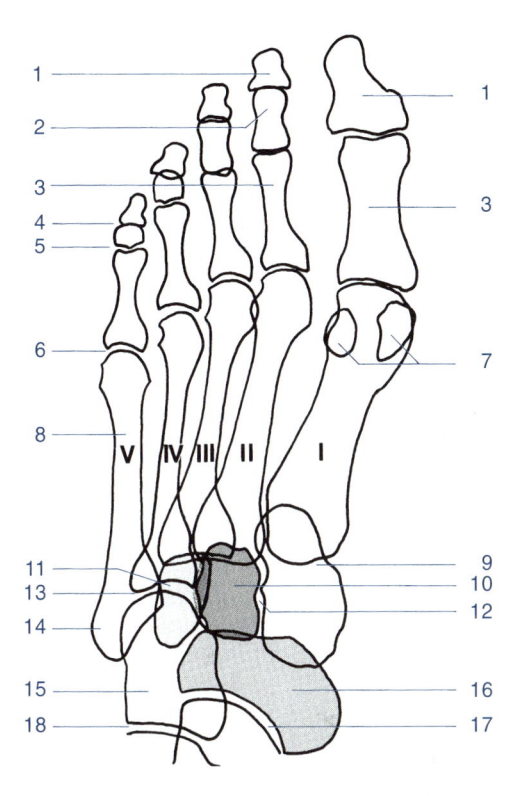

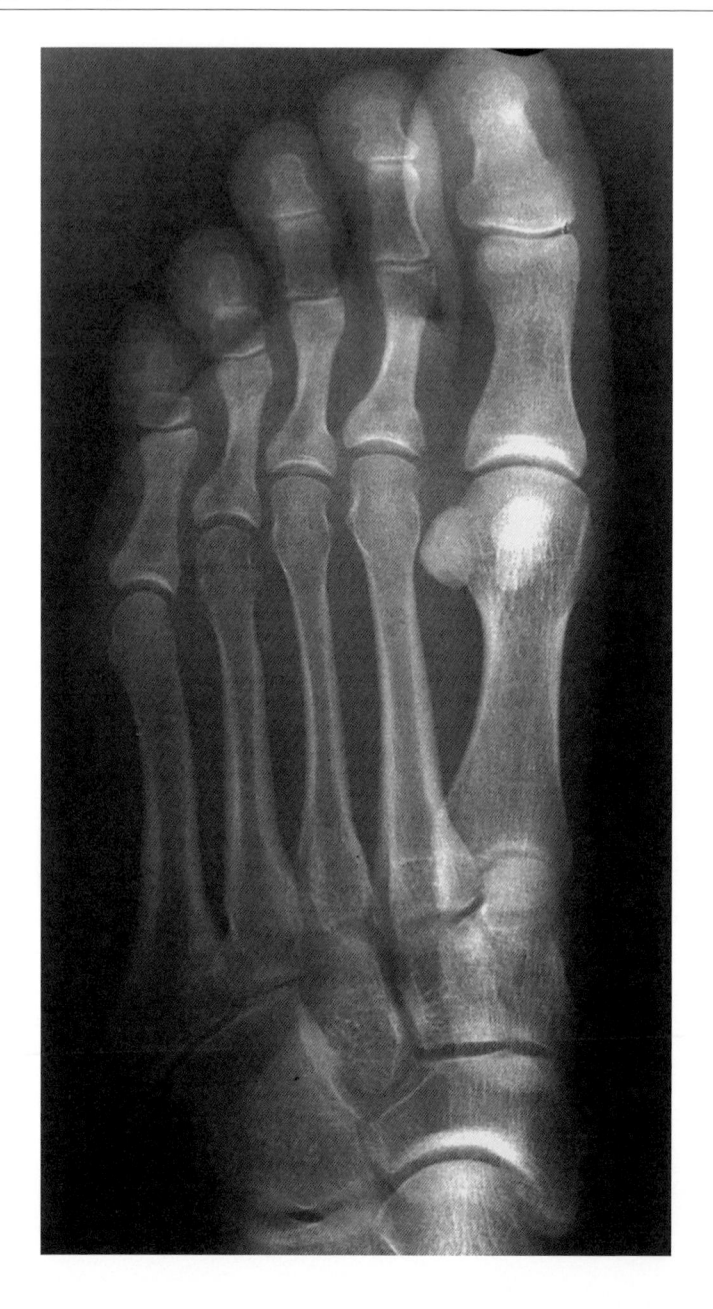

下 肢

前足部 斜位

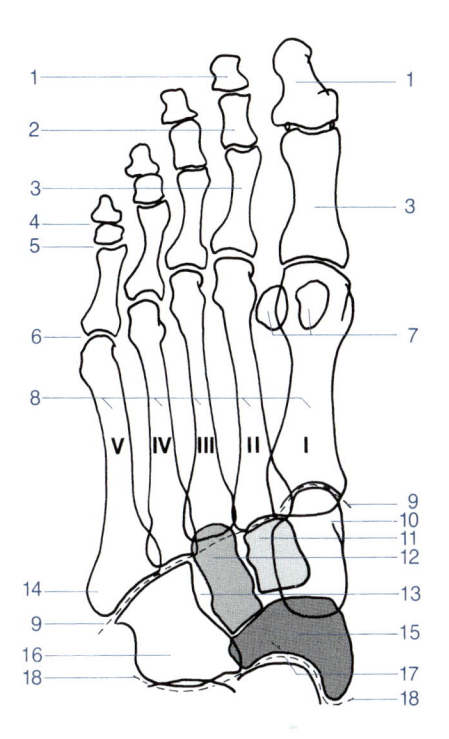

1. 末節骨 Distal phalanx
2. 中節骨 Middle phalanx
3. 基節骨 Proximal phalanx
4. 遠位指節間関節（DIP関節）Distal interphalangeal joint
5. 近位指節間関節（PIP関節）Proximal interphalangeal joint
6. 中足指節関節（MP関節）Metatarsophalangeal joint
7. 種子骨 Sesamoids
8. 中足骨 Metatarsals
9. 足根中足関節 Tarsometatarsal joint（**Lisfranc関節** Lisfranc's joint）
10. 内側楔状骨 Medial cuneiform
11. 中間楔状骨 Intermediate cuneiform
12. 外側楔状骨 Lateral cuneiform
13. 足根間関節 Intertarsal joint
14. 第5中足骨底 Base of the fifth metatarsal
15. 舟状骨 Navicular
16. 立方骨 Cuboid
17. 距踵舟関節 Talocalcaneonavicular joint
18. 横足根関節 Transverse tarsal joint（**Chopart関節**：距骨，踵骨，舟状骨，立方骨で形成される関節線）

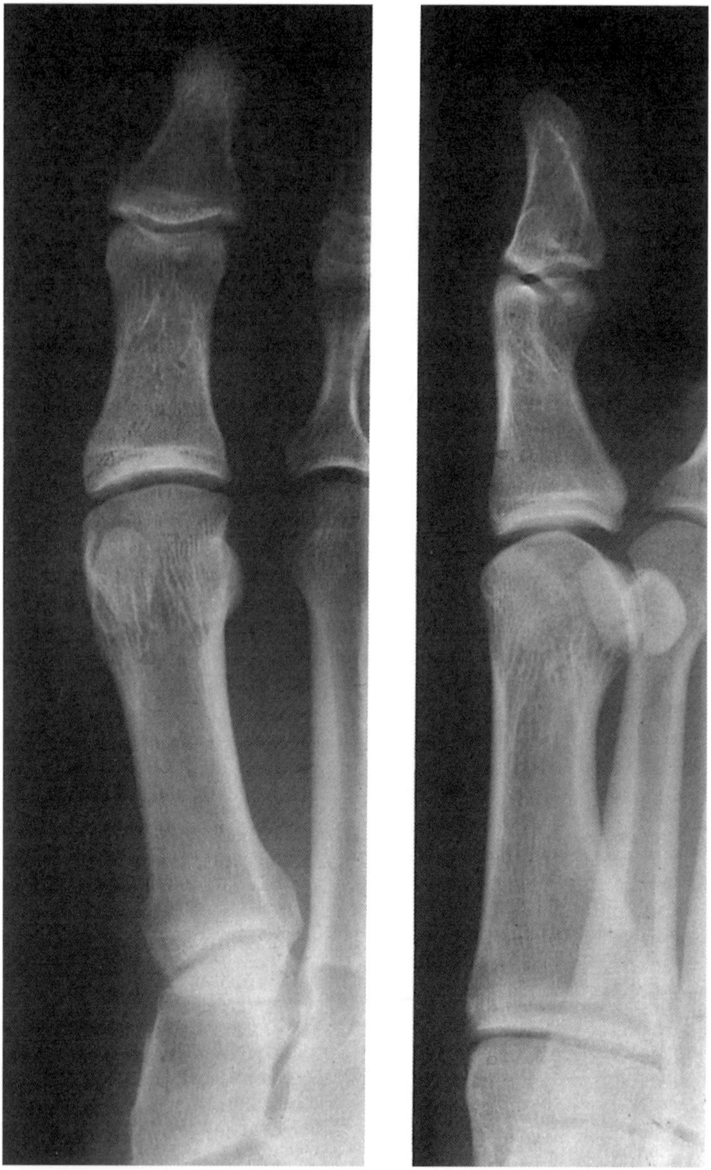

母趾　正面(前後)および側面　　205

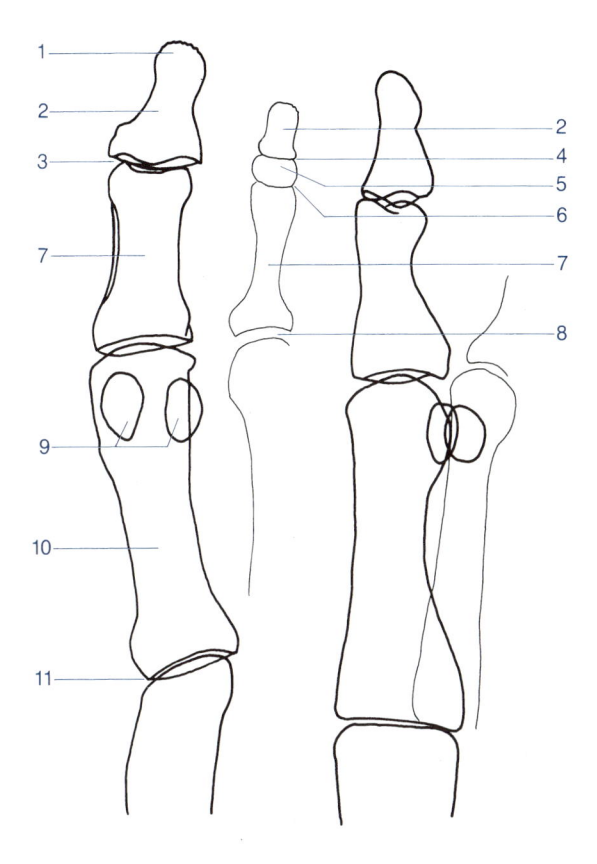

1　末節骨　Distal phalanx (tuft)
2　末節骨　Distal phalanx
3　母指指節間関節(IP関節)
　　Interphalangeal joint of the great toe
4　遠位指節間関節(DIP関節)　Distal interphalangeal joint
5　中節骨　Middle phalanx
6　近位指節間関節(PIP関節)　Proximal interphalangeal joint
7　基節骨　Proximal phalanx
8　中足指節関節(MP関節)
　　Metatarsophalangeal joint
9　種子骨　Sesamoids
10　第1中足骨　First metatarsal
11　足根中足関節　Tarsometatarsal joint

いろいろな単純写真解剖

単純X線写真　208
スポット像　224
断層撮影　232

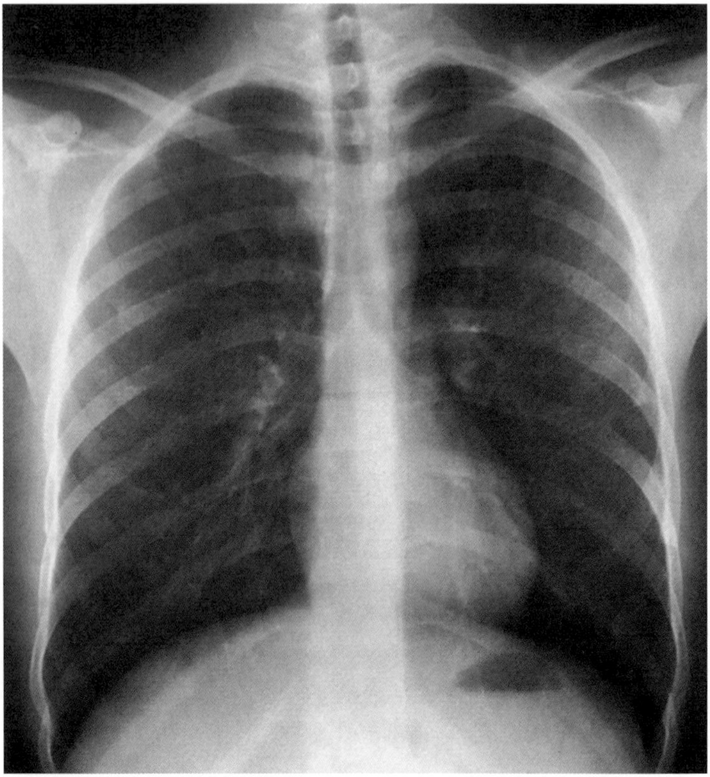

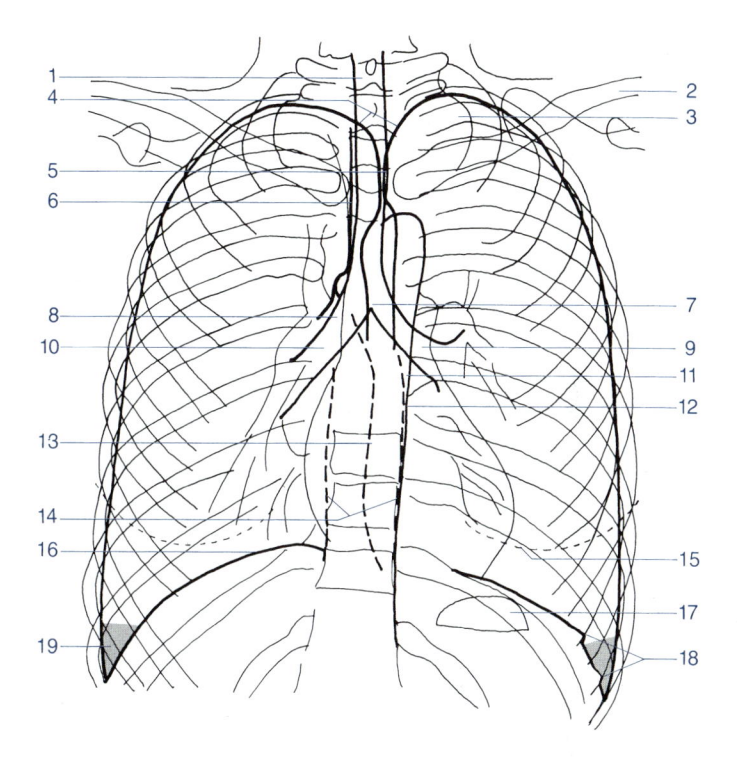

胸部　正面（後前）

1　気管　Trachea	10　中間気管支　Intermediate bronchus
2　鎖骨　Clavicle	11　大動脈傍線　Paraaortic stripe
3　肺尖　Apex of the lung	12　下行大動脈　Descending aorta
4　肺尖上縁　Curve of the apex of the lung	13　奇静脈食道線　Azygoesophageal stripe
5　両肺間の後接合線　Posteriorz border between the right and left lungs	14　傍脊椎線　Paraspinal stripe
	15　乳房影　Shadow of the breast
6　右気管傍線　Right paratracheal stripe	16　横隔膜のドーム　Dome of the diaphragm
7　気管分岐部　Carina of the trachea	17　胃泡　Gastric bubble
8　右主気管支　Right main bronchus	18　横隔膜筋束影　Insertions of the diaphragm
9　左主気管支　Left main bronchus	19　肋骨横隔膜角　Costodiaphragmatic recess (costophrenic angle)

210　単純X線写真

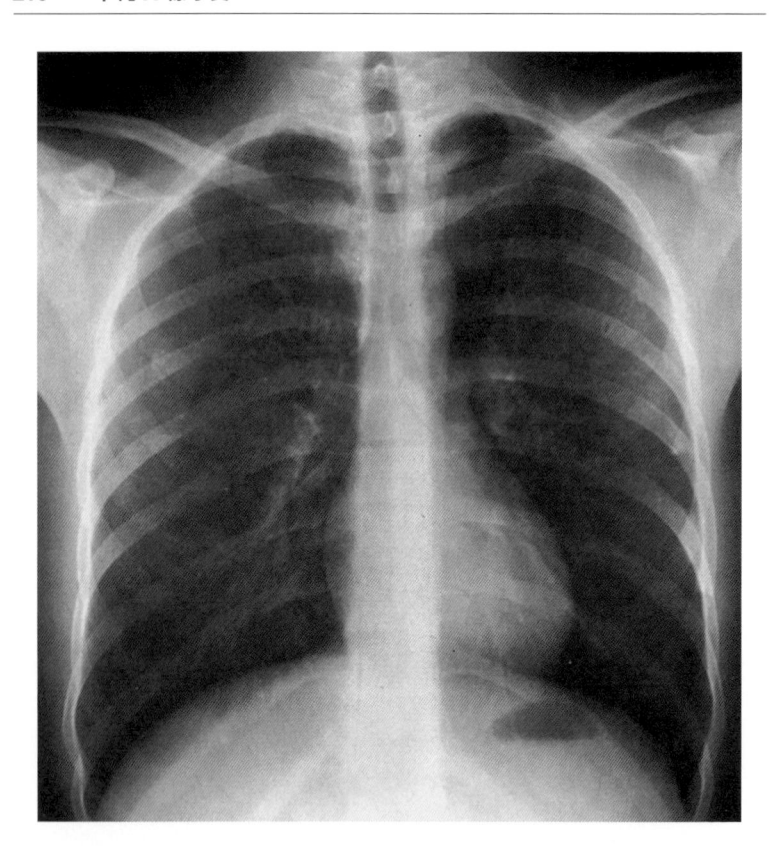

胸部　正面(後前)　(心臓・脈管)

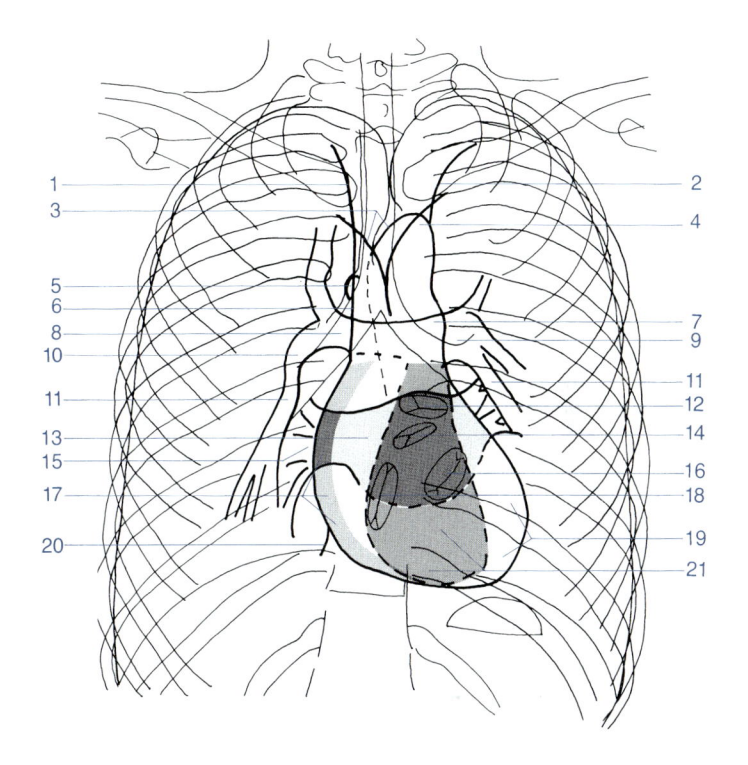

1　右腕頭静脈縁 Contour of the right brachiocephalic vein	11　下葉肺動脈 Inferior lobar branch of the pulmonary artery
2　鎖骨下動脈縁 Contour of the subclavian artery	12　肺動脈弁 Pulmonic valve
3　鎖骨下動脈と大動脈弓 Subclavian and aortic arches	13　左心房 Left atrium
4　大動脈弓 Aortic arch	14　大動脈弁 Aortic valve
5　奇静脈 Azygos vein	15　肺静脈合流部 Venous confluence
6　上大静脈 Superior vena cava	16　僧帽弁 Mitral valve
7　肺動脈幹 Main pulmonary artery segment	17　右心房 Right atrium
8　右肺動脈 Right pulmonary artery	18　三尖弁 Tricuspid valve
9　左肺動脈 Left pulmonary artery	19　左心室 Left ventricle
10　葉間肺動脈 Interlobar part of pulmonary artery	20　下大静脈 Inferior vena cava
	21　右心室 Right ventricle

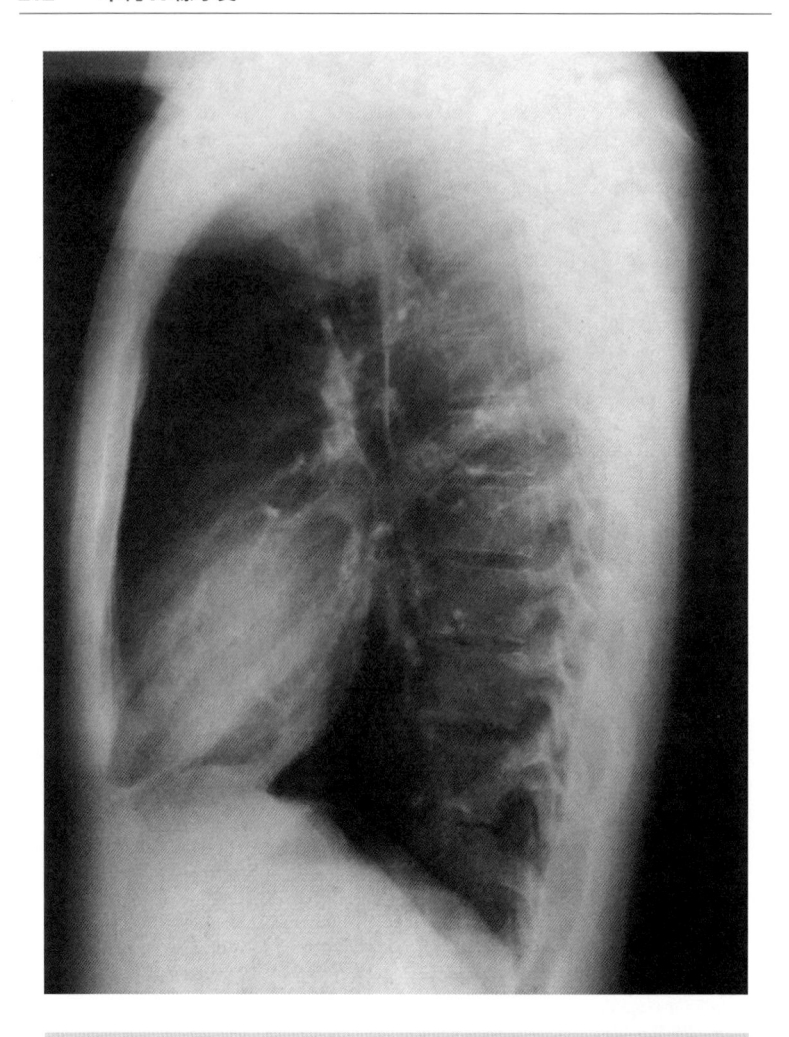

1	肩の軟部組織 Soft tissues of the shoulder	9	右上葉気管支 Right upper lobe bronchus
2	気管 Trachea	10	胸骨後腔 Retrosternal space
3	肩甲骨 Scapula	11	左上葉気管支 Left upper lobe bronchus
4	胸骨角 Sternal angle	12	肺動脈幹 Main pulmonary artery
5	大動脈弓 Aortic arch	13	下行大動脈 Descending aorta
6	胸骨体 Body of the sternum	14	肺動脈弁 Pulmonic valve
7	大動脈肺動脈窓 Aortopulmonary window	15	肺静脈 Pulmonary veins
8	上行大動脈 Ascending aorta		

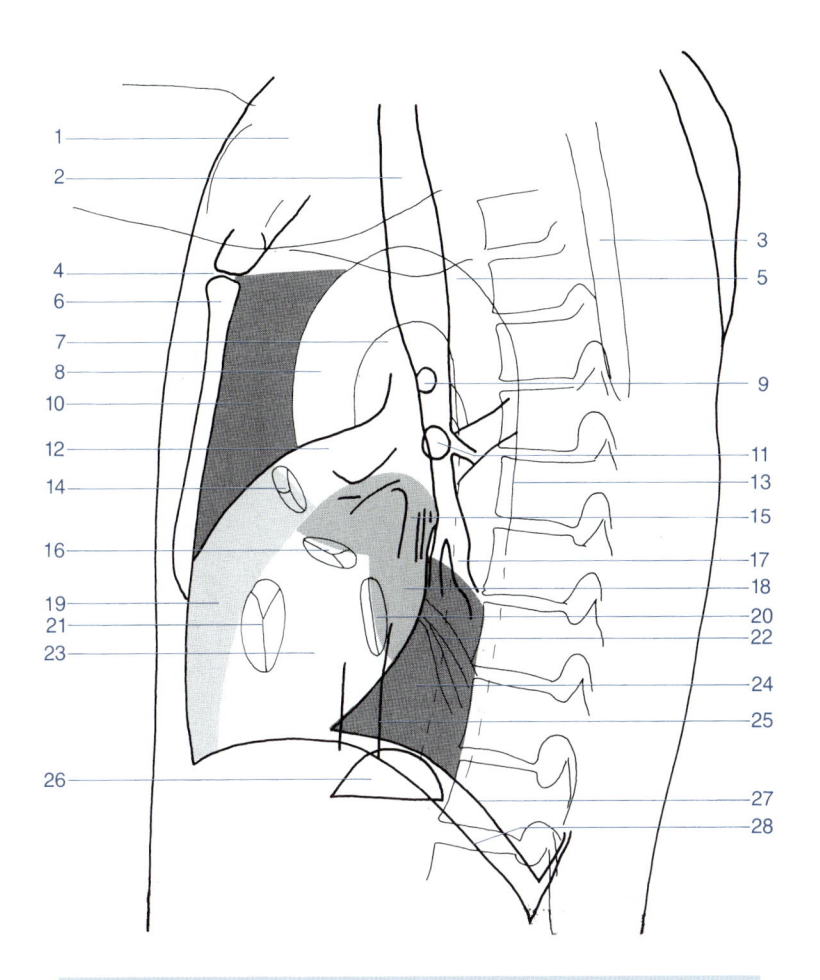

16	大動脈弁 Aortic valve	24	後心腔 Retrocardiac space
17	下葉気管支 Lower lobe bronchus	25	下大静脈 Inferior vena cava
18	左心房 Left atrium	26	胃泡 Gastric bubble
19	右心室 Right ventricle	27	左横隔膜 Left hemidiaphragm
20	僧帽弁 Mitral valve		胃包の接線と心陰影端
21	三尖弁 Tricuspid valve	28	右横隔膜 Right hemidiaphragm
22	肺静脈 Pulmonary veins		
23	左心室 Left ventricle		

214　単純 X 線写真

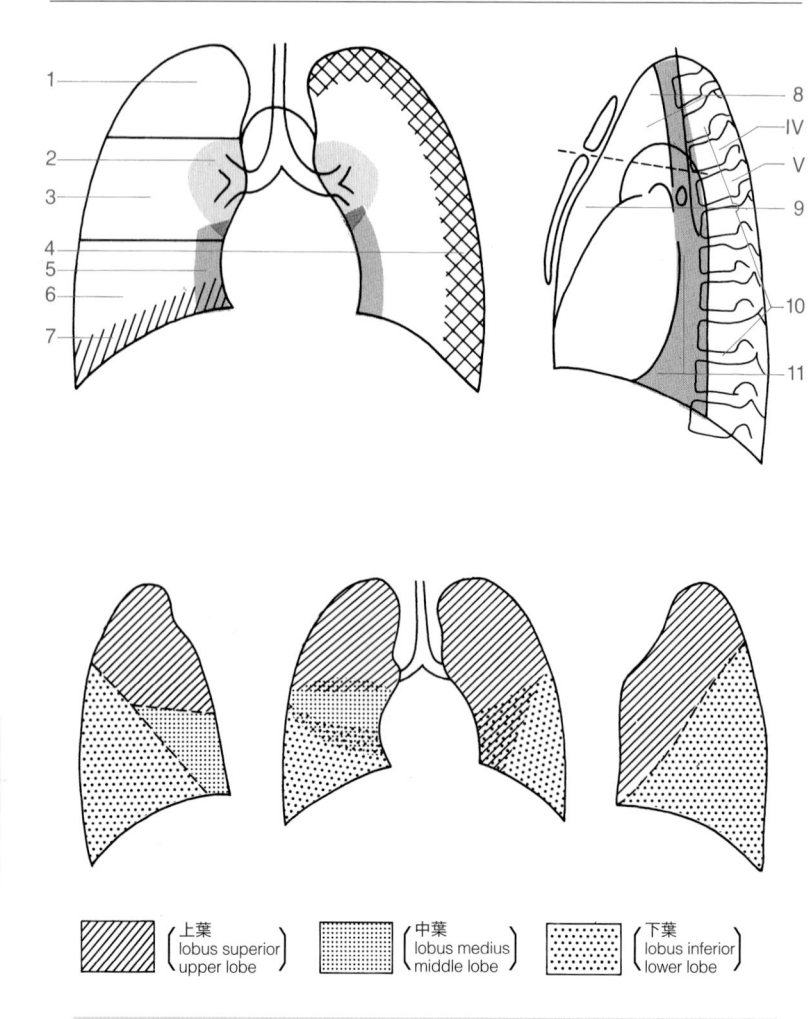

上葉 (lobus superior / upper lobe)	中葉 (lobus medius / middle lobe)	下葉 (lobus inferior / lower lobe)

1　上肺野　Upper region of the lung	7　横隔膜上部　Supradiaphragmatic region
2　肺門部　Perihilar region	8　前縦隔上部　Superior anterior mediastinum
3　中肺野　Middle region of the lung	9　前縦隔下部　Inferior anterior mediastinum
4　胸壁　Chest wall	10　後縦隔　Posterior mediastinum
5　心膜部　Pericardiac region	11　中縦隔　Middle mediastinum
6　下肺野　Lower region of the lung	

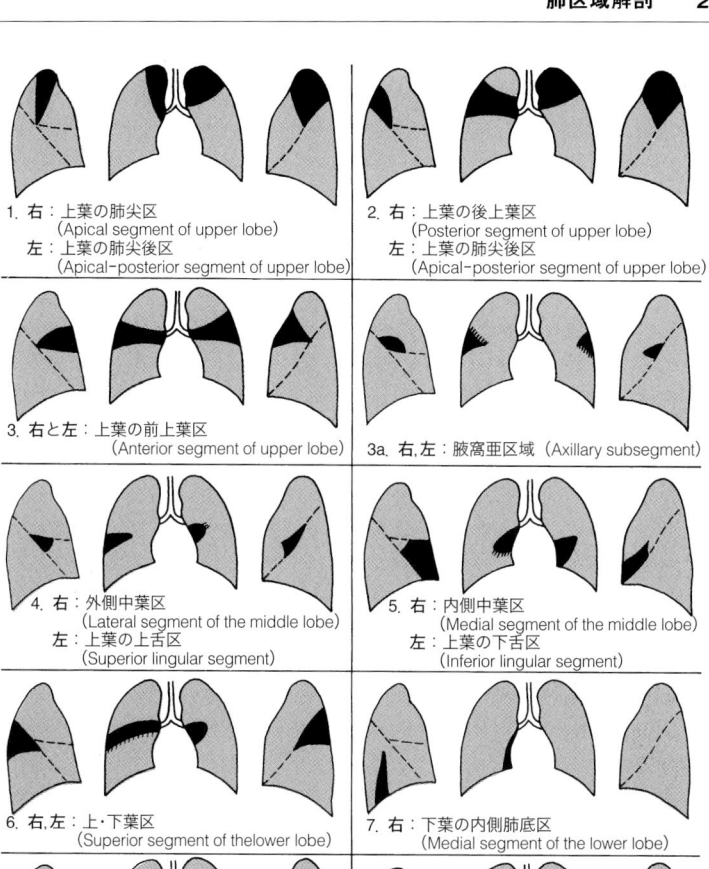

肺区域解剖 215

1. 右：上葉の肺尖区 (Apical segment of upper lobe)
   左：上葉の肺尖後区 (Apical-posterior segment of upper lobe)

2. 右：上葉の後上葉区 (Posterior segment of upper lobe)
   左：上葉の肺尖後区 (Apical-posterior segment of upper lobe)

3. 右と左：上葉の前上葉区 (Anterior segment of upper lobe)

3a. 右,左：腋窩亜区域 (Axillary subsegment)

4. 右：外側中葉区 (Lateral segment of the middle lobe)
   左：上葉の上舌区 (Superior lingular segment)

5. 右：内側中葉区 (Medial segment of the middle lobe)
   左：上葉の下舌区 (Inferior lingular segment)

6. 右,左：上・下葉区 (Superior segment of the lower lobe)

7. 右：下葉の内側肺底区 (Medial segment of the lower lobe)

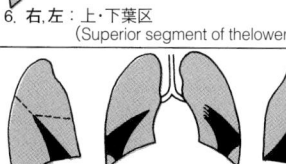

8. 右,左：下葉の前肺底区 (Anterior basal segment of the lower lobe)

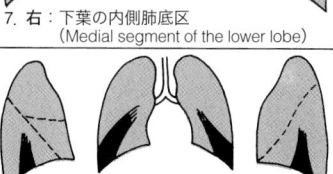

9. 右,左：下葉の外側肺底区 (Lateral basal segment of the lower lobe)

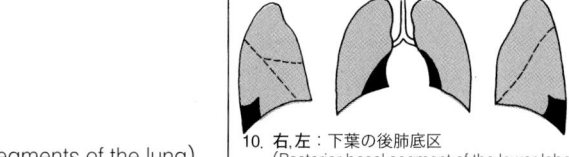

10. 右,左：下葉の後肺底区 (Posterior basal segment of the lower lobe)

肺区域 (Segments of the lung)

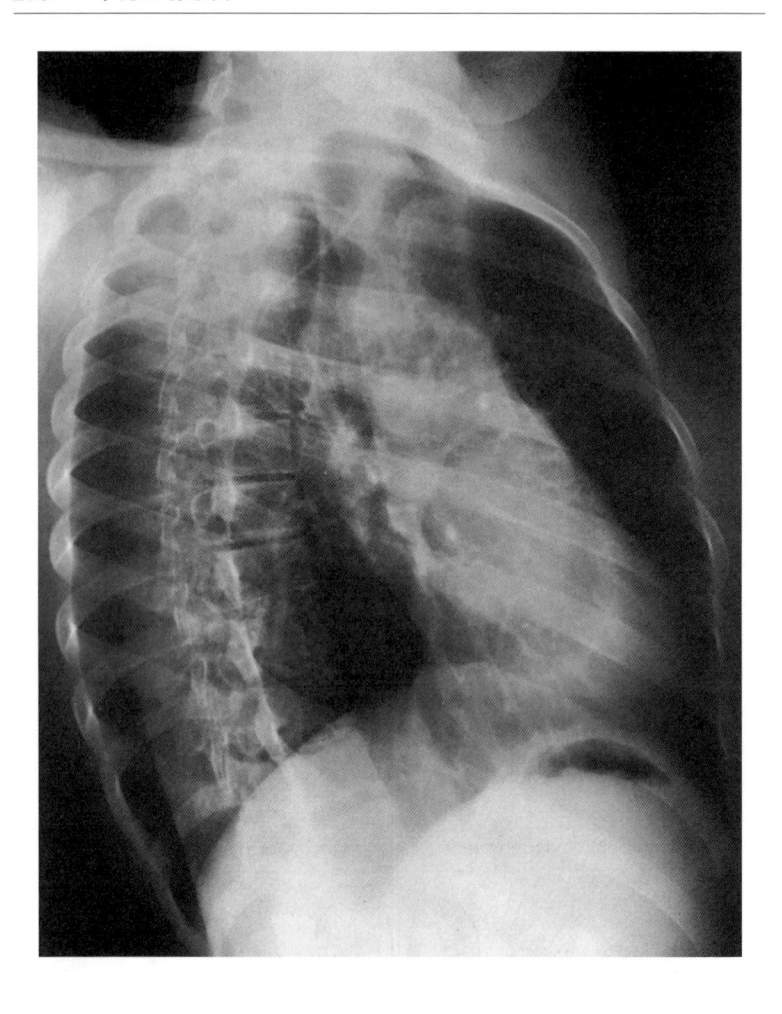

単純 X 線写真

胸部　右前斜位　217

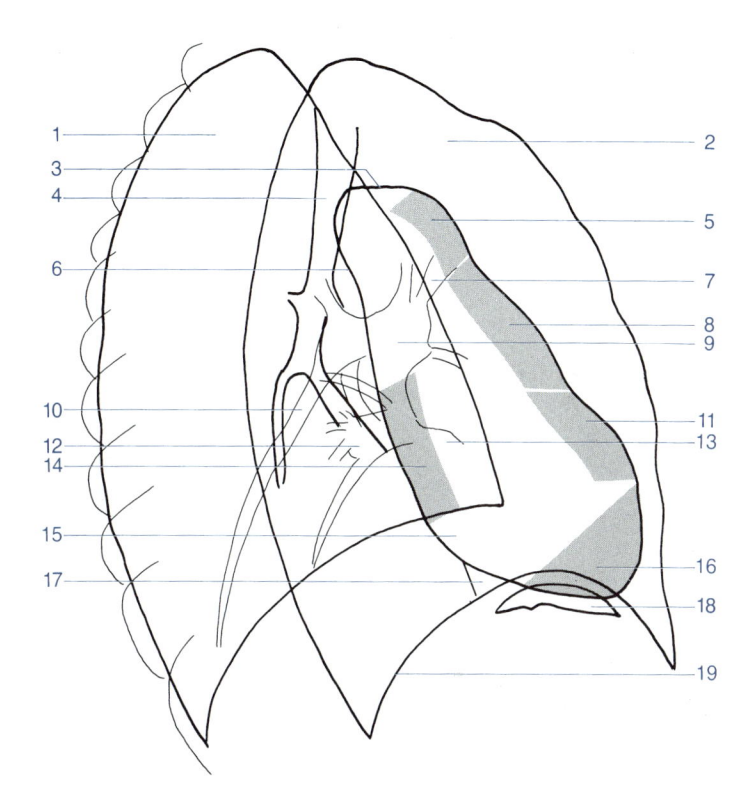

1　右肺　Right lung	10　右下葉動脈　Right inferior lobar brabch of the pulmonary artery
2　左肺　Left lung	11　漏斗部　Infundibulum
3　大動脈弓　Aortic arch	12　右下肺静脈　Inferior right pulmonary vein
4　気管　Trachea	13　左下肺静脈　Inferior left pulmonary vein
5　上行大動脈　Ascending aorta	14　左心房　Left atrium
6　下行大動脈　Descending aorta	15　右心房　Right atrium
7　左上葉肺動脈, 静脈, 気管支　Left upper lobe pulmonary vein, artery, and bronchus	16　左心室　Left ventricle
8　肺動脈幹　Main pulmonary artery	17　下大静脈　Inferior vena cava
9　左肺動脈　Left pulmonary artery	18　胃泡　Gastric bubble
	19　横隔膜　Diaphragm

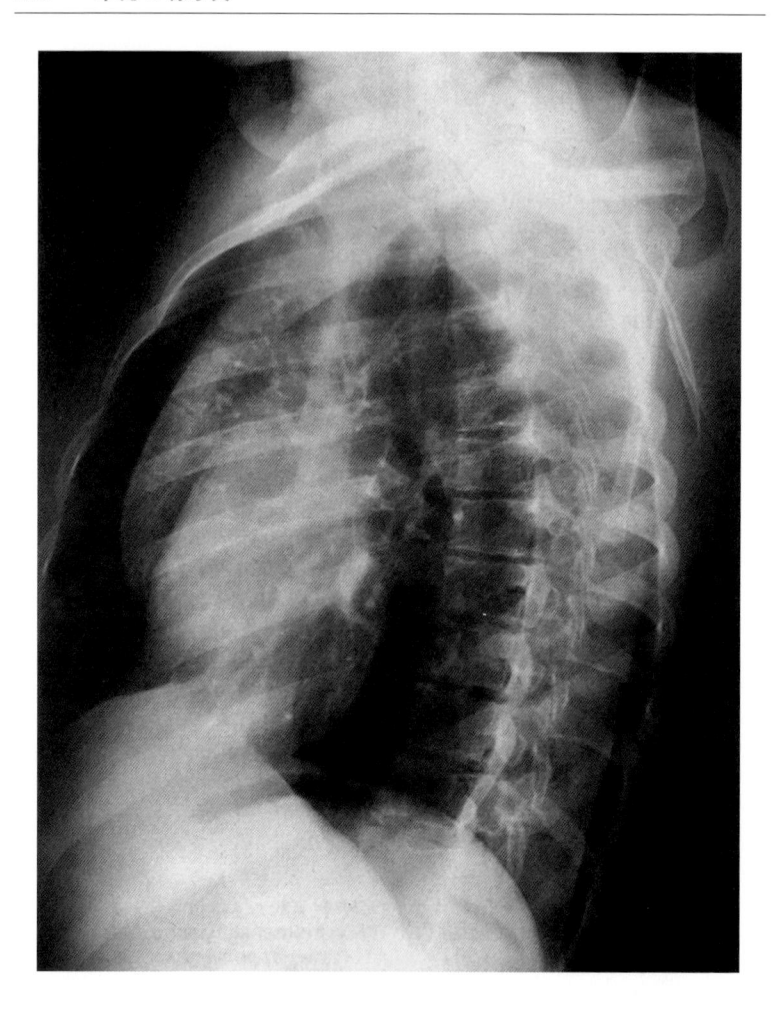

単純 X 線写真

胸部 左前斜位

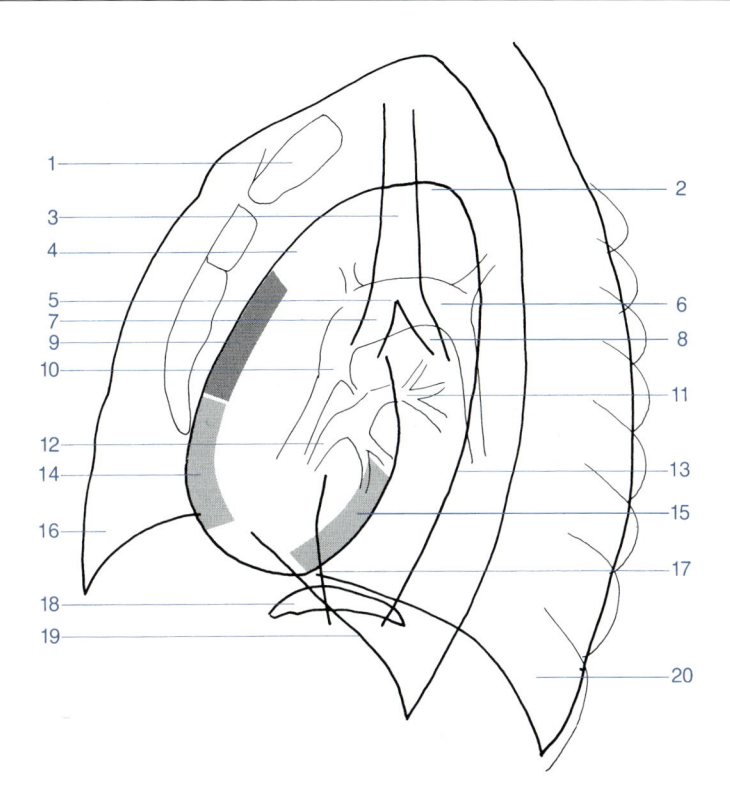

1	胸骨 Sternum	12	右肺静脈 Right pulmonary vein
2	大動脈弓 Aortic arch	13	下行大動脈 Descending aorta
3	気管 Trachea	14	右心室 Right ventricle
4	上行大動脈 Ascending aorta	15	左心室 Left ventricle
5	気管分岐部 Carina of the trachea	16	右肺 Right lung
6	左肺動脈 Left pulmonary artery	17	下大静脈 Inferior vena cava
7	右主気管支 Right main bronchus	18	胃泡（左横隔膜）Gastric bubble (left hemidiaphragm)
8	左主気管支 Left main bronchus	19	右横隔膜 Right hemidiaphragm
9	右心房 Right atrium	20	左肺 Left lung
10	右肺動脈 Right pulmonary artery		
11	左肺静脈 Left pulmonary vein		

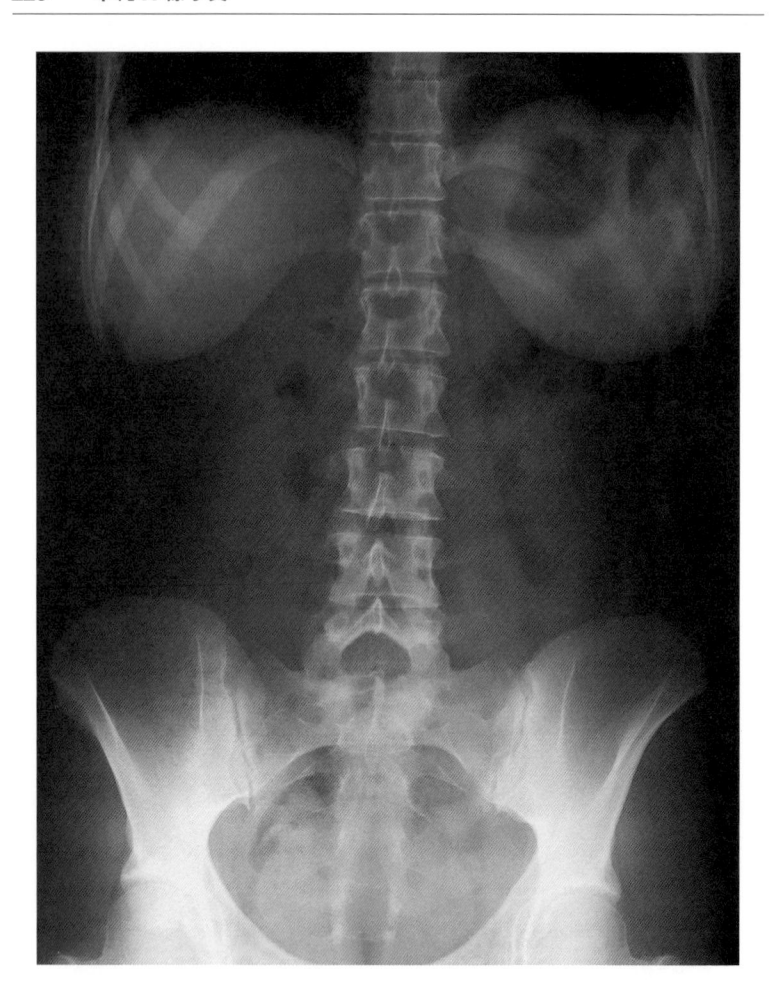

単純X線写真

腹部　立位正面

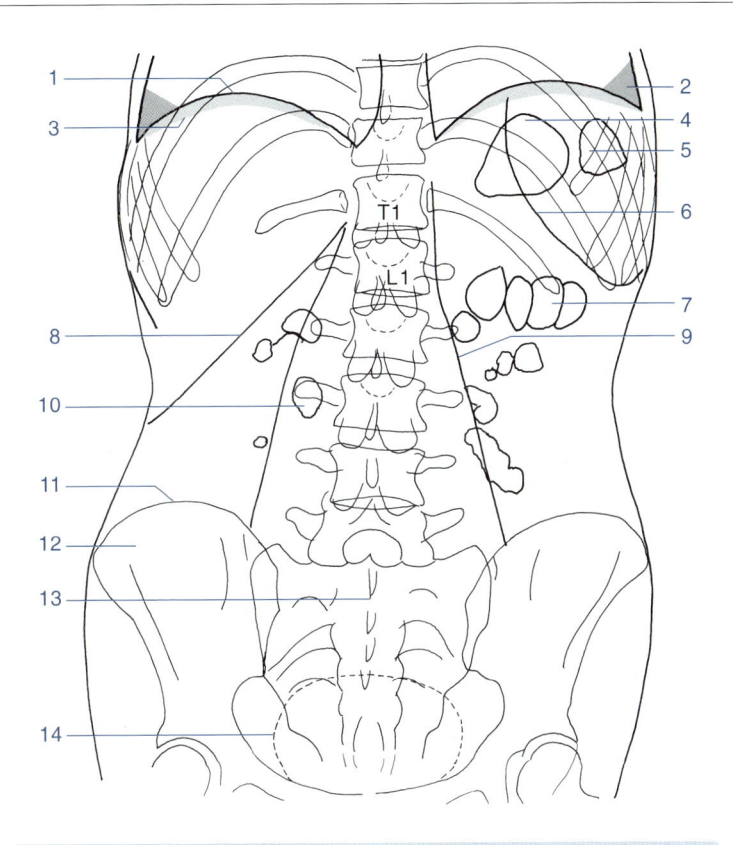

1 横隔膜　Diaphragm
2 肋骨横隔膜角　Costodiaphragmatic recess (costophrenic angle)
3 横隔膜下腔　Subphrenic space
4 胃泡　Gastric bubble
5 結腸脾弯曲部の空気　Gas in the splenic flexure of the colon
6 脾臓下縁　Lower margin of the spleen
7 横行結腸の空気　Gas in the transverse colon
8 肝下縁　Inferior margin of the liver
9 腸腰筋縁　Margin of the psoas muscle
10 小腸の空気　Gas in the small intestine
11 腸骨稜　Iliac crest
12 腸骨　Ilium
13 仙骨　Sacrum
14 膀胱　Urinary bladder

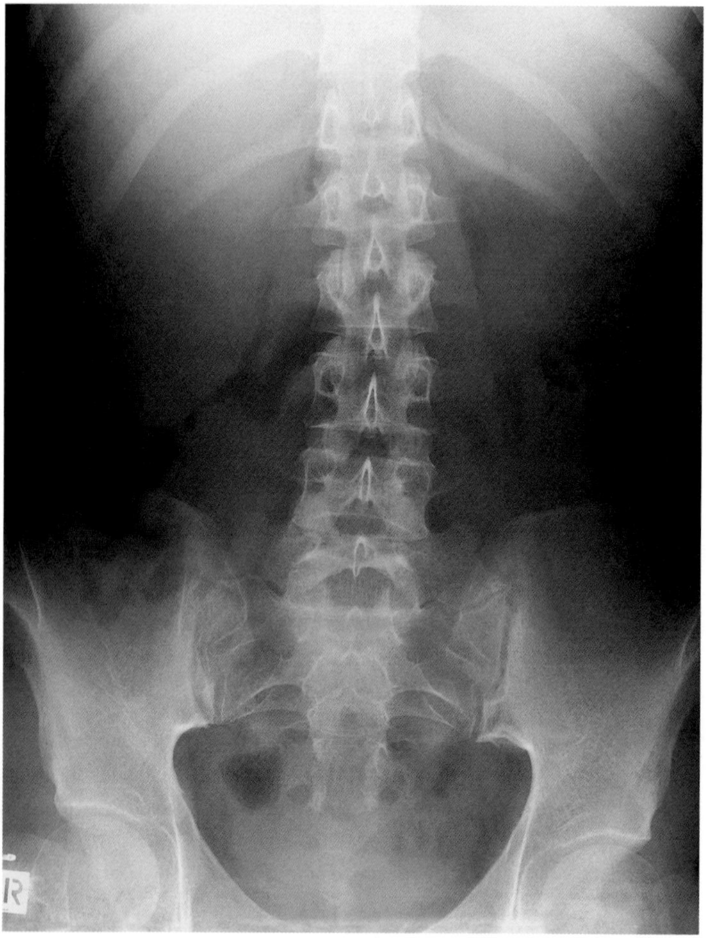
R

腹部　背臥位正面

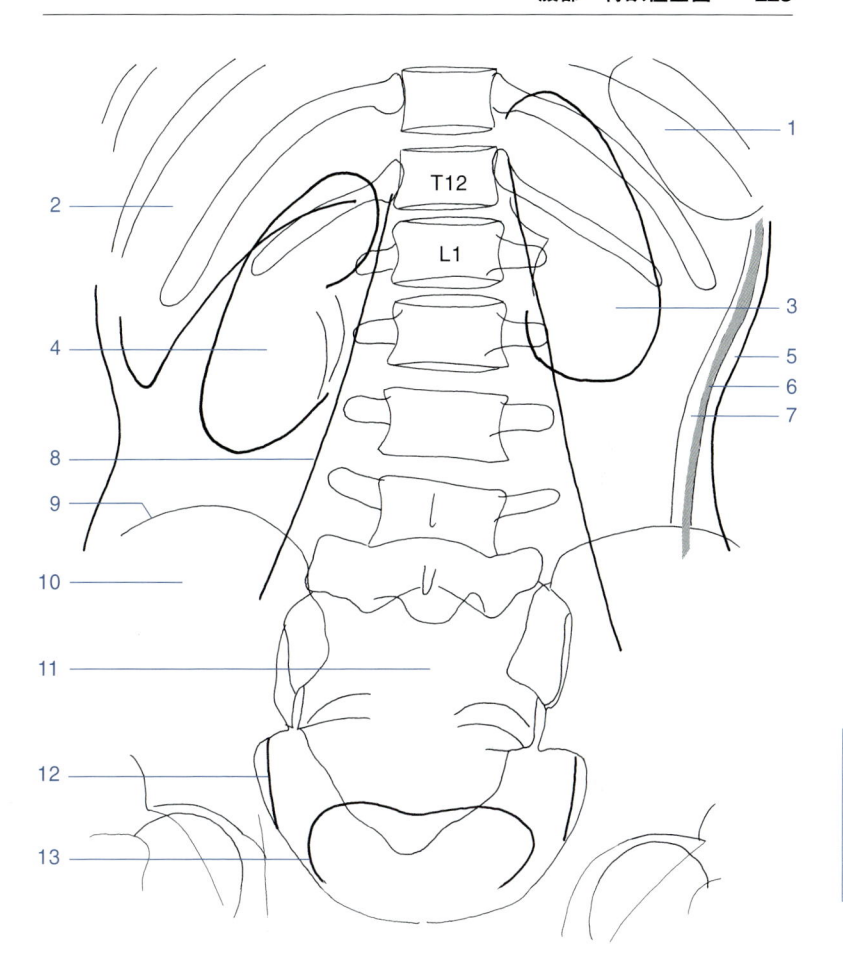

1　脾臓 Spleen	8　腸腰筋 Psoas muscle
2　肝臓 Liver	9　腸骨稜 Iliac crest
3　左腎 Left kidney	10　腸骨 Ilium
4　右腎 Right kidney	11　仙骨 Sacrum
5　皮下脂肪 Subcutaneous fat	12　内閉鎖筋 Obturator internus muscle
6　腹筋 Abdominal muscles	13　膀胱 Urinary bladder
7　腹膜前脂肪 Properitoneal fat	

スポット像

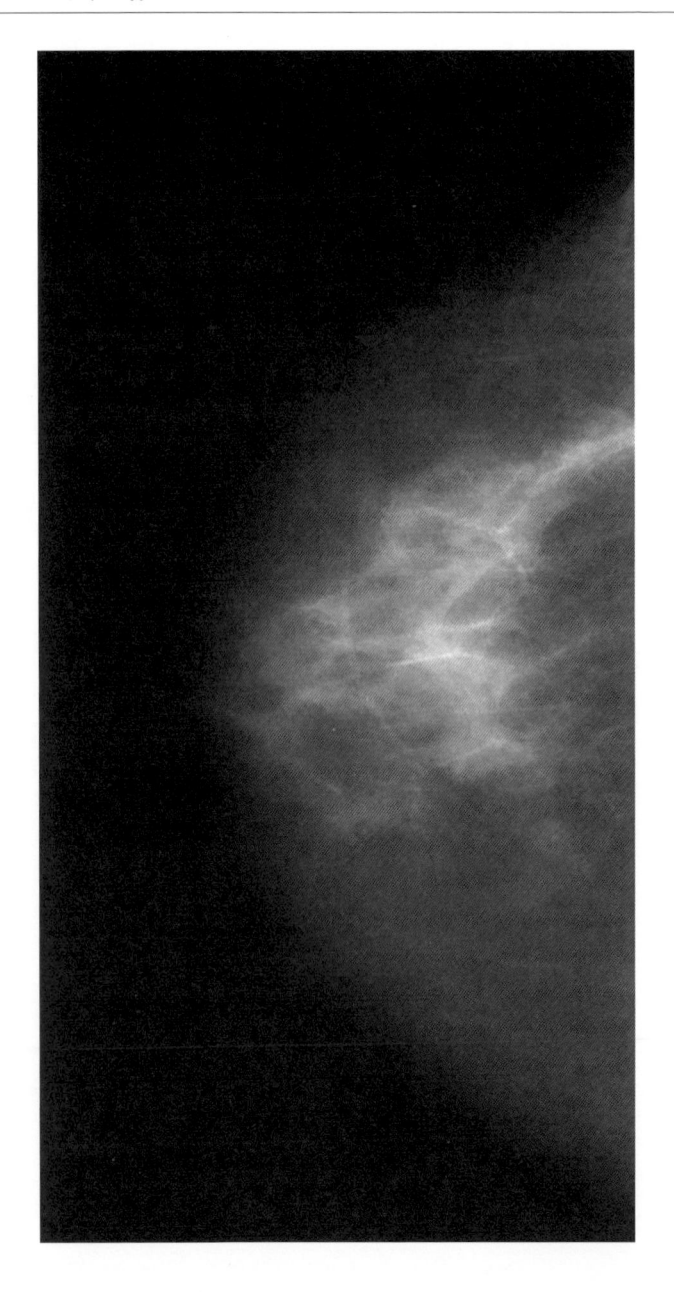

マンモグラフィー CC（頭尾方向）

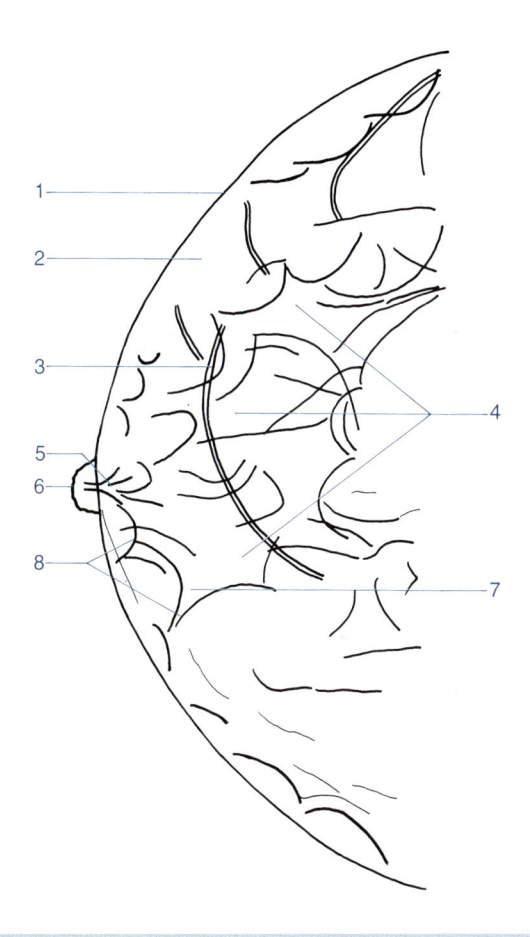

1 皮膚 Skin
2 皮下脂肪 Subcutaneous fat
3 静脈 Veins
4 腺組織 Glandular tissue
5 乳頭後方の乳管 Lactiferous duct posterior to the nipple
6 乳頭 Nipple
7 小葉縁 Contour of a lobule
8 Cooper 靭帯 Cooper's ligaments

スポット像

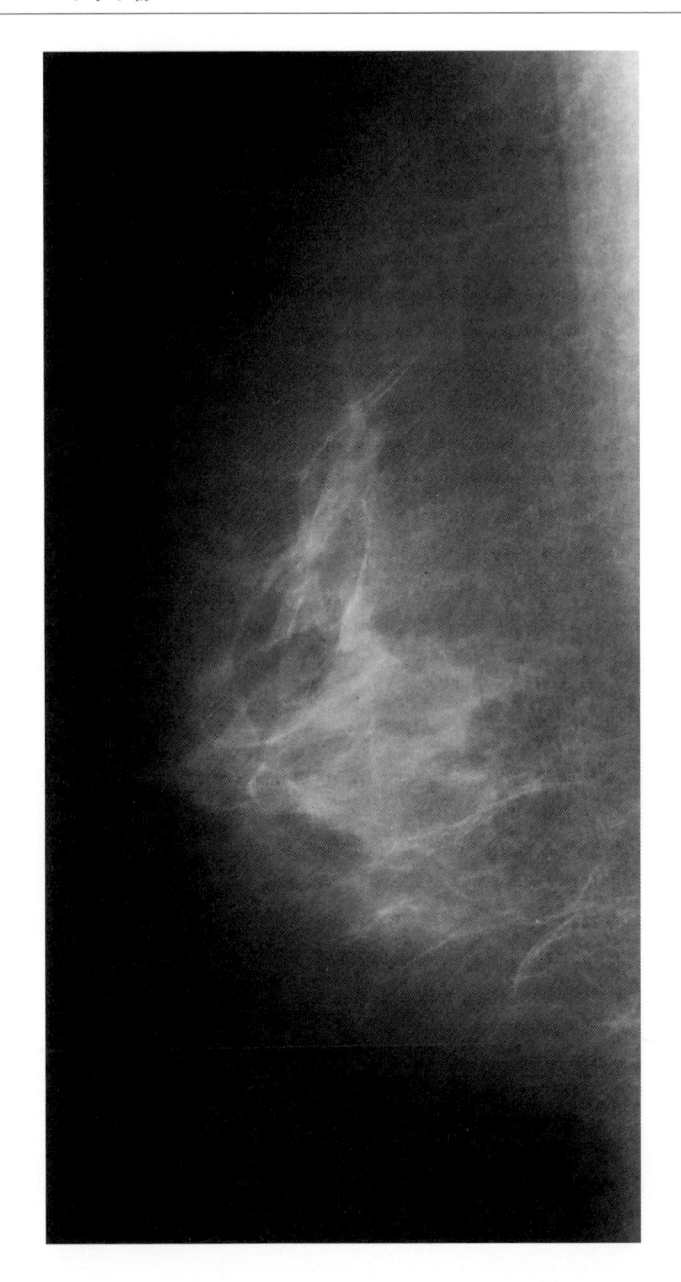

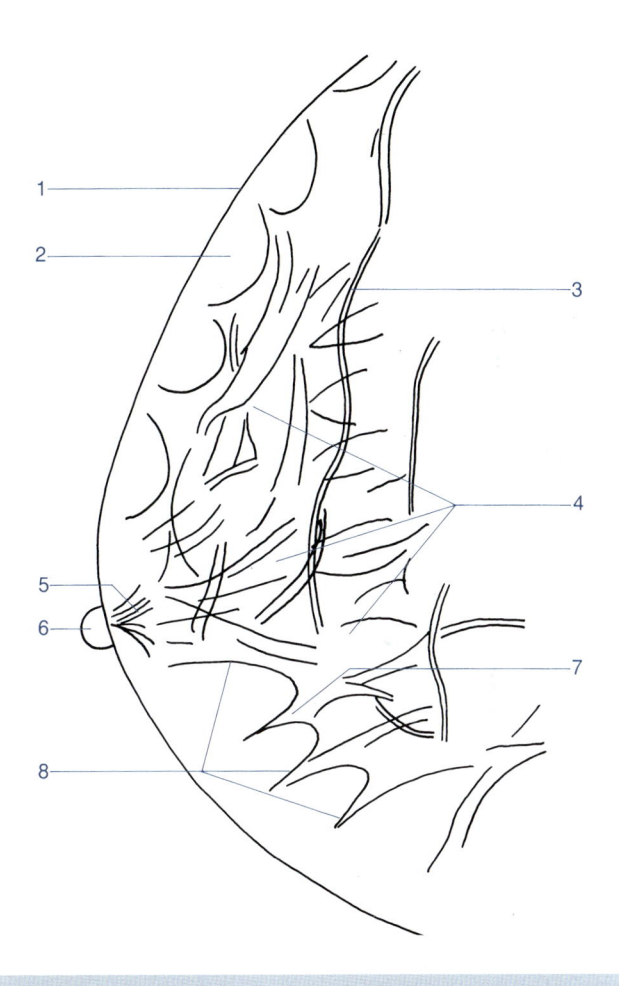

マンモグラフィー **ML**（内外側方向） **227**

1 皮膚 Skin
2 皮下脂肪 Subcutaneous fat
3 静脈 Veins
4 腺組織 Glandular tissue
5 乳頭後方の乳管 Lactiferous duct posterior to the nipple
6 乳頭 Nipple
7 小葉縁 Contour of a lobule
8 **Cooper** 靭帯 Cooper's ligaments

228　スポット像

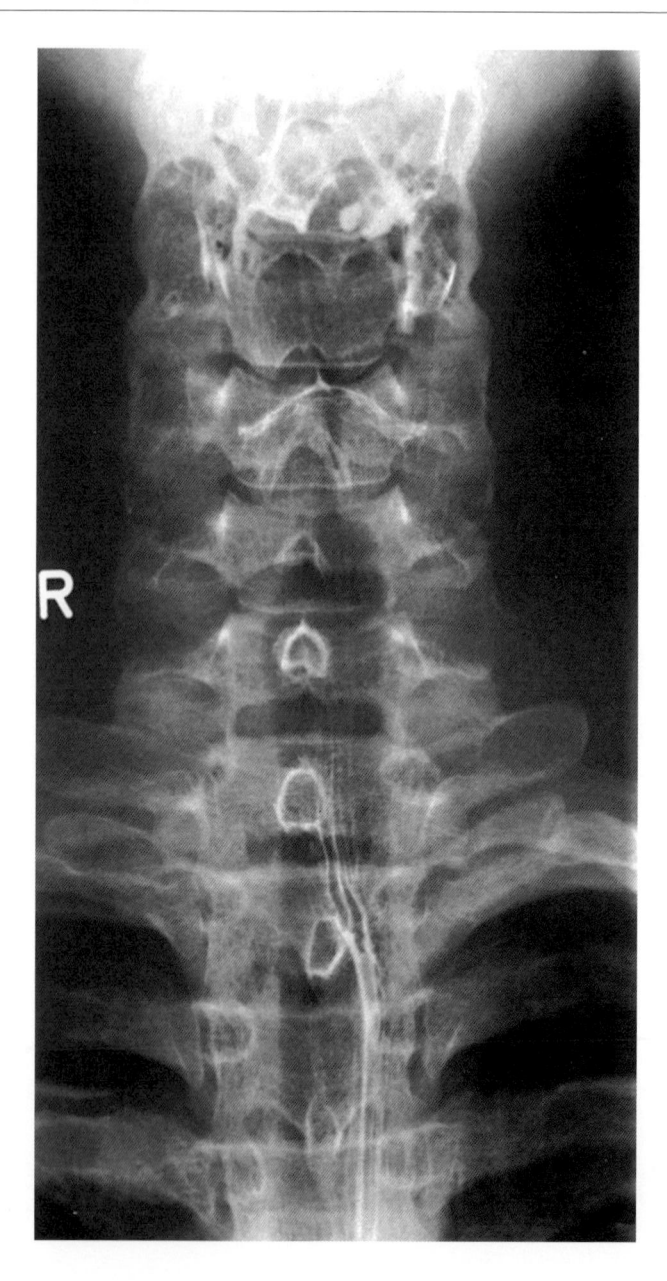

気管　正面（前後）　229

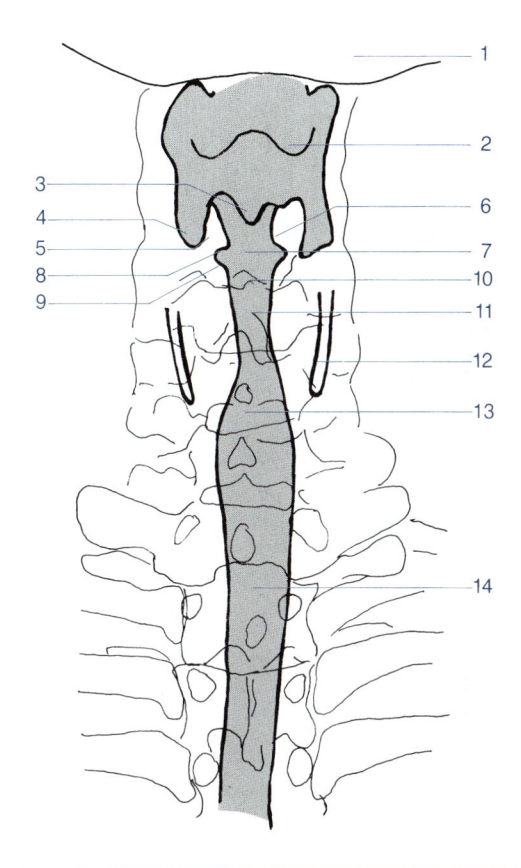

1	下顎骨 Mandible	8	喉頭室 Ventricle of the larynx
2	喉頭蓋谷 Floor of the vallecula	9	声帯 Vocal fold (true vocal cord)
3	披裂間切痕 Interarytenoid notch	10	声門裂 Rima glottidis
4	梨状陥凹 Piriform recess	11	声門下腔 Subglottic space
5	披裂軟骨 Arytenoid cartilage	12	甲状軟骨 Thyroid cartilage
6	前庭ひだ Vestibular fold (仮声帯 False vocal cord)	13	気管近位部 Proximal trachea
7	喉頭前庭 Vestibule of the larynx	14	気管遠位部 Distal trachea

スポット像

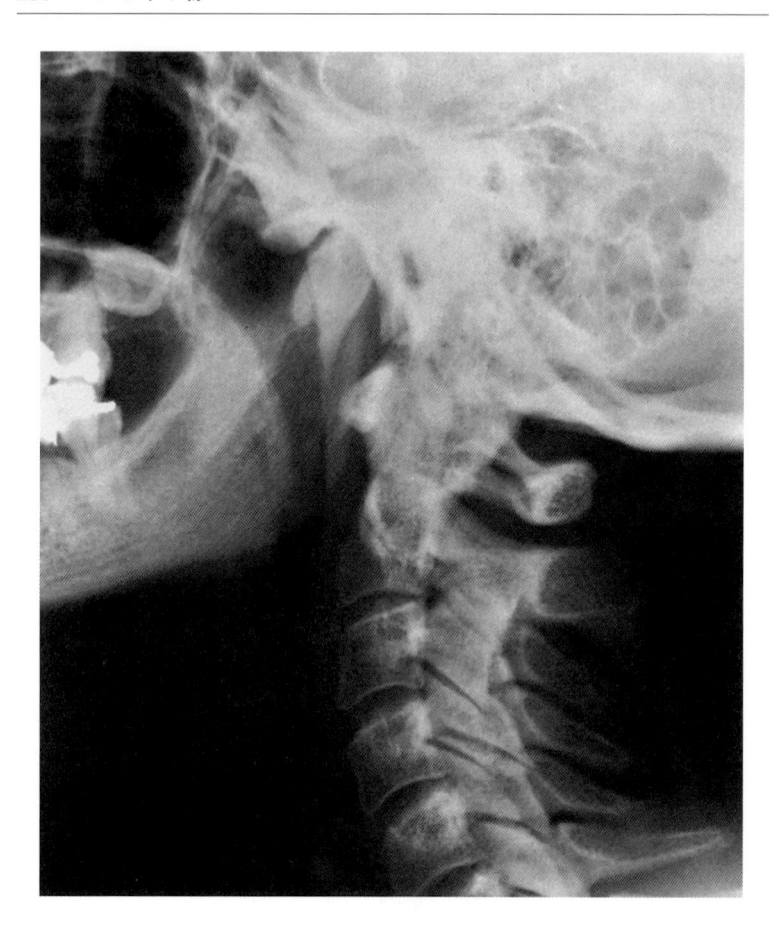

気管　側面　231

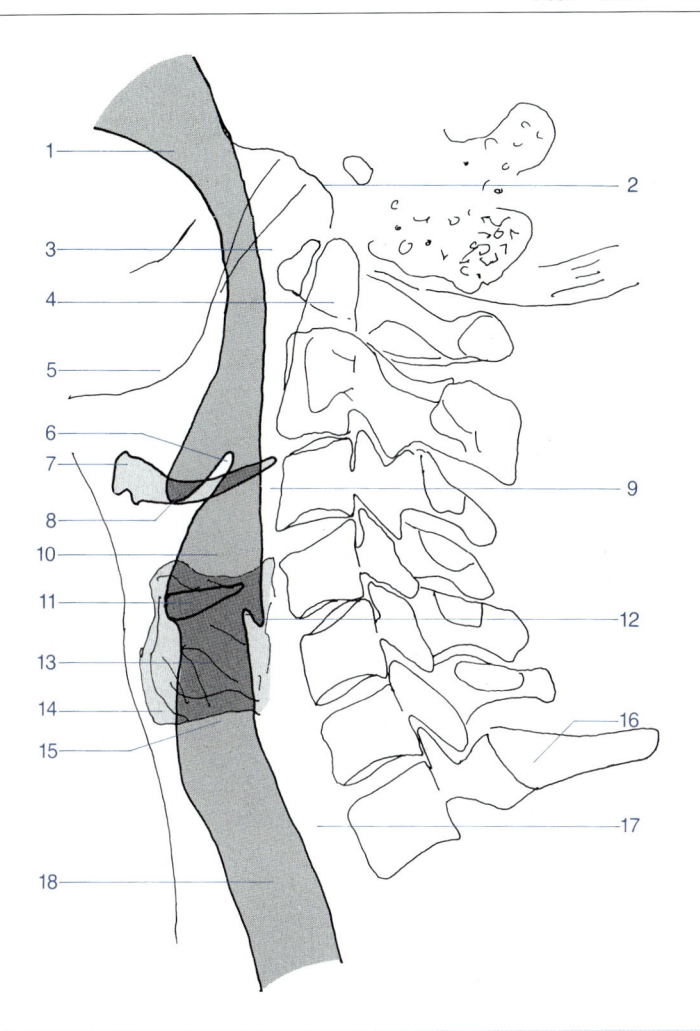

1　口腔　Oral cavity	11　喉頭室　Ventricle of the larynx
2　頭蓋底　Base of the skull	12　梨状陥凹後下面　Inferior posterior margin of the piriform sinus
3　咽頭後隙　Posterior nasopharynx	13　声門下腔　Subglottic space
4　歯突起　Dens of the axis	14　甲状軟骨　Thyroid cartilage
5　下顎骨　Mandible	15　気管近位部　Proximal trachea
6　喉頭蓋　Epiglottis	16　第7頸椎　Vertebra C7
7　舌骨　Hyoid bone	17　食道　Esophagus
8　喉頭蓋谷　Floor of the vallecula	18　気管遠位部　Distal trachea
9　後咽頭腔　Retropharyngeal space	
10　喉頭前庭　Vestibule of the larynx	

232 断層撮影

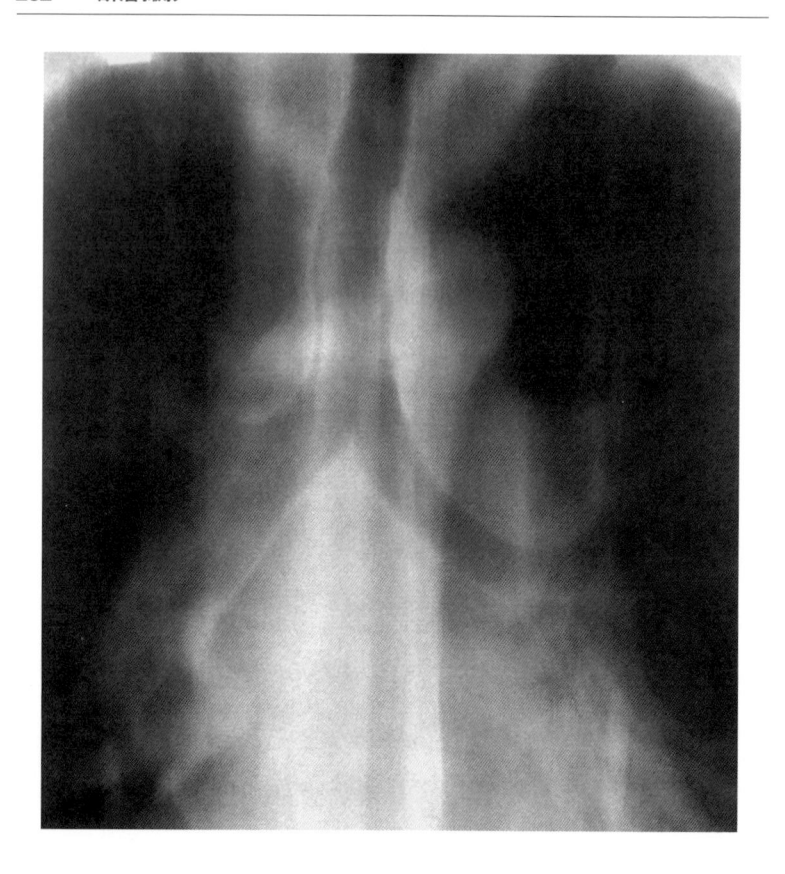

肺門部 前後断層

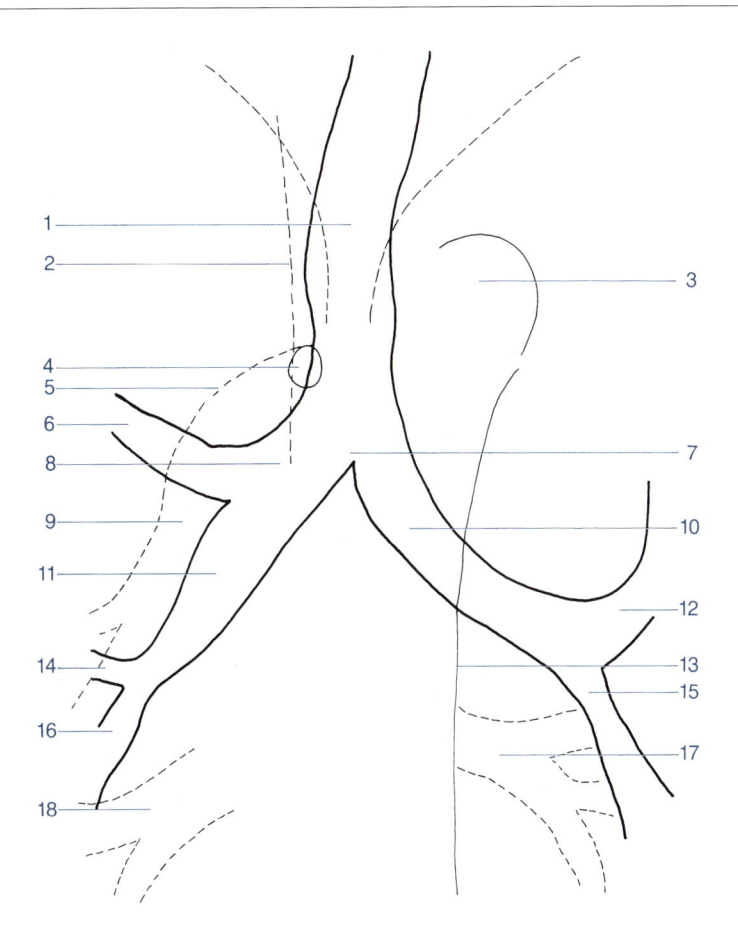

1	気管 Trachea	10	左主気管支 Left main bronchus
2	上大静脈 Superior vena cava	11	中間気管支 Intermediate bronchus
3	大動脈弓 Aortic arch	12	左上葉気管支 Left upper lobe bronchus
4	奇静脈 Azygos vein	13	下行大動脈 Descending aorta
5	右肺動脈 Right pulmonary artery	14	中葉気管支 Middle lobe bronchus
6	右上葉気管支 Right upper lobe bronchus	15	左下葉気管支 Left lower lobe bronchus
7	気管分岐部 Bifurcation of the trachea	16	右下葉気管支 Right lower lobe bronchus
8	右主気管支 Right main bronchus	17	左下葉肺静脈 Left lower lobe pulmonary veins
9	下葉肺動脈 Inferior lobar branch of the pulmonary artery	18	右下葉肺静脈合流部 Venous confluence

断層撮影

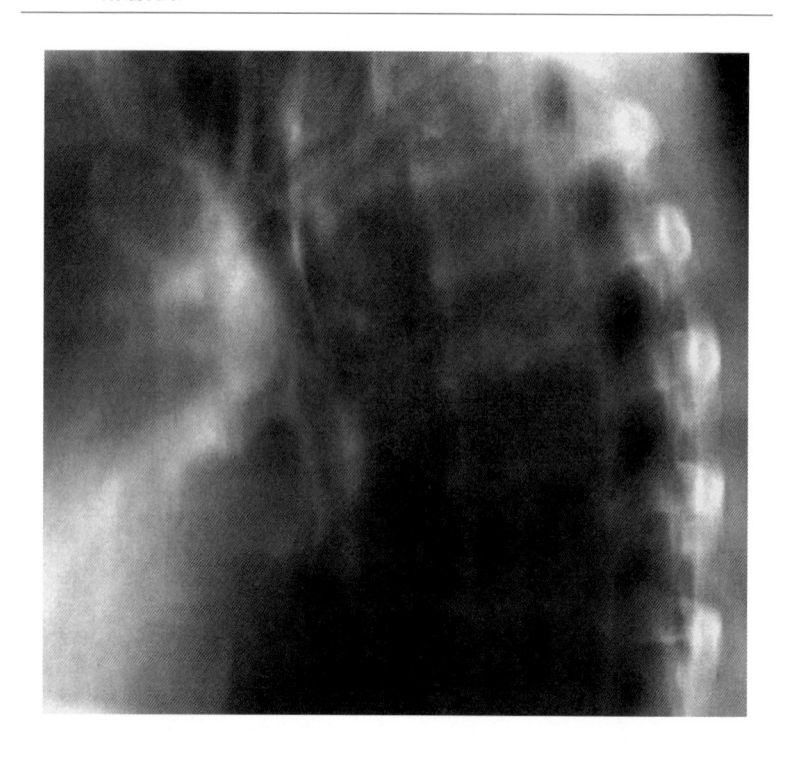

右肺門部　側面断層　235

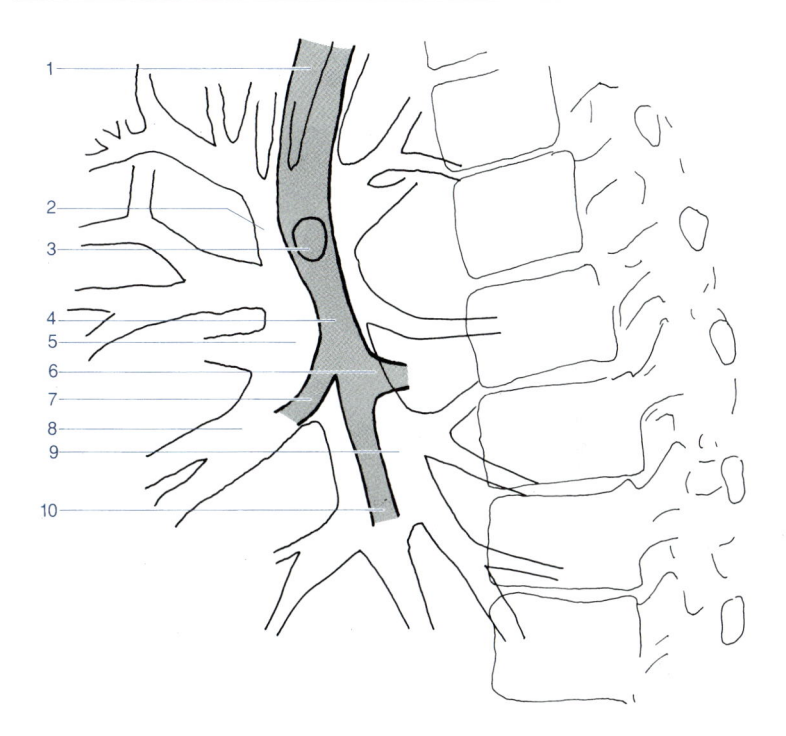

1　気管 Trachea
2　肺動脈肺尖枝 Superior lobar branch of the pulmonary artery
3　上葉気管支起始部 Origin of the upper lobe bronchus
4　中間気管支 Intermediate bronchus
5　右肺動脈 Right pulmonary artery
6　下葉気管支区域枝 Segmental bronchus of the lower lobe
7　中葉気管支 Middle lobe bronchus
8　肺動脈中葉枝 Middle lobar branch of the pulmonary artery
9　下葉肺動脈 Inferior lobar branch of the pulmonary artery
10　下葉気管支 Lower lobe bronchus

236　断層撮影

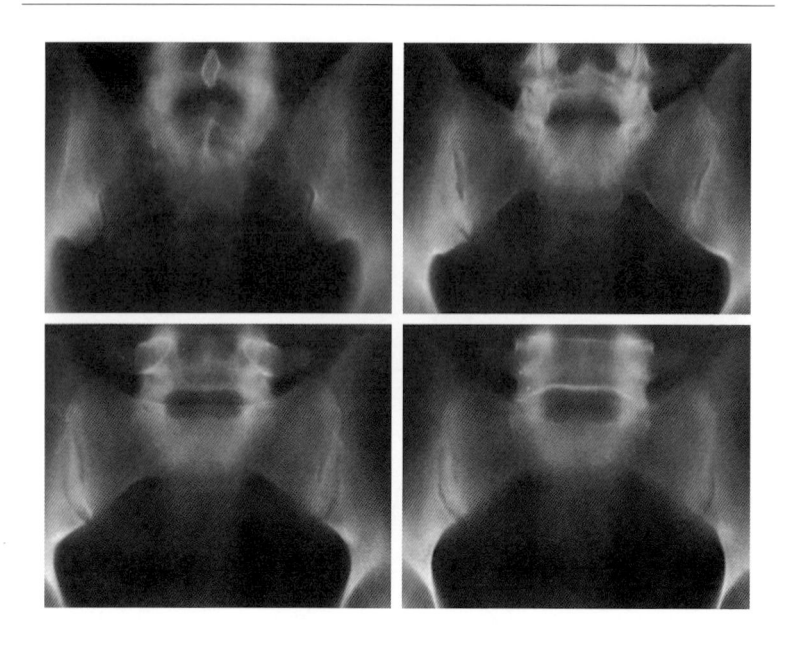

仙腸関節

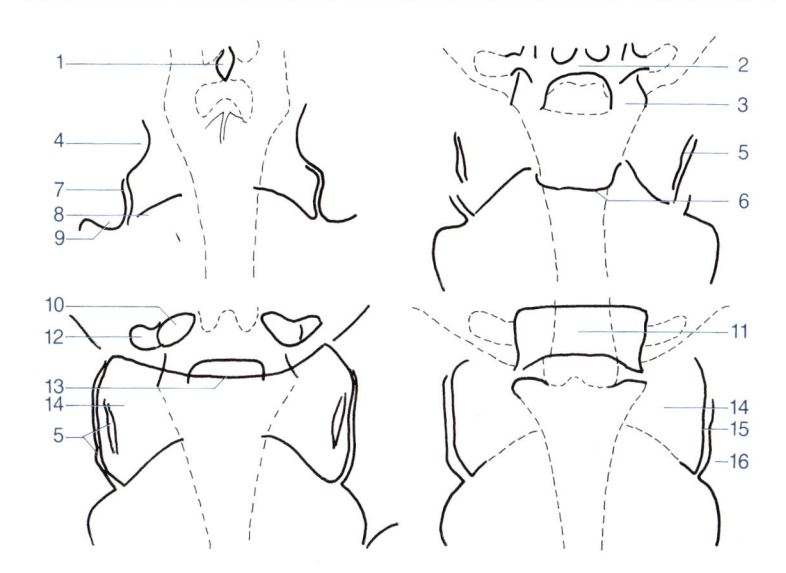

1 棘突起 Spinous process
2 椎弓板 Lamina
3 下関節突起 Inferior articular process
4 上後腸骨棘 Posterior superior iliac spine
5 仙腸関節内側面 Middle portion of the sacroiliac joint
6 仙骨前面 Anterior aspect of the sacrum
7 仙腸関節の後下面 Posterior inferior aspect of the sacroiliac joint
8 仙骨孔 Sacral foramina
9 下後腸骨棘 Posterior inferior iliac spine
10 椎弓根 Pedicle
11 第5腰椎 L5
12 横突起 Transverse process
13 岬骨 Promontory
14 仙骨翼 Sacral ala
15 仙腸関節前面 Anterior aspect of the sacroiliac joint
16 腸骨 Ilium(Iliac bone)

造影検査

消化管　240
経静脈造影検査　264
関節造影　268
動脈造影　280
静脈造影　326

240　消化管

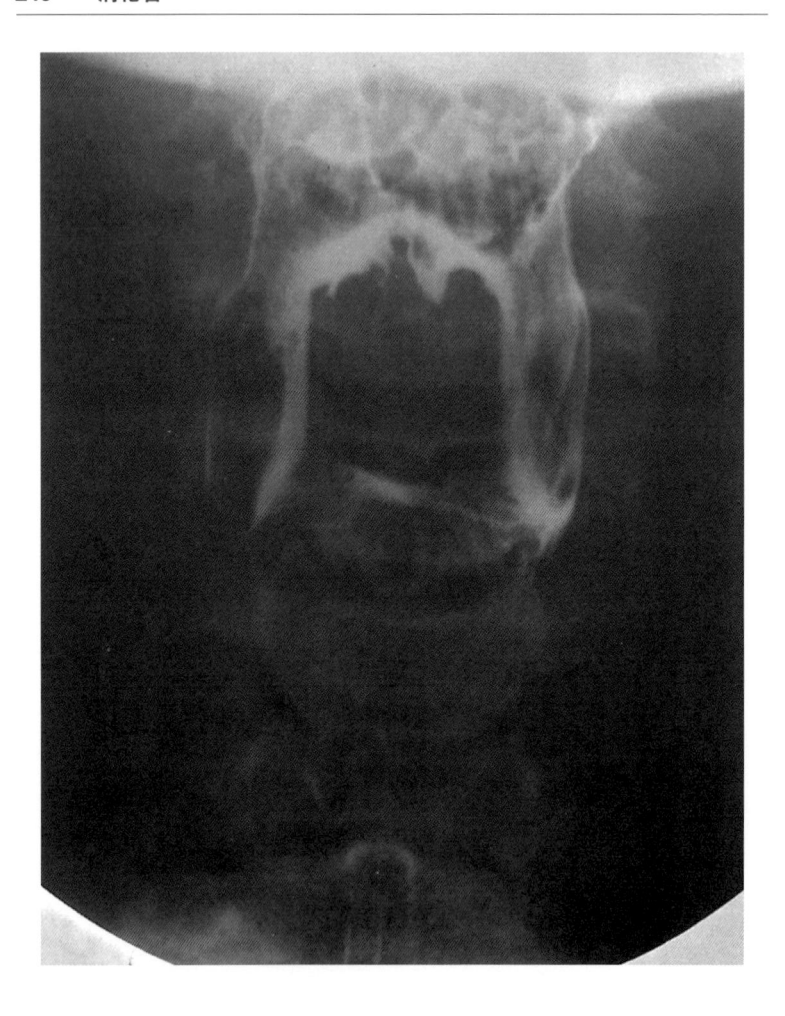

下咽頭　正面（前後）　241

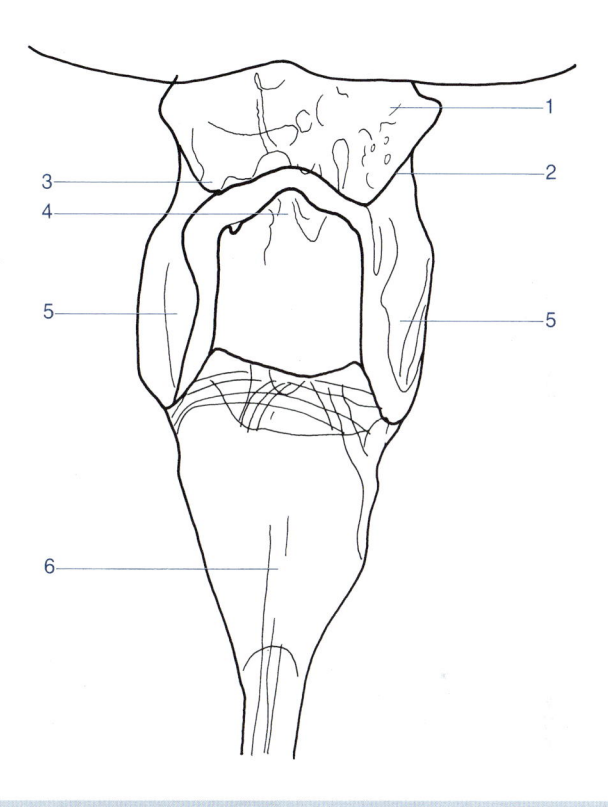

1　咽頭　Pharynx
2　外側舌喉頭蓋ヒダ　Lateral glossoepiglottic fold
3　喉頭蓋谷　Vallecula
4　喉頭蓋　Epiglottis
5　梨状陥凹　Piriform sinus
6　食道　Esophagus

242　消化管

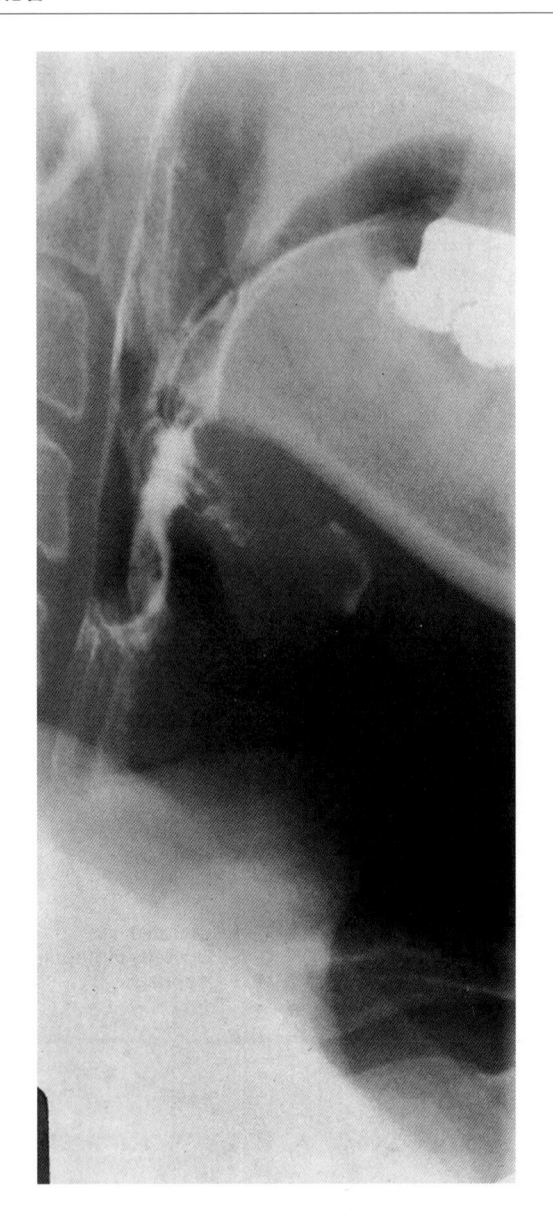

下咽頭 側面

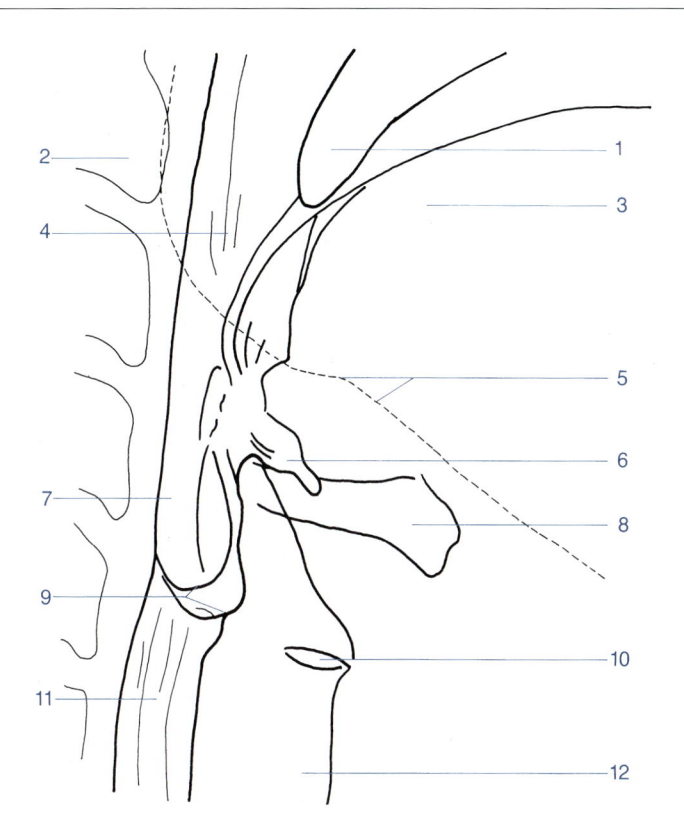

1 口蓋垂 Uvula	7 喉頭 Larynx
2 第2頸椎 Cervical spine (軸椎 Axis)	8 舌骨 Hyoid bone
3 舌根 Base of tongue	9 梨状陥凹 Piriform recess
4 中咽頭 Oropharynx	10 喉頭室 Ventricle of the larynx
5 下顎骨 Mandible	11 食道 Esophagus
6 喉頭蓋谷 Vallecula	12 気管 Trachea

244　消化管

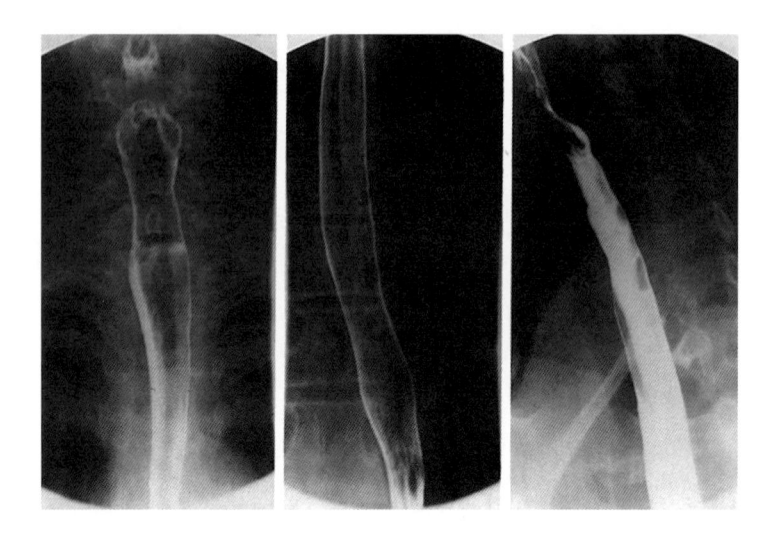

食道　245

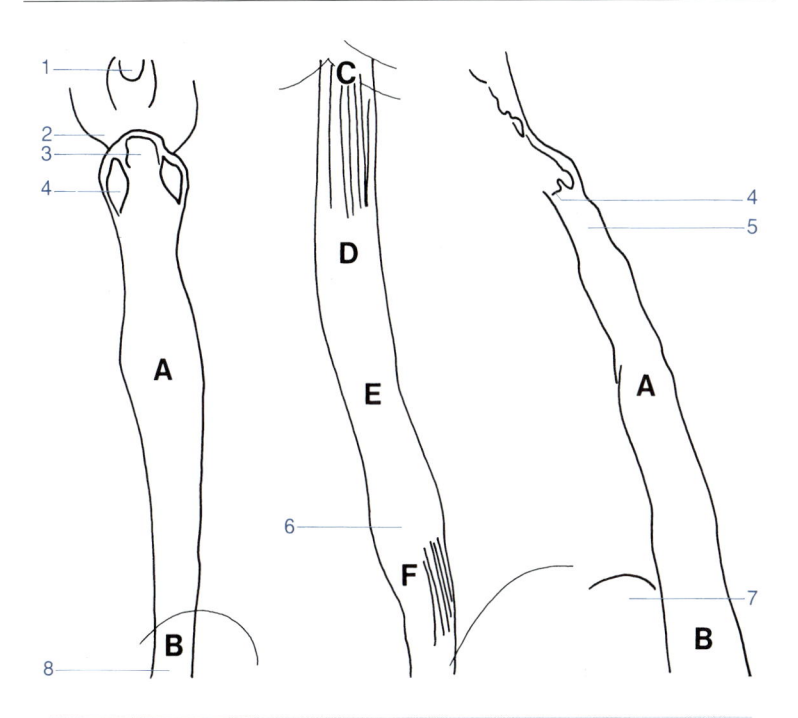

1	口蓋垂 Uvula
2	外側舌喉頭蓋ヒダ Lateral glossoepiglottic fold
3	喉頭蓋 Epiglottis
4	梨状陥凹 Piriform sinus
5	上部食道括約筋 Upper esophageal sphincter
6	食道体部 Body of the esophagus
7	大動脈弓 Aortic arch
8	食道の大動脈, 気管支間部分 Bronchial and aortic segment
A	気管周囲部 Paratracheal segment
B	大動脈部 Aortic segment
C	気管支部 Bronchial segment
D	気管支間部 Interbronchial segment
E	心臓後部 Retrocardiac segment
F	横隔膜上部 Epiphrenic segment

246 消化管

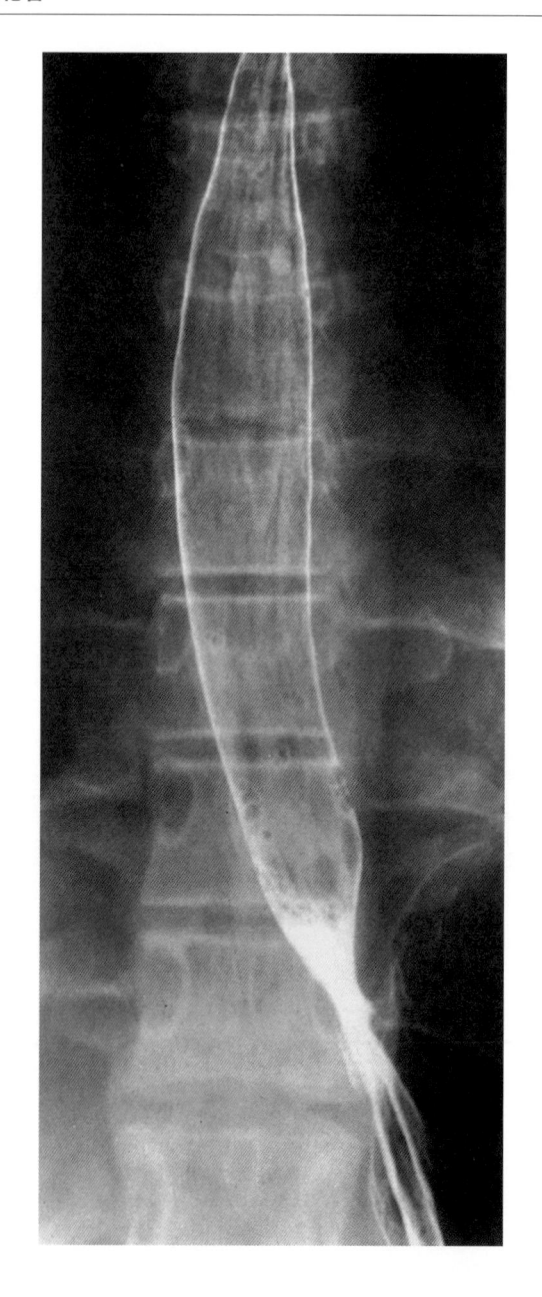

胃（食道） **247**

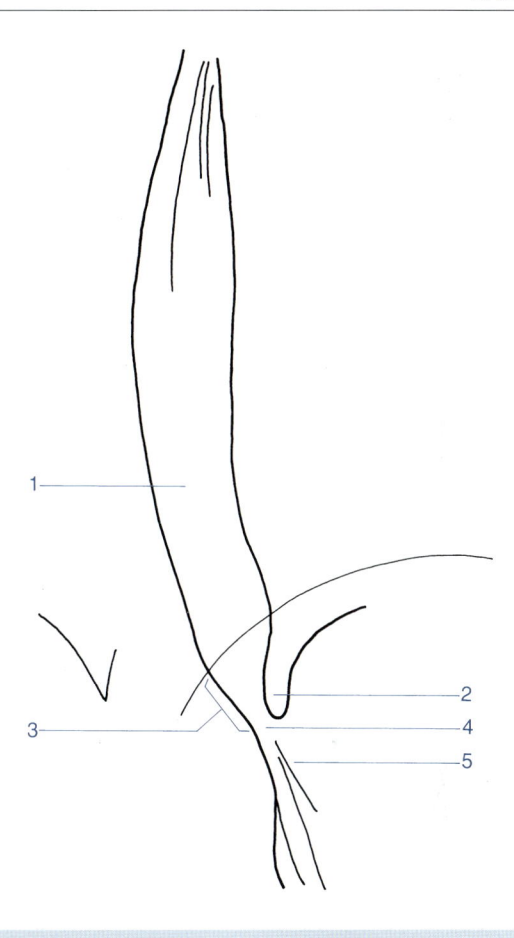

1 食道遠位部 Distal esophagus	4 食道裂孔 Esophageal hiatus
2 胃食道角 Gastroesophageal angle	5 噴門 Cardia
3 腹部食道 Abdominal esophagus	

248　消化管

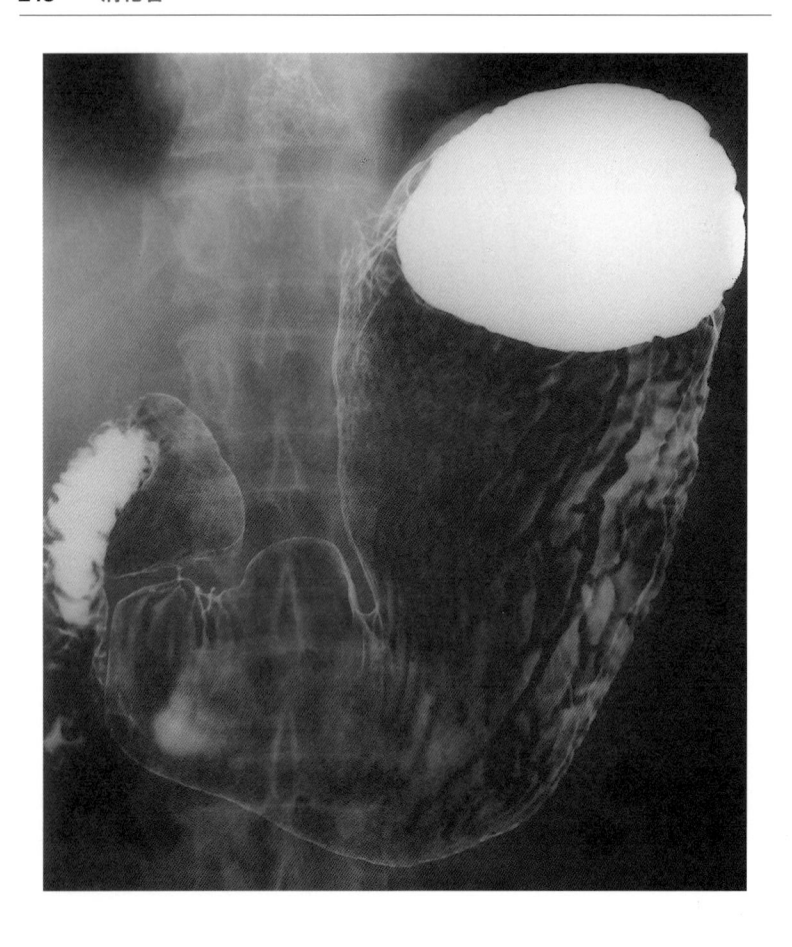

胃 249

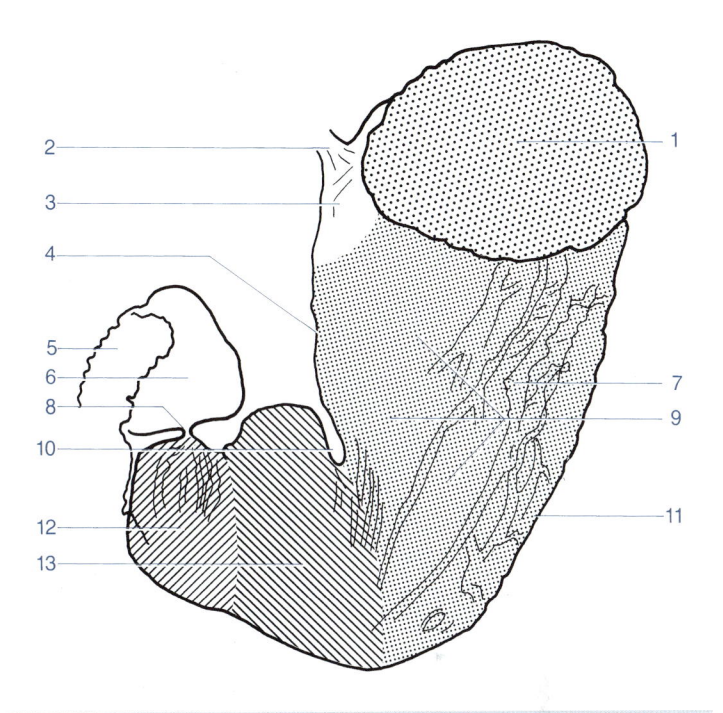

1 胃底 Fundus
2 腹部食道 Abdominal esophagus
3 噴門 Cardia
4 小弯 Lesser curvature
5 十二指腸下行部 Descending part of the duodenum
6 十二指腸球部 Duodenal bulb
7 胃のヒダ（後壁） Gastric folds (posterior wall)
8 幽門 Pylorus
9 胃体 Body of the stomach
10 角切痕 Angular notch
11 大弯 Greater curvature
12 幽門洞 Pyloric antrum
13 胃遠位部 Distal stomach

250 消化管

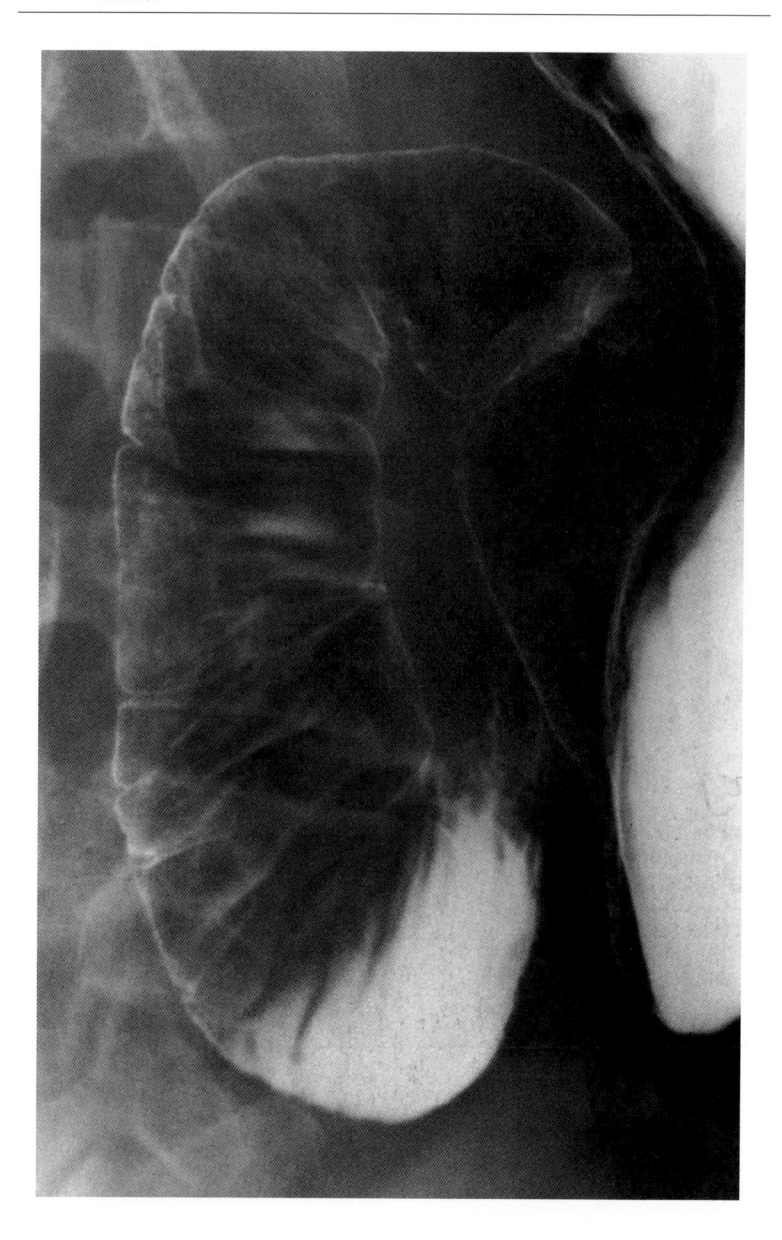

胃（十二指腸） 251

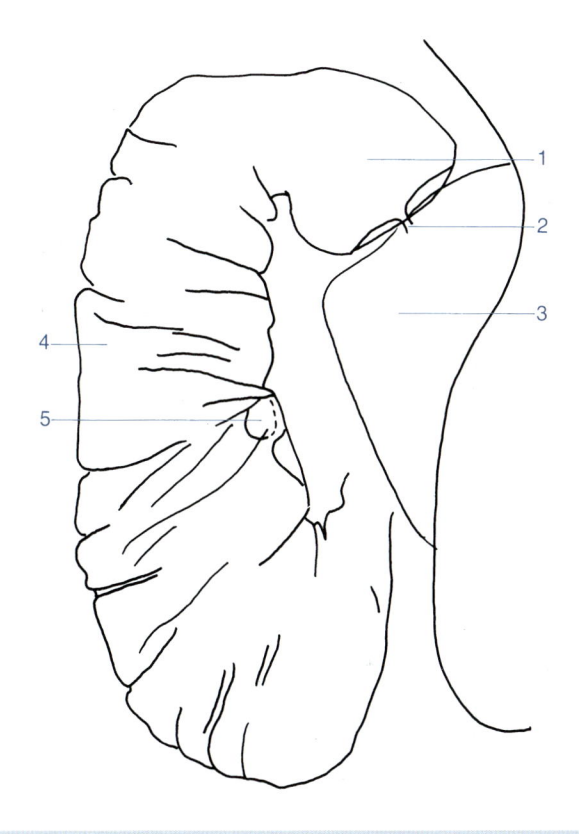

1 十二指腸球部 Duodenal bulb
2 幽門 Pylorus
3 幽門洞 Pyloric antrum
4 十二指腸下行部 Descending part of the duodenum
5 Vater乳頭 Papilla of Vater
（十二指腸乳頭 Duodenal papilla）

252　消化管

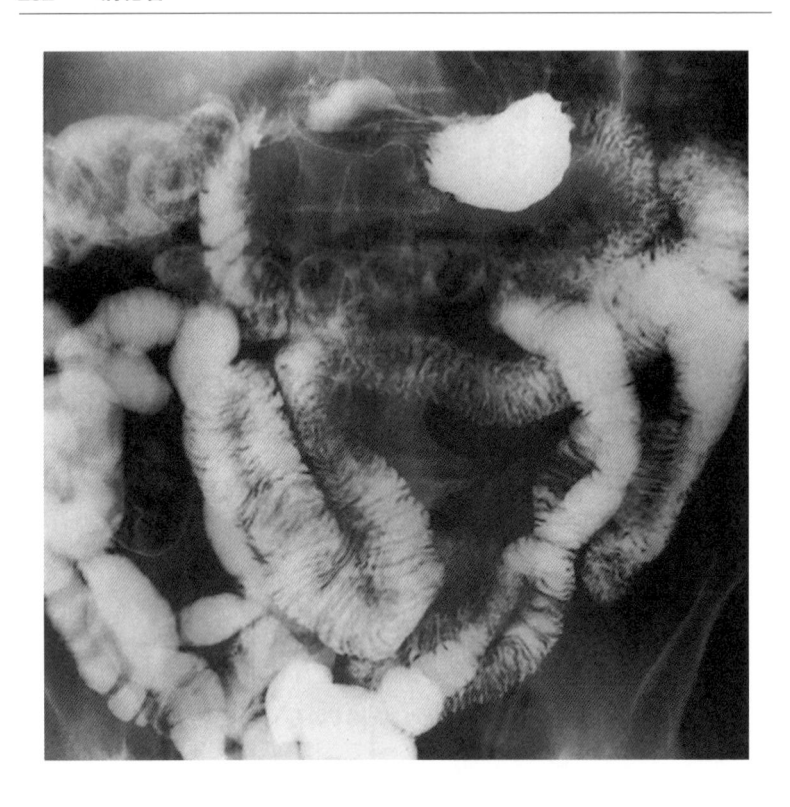

胃・小腸 **253**

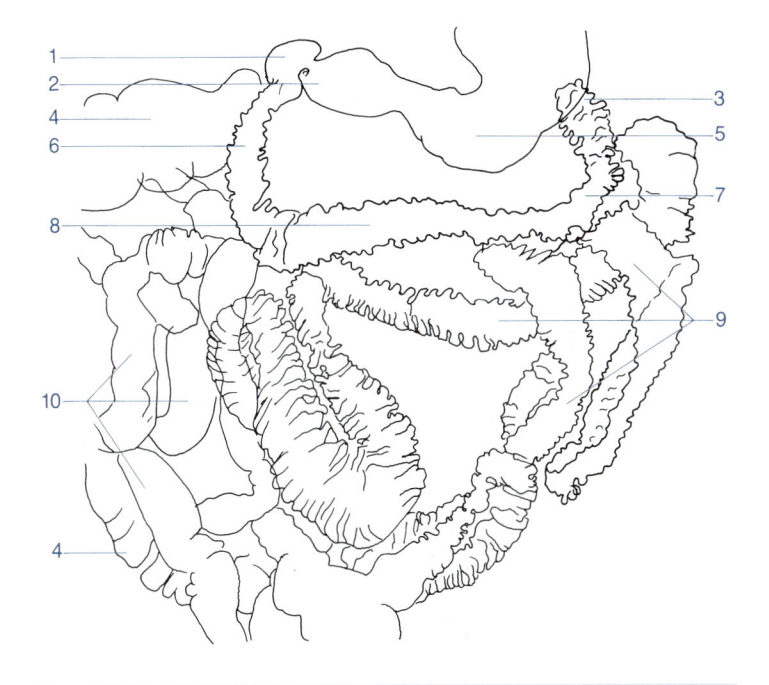

1 十二指腸球部 Duodenal bulb
2 幽門洞 Pyloric antrum
3 十二指腸空腸移行部 Duodenojejunal junction
4 結腸 Colon
5 胃体 Body of the stomach
6 十二指腸下行部 Descending part of the duodenum
7 十二指腸上行部 Ascending part of the duodenum
8 十二指腸水平部 Horizontal part of duodenum
9 空腸 Jejunum
10 回腸 Ileum

254 消化管

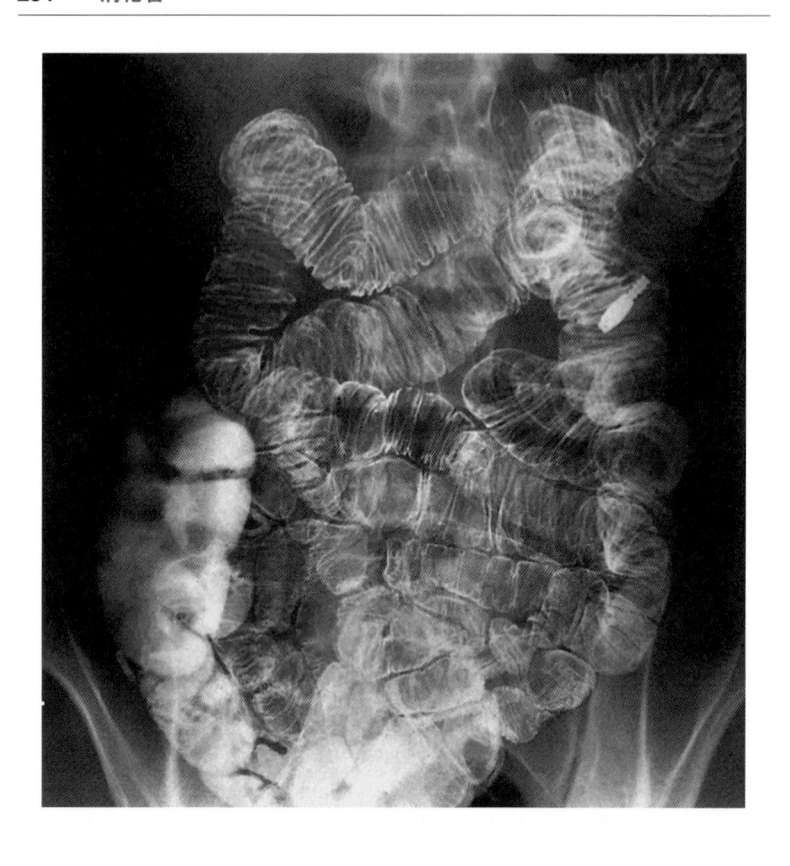

小　腸　255

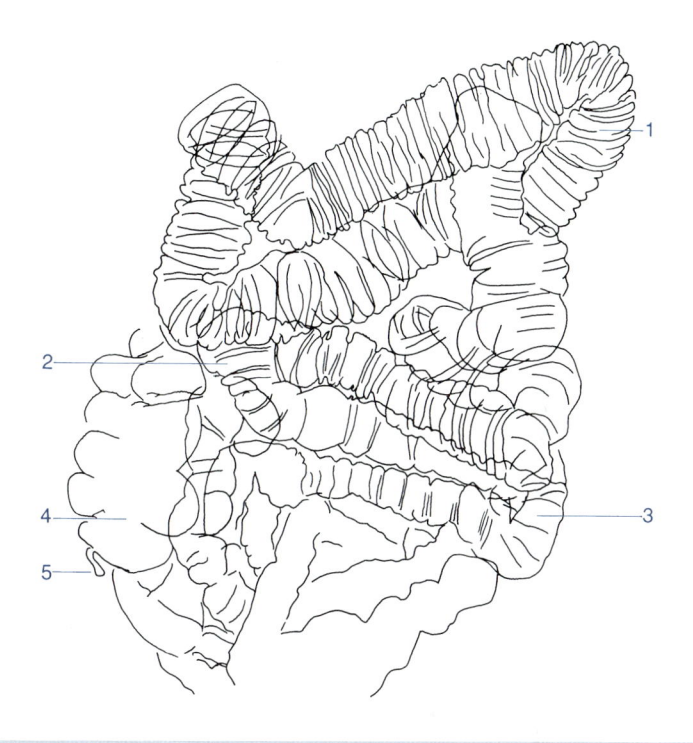

1 空腸 Jejunum
2 空回腸移行部 Junction of ileum and jejunum
3 回腸 Ileum
4 盲腸 Cecum
5 虫垂 Appendix

256　消化管

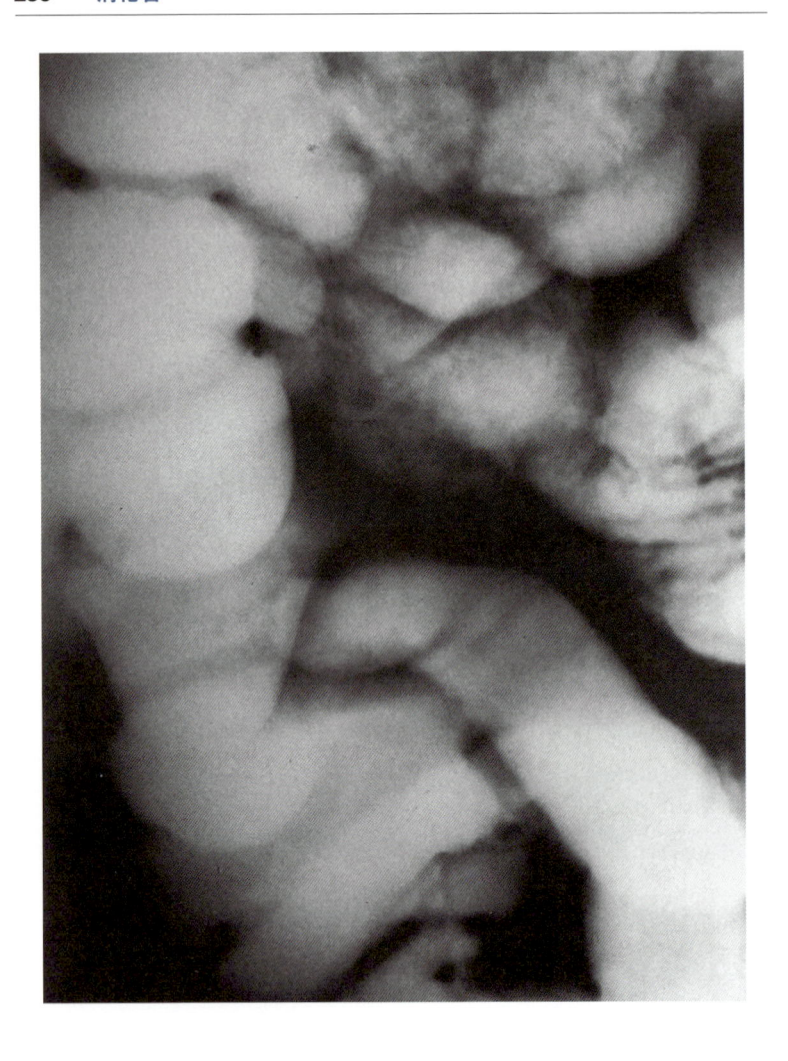

回盲部　圧迫スポット像　*257*

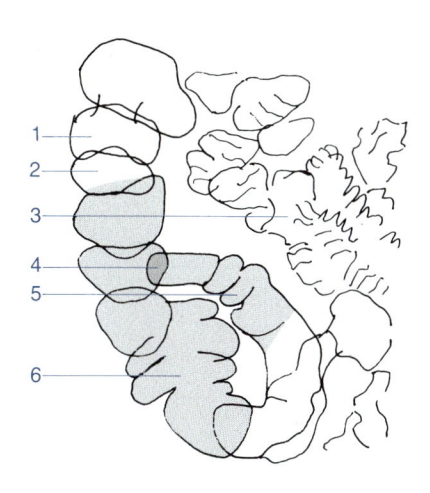

1　結腸ハウストラ Haustra of the colon	4　回盲弁 Ileocecal valve
2　上行結腸 Ascending colon	5　回腸末端部 Terminal ileum
3　回腸 Ileum	6　盲腸 Cecum

258 消化管

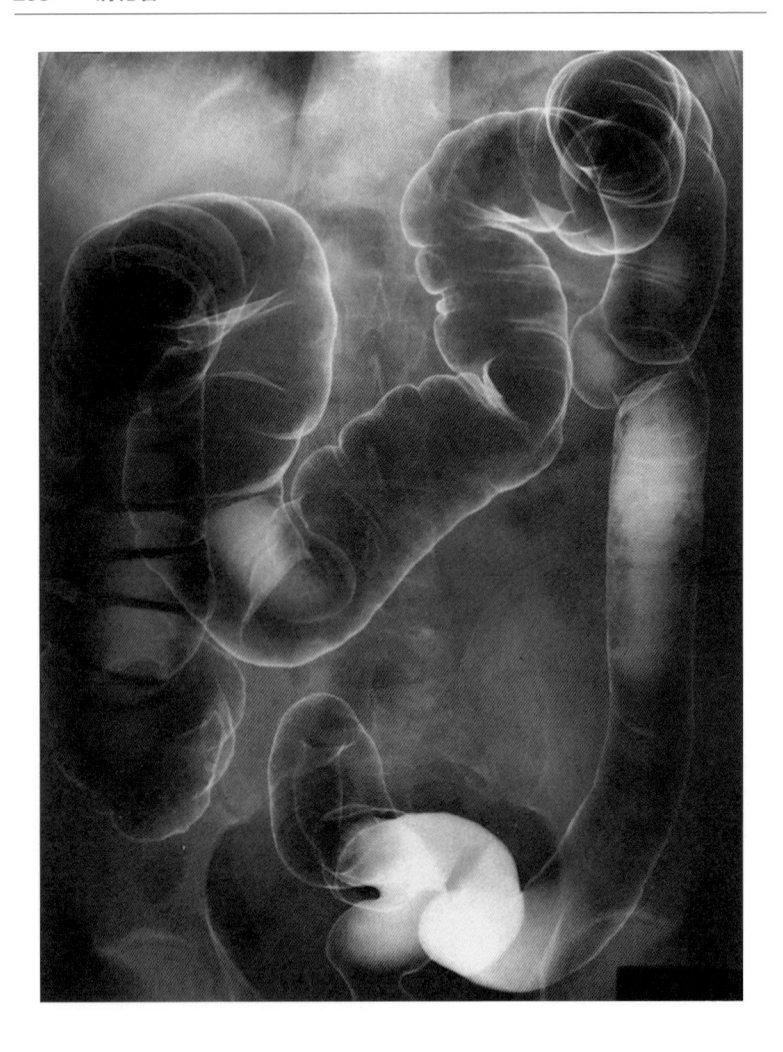

結　腸

1	結腸脾弯曲部 Splenic flexure of the colon	7	回盲弁 Ileocecal valve
2	結腸肝弯曲部 Hepatic flexure of the colon	8	盲腸 Cecum
3	上行結腸 Ascending colon	9	S状結腸 Sigmoid colon
4	横行結腸 Transverse colon	10	虫垂 Appendix
5	下行結腸 Descending colon	11	直腸 Rectum
6	ハウストラ Haustra		

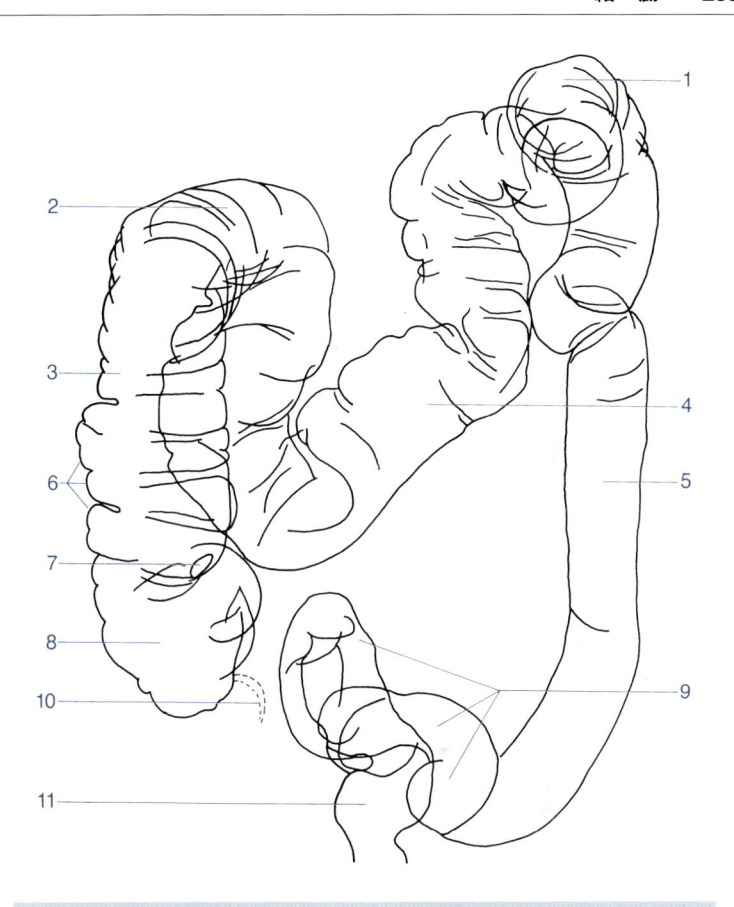

260　消化管

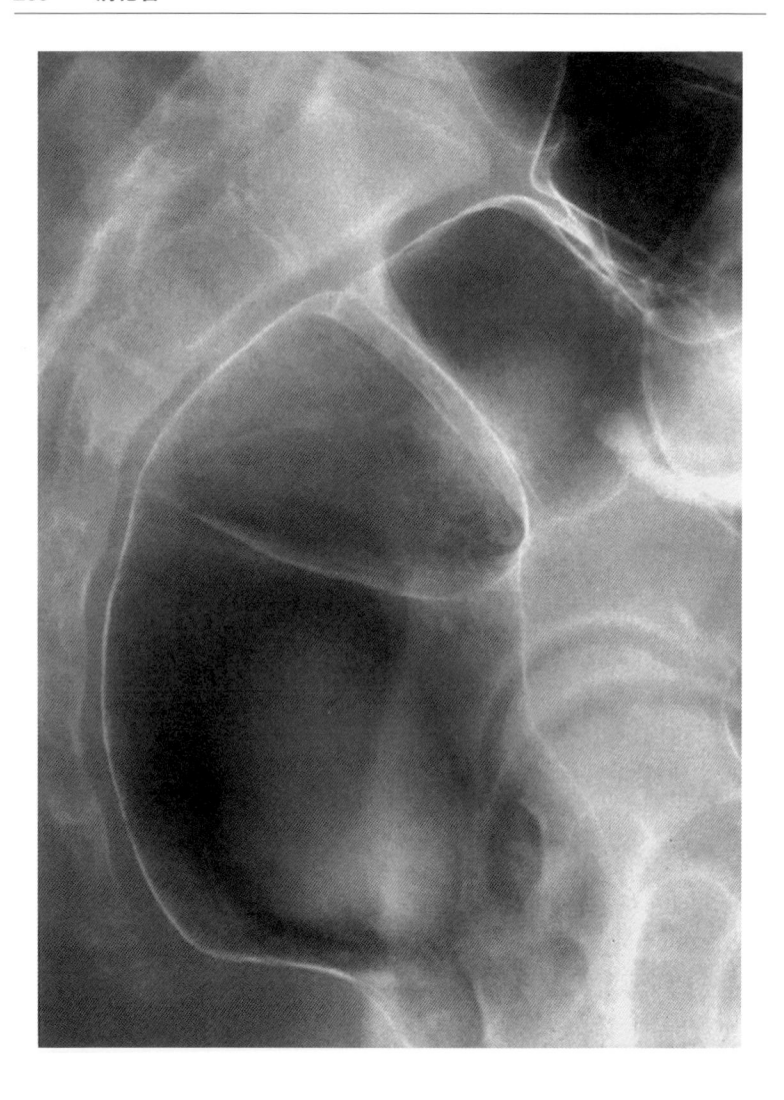

直　腸　**261**

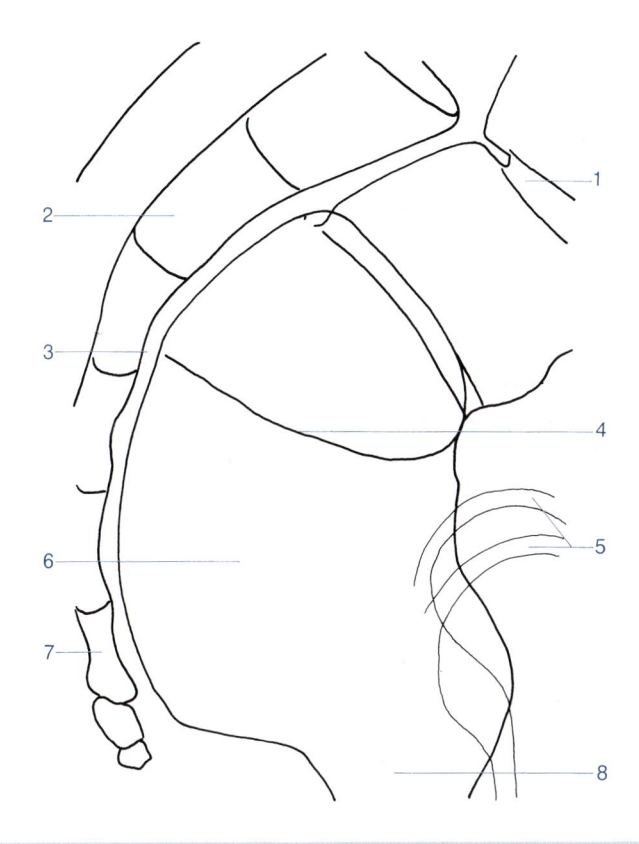

1 直腸S状結腸移行部 Rectosigmoid junction	5 大腿骨頭 Femoral head
2 仙骨 Sacrum	6 直腸膨大部 Rectal ampulla
3 後直腸腔 Retrorectal space	7 尾骨 Coccyx
4 直腸横ヒダ Transverse rectal fold (**Houston**弁 Valve of Houston)	8 肛門直腸接合部 Anorectal junction

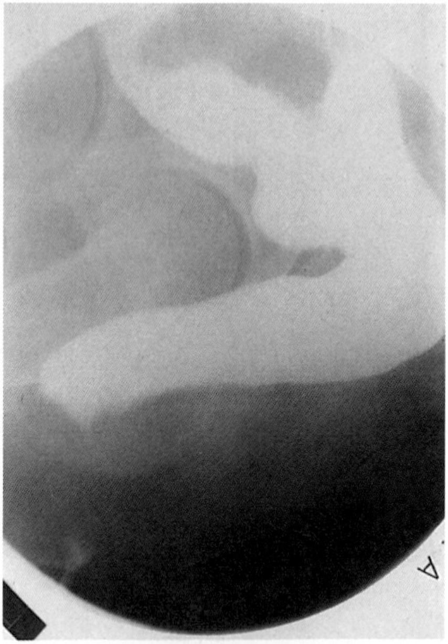

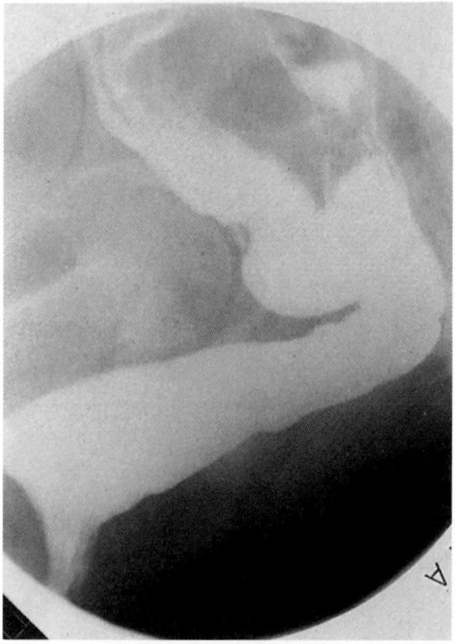

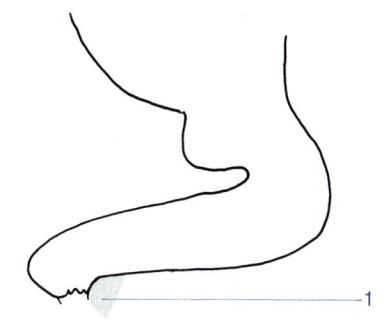

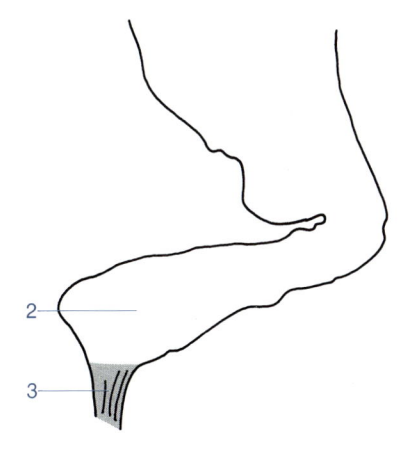

| 1 | 恥骨直腸筋 Puborectalis muscle | 3 | 肛門管 Anal canal |
| 2 | 直腸膨大部 Rectal ampulla | | |

264　経静脈造影検査

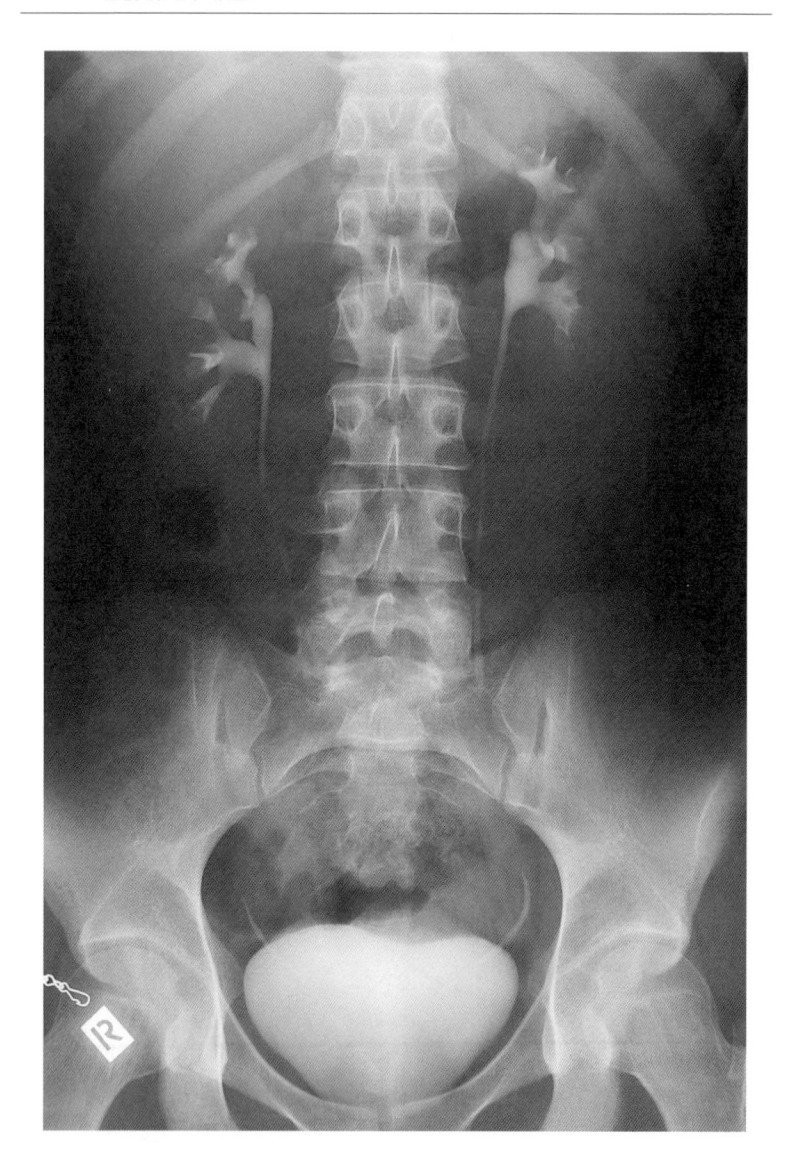

排泄性尿路造影 **265**

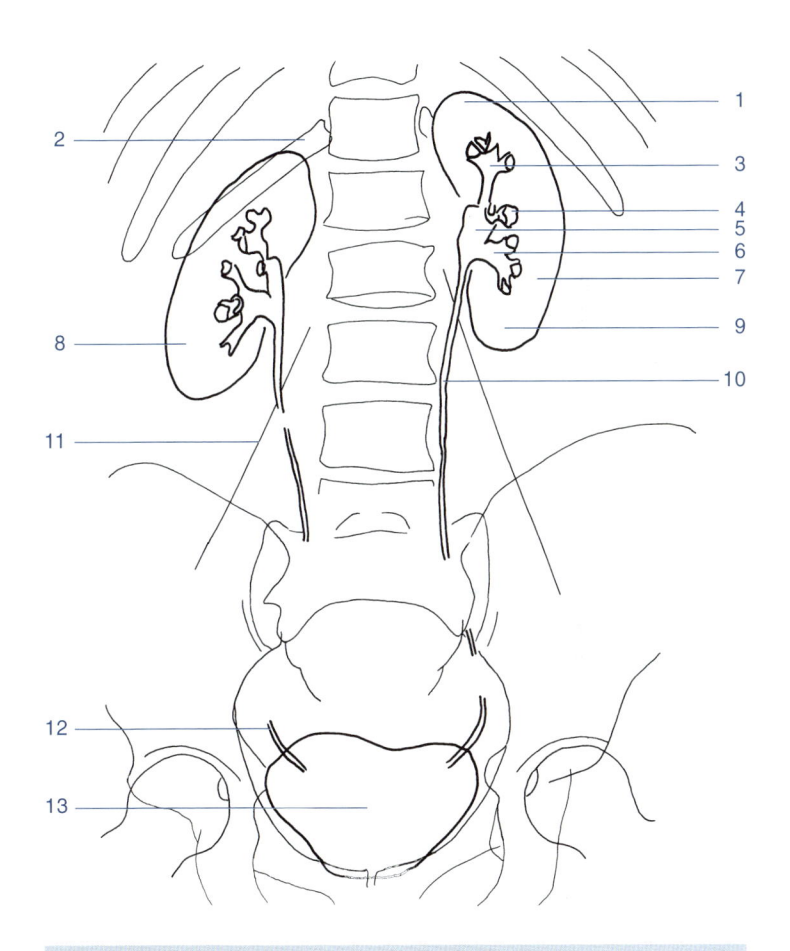

1 腎上極 Superior pole of the kidney
2 第12肋骨 Twelfth rib
3 上部腎杯 Superior calyces
4 中部腎杯 Middle calyces
5 腎盂 Renal pelvis
6 下部腎杯 Inferior calyces
7 左腎 Left kidney
8 右腎 Right kidney
9 腎下極 Inferior pole of the kidney
10 尿管 Ureter
11 腸腰筋縁 Margin of the psoas muscle
12 遠位尿管 Distal ureter
13 膀胱 Urinary bladder

経静脈造影検査

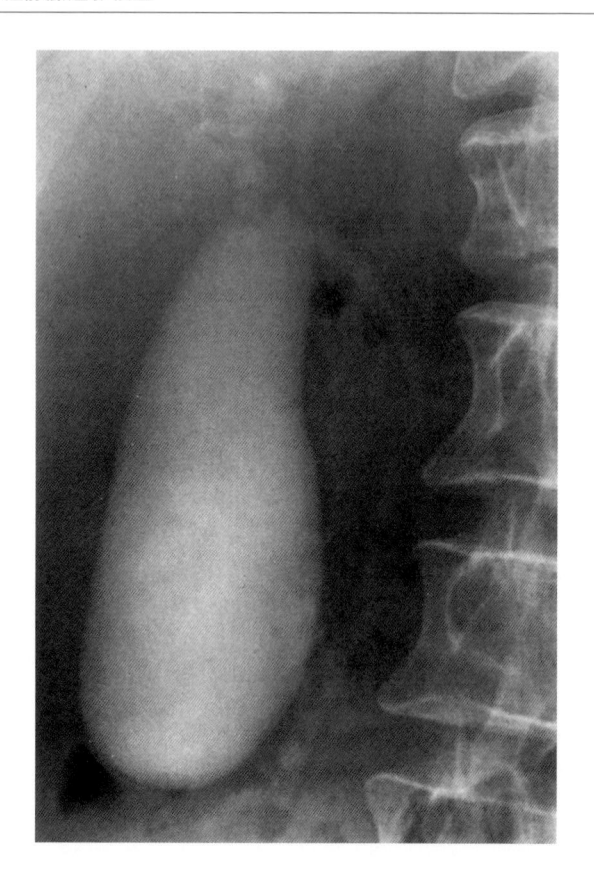

静脈性胆囊胆管造影

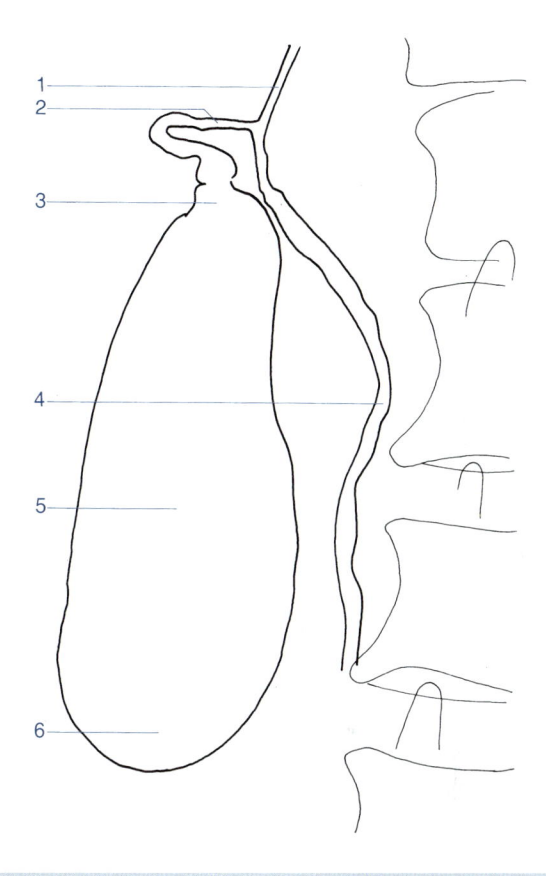

1 総肝管 Common hepatic duct	4 総胆管 Common bile duct
2 胆囊管 Cystic duct	5 胆囊体部 Body of the gallbladder
3 胆囊頸部 Neck of the gallbladder	6 胆囊底部 Fundus of the gallbladder

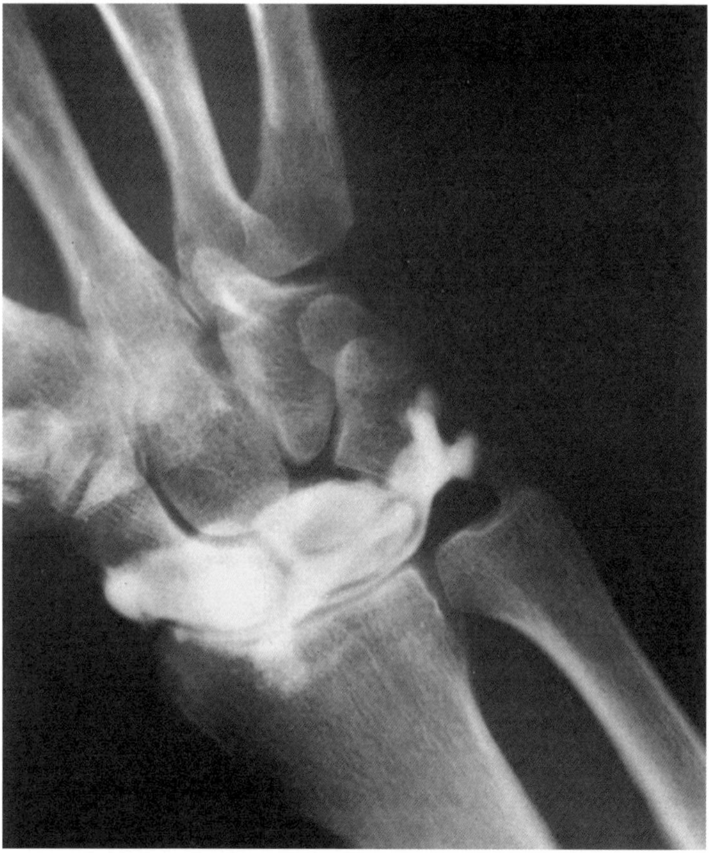

手関節造影　正面（前後）

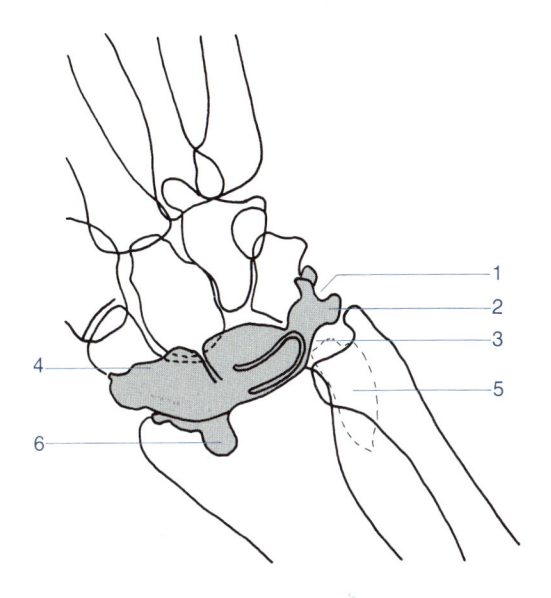

1　半月圧痕　Meniscus
2　尺骨陥凹　Ulnar recess
3　三角線維軟骨　Triangular fibrocartilage
4　背側陥凹　Extensor recess
5　嚢状陥凹　Saccular recess
6　掌側陥凹　Flexor recess

270 関節造影

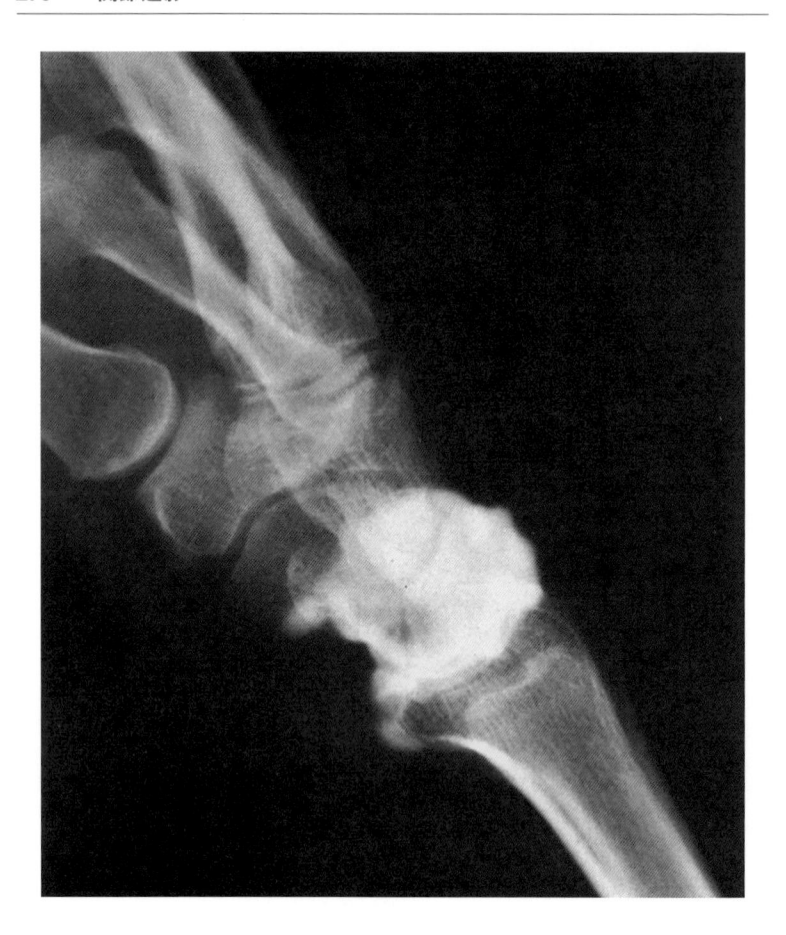

手関節造影 側面

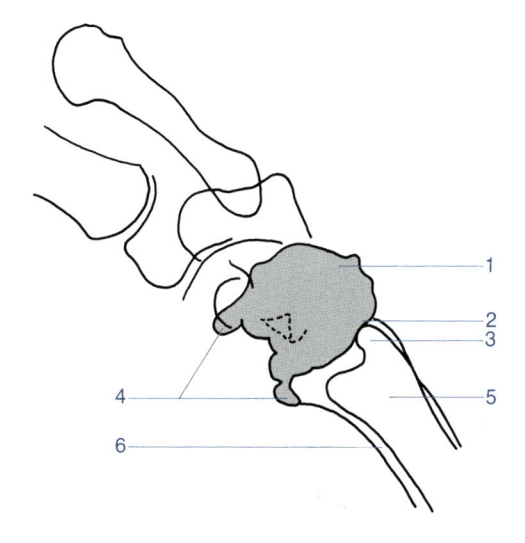

1 背側陥凹 Extensor recess
2 尺骨陥凹 Ulnar recess
3 尺骨茎状突起 Ulnar styloid process
4 掌側陥凹 Flexor recess
5 尺骨 Ulna
6 橈骨 Radius

272 関節造影

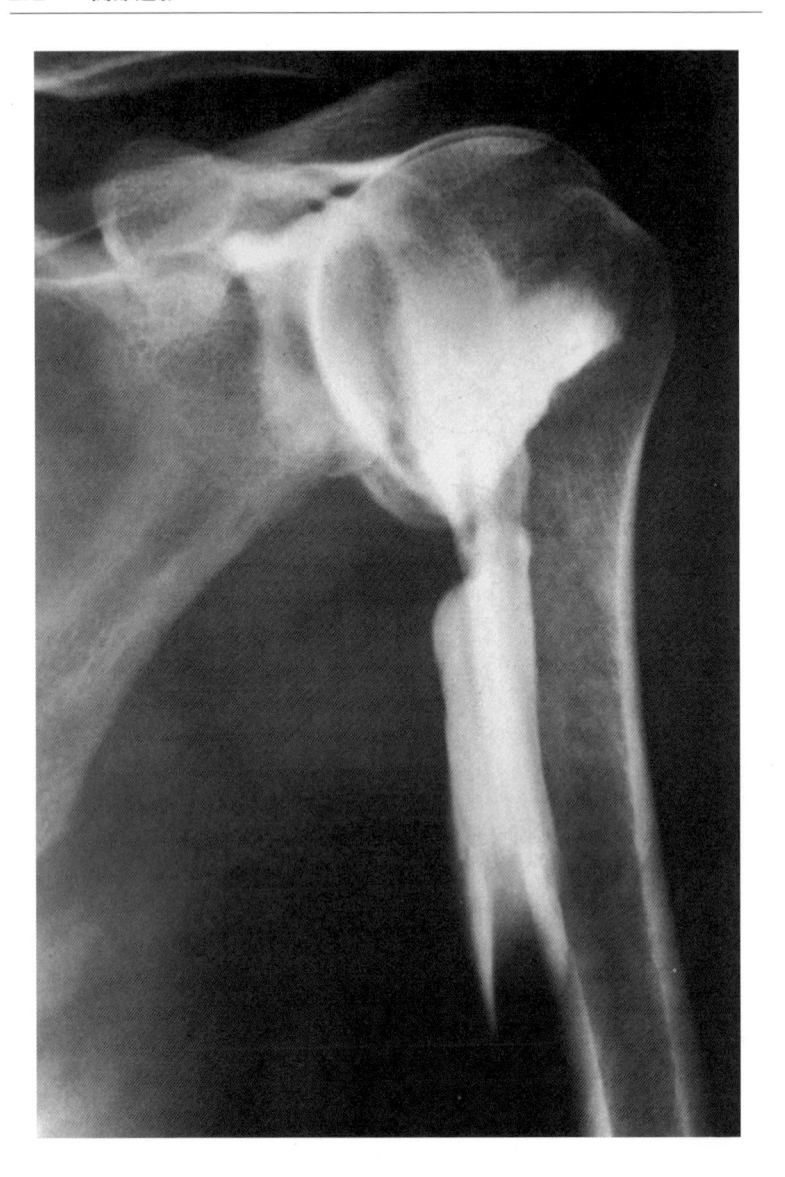

肩関節造影　正面（前後）

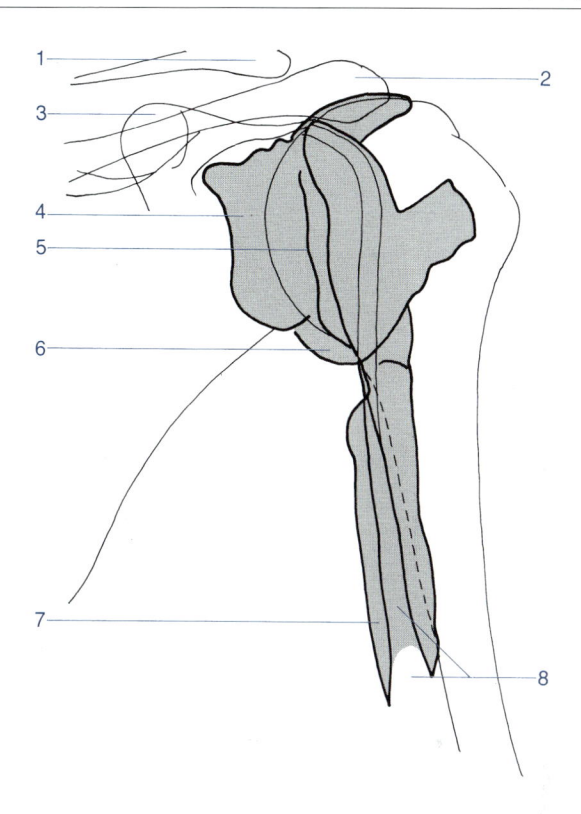

1 鎖骨 Clavicle
2 肩峰 Acromion
3 烏口突起 Coracoid process
4 肩甲下滑液包 Subscapular bursa
5 肩甲骨関節唇 Glenoid labrum
6 腋窩陥凹 Axillary recess
7 結節間腱鞘 Intertubercular sheath
8 上腕二頭筋長頭の腱鞘 Tendon sheath of the long head of the biceps

274 関節造影

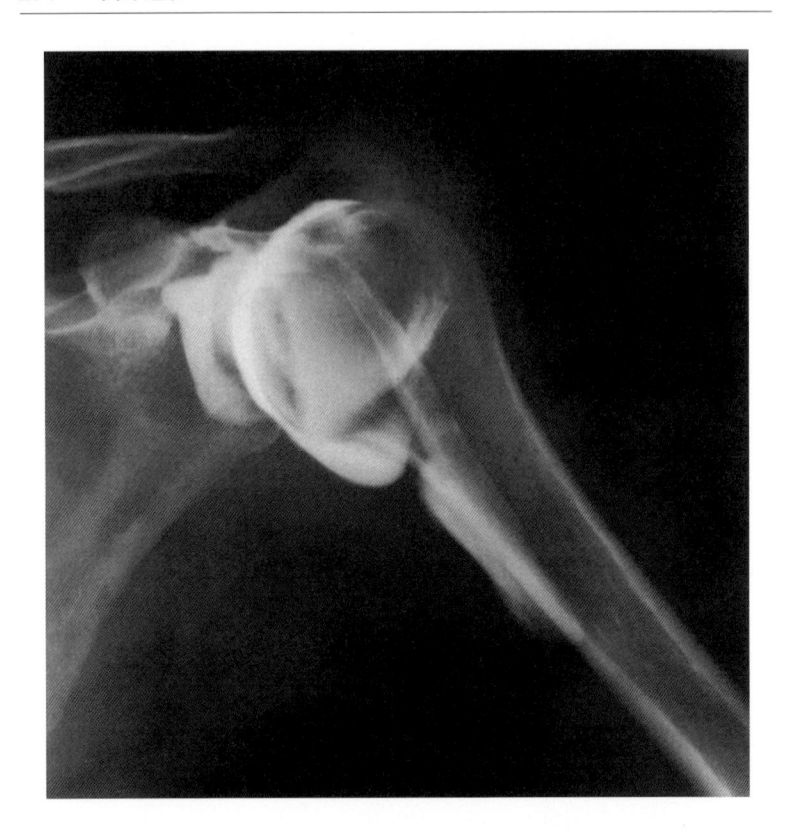

肩関節造影 斜位

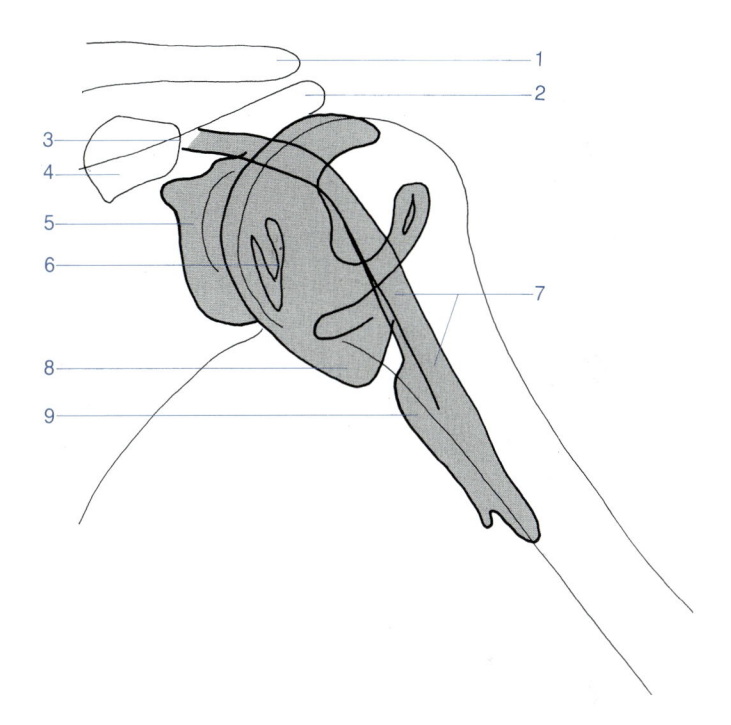

1 鎖骨 Clavicle
2 肩峰 Acromion
3 上腕二頭筋起始部 Insertion of the biceps tendon
4 烏口突起 Coracoid process
5 肩甲下滑液包 Subscapular bursa
6 肩甲骨の関節唇 Glenoid labrum
7 上腕二頭筋長頭の腱鞘 Tendon sheath of the long head of the biceps
8 腋窩陥凹 Axillary recess
9 結節間腱鞘 Intertubercular sheath

関節造影

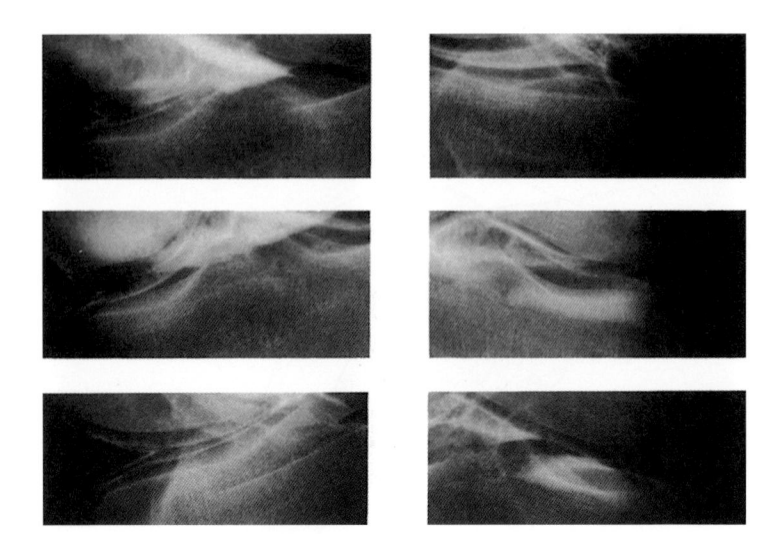

膝関節造影　277

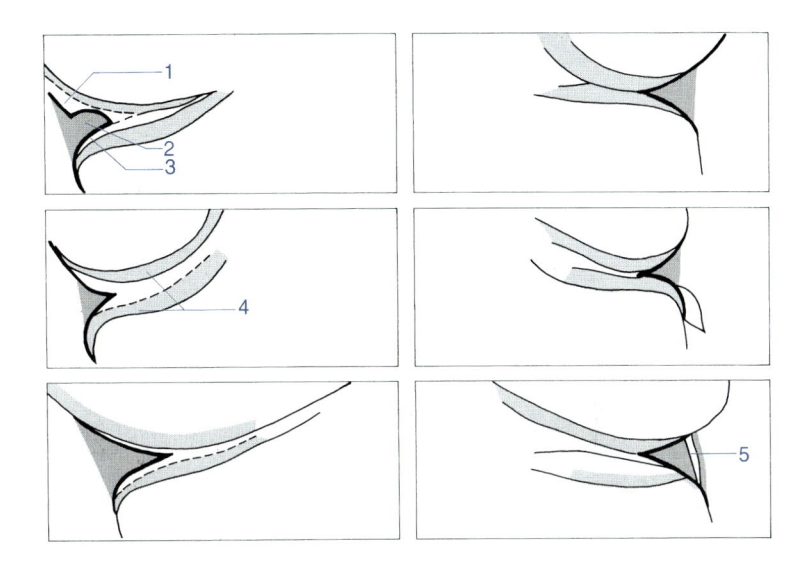

1　上陥凹　Superior capsular recess
2　半月板　Meniscus
3　下陥凹　Inferior capsular recess
4　軟骨　Cartilage
5　膝窩陥凹　Popliteal bursa

関節造影

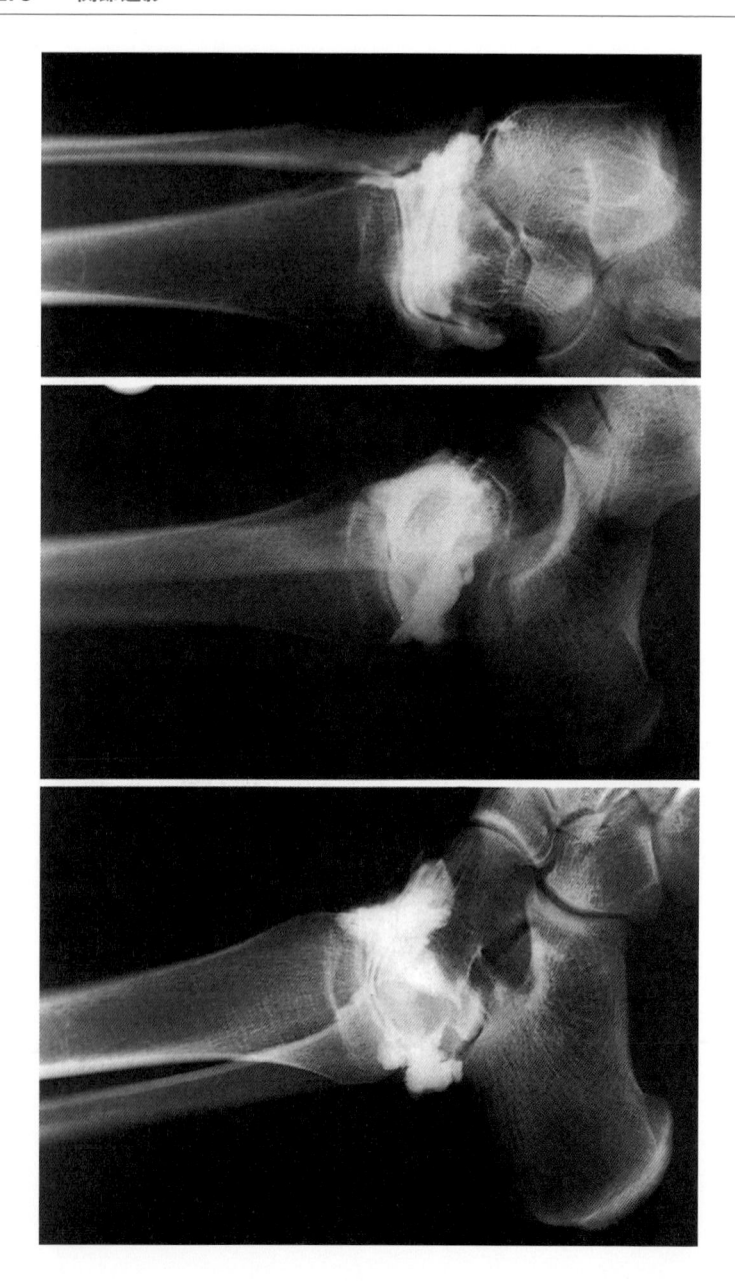

足関節造影 279

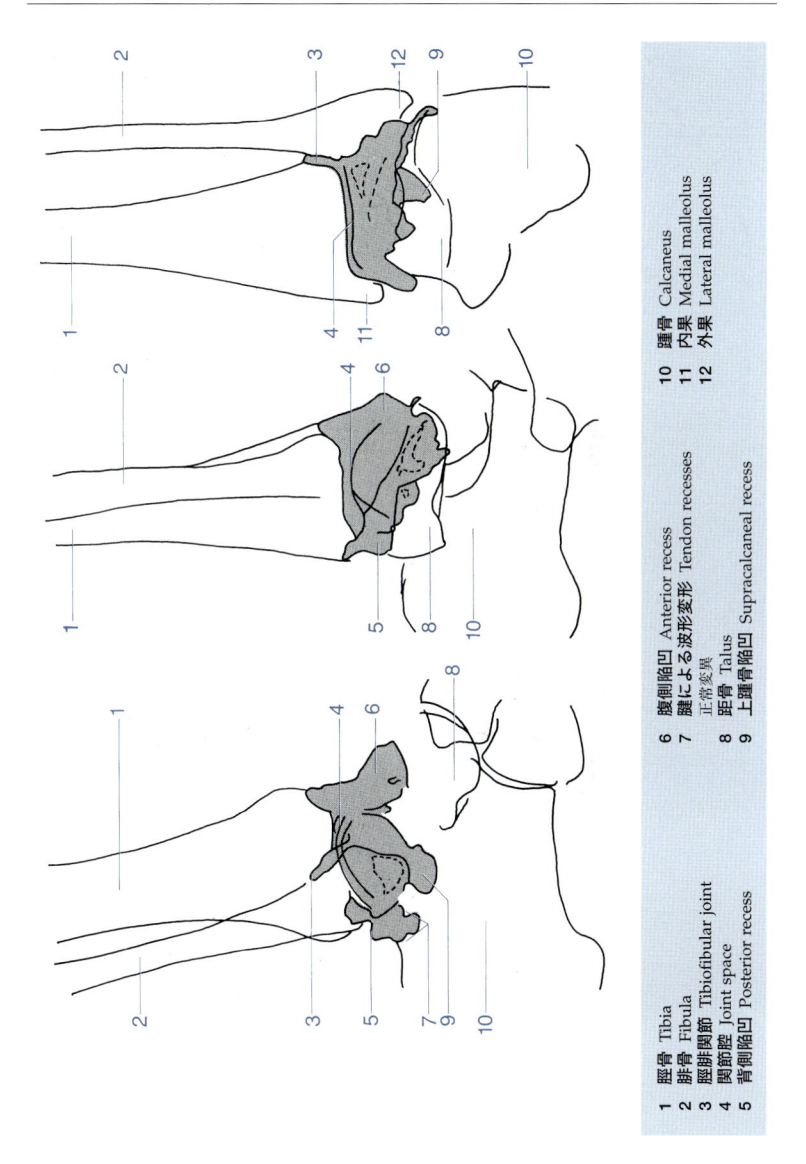

1 脛骨 Tibia
2 腓骨 Fibula
3 脛腓関節 Tibiofibular joint
4 関節腔 Joint space
5 背側陥凹 Posterior recess
6 腹側陥凹 Anterior recess
7 腱による波形変形 Tendon recesses
8 正常変異
9 距骨 Talus
9 上踵骨陥凹 Supracalcaneal recess
10 踵骨 Calcaneus
11 内果 Medial malleolus
12 外果 Lateral malleolus

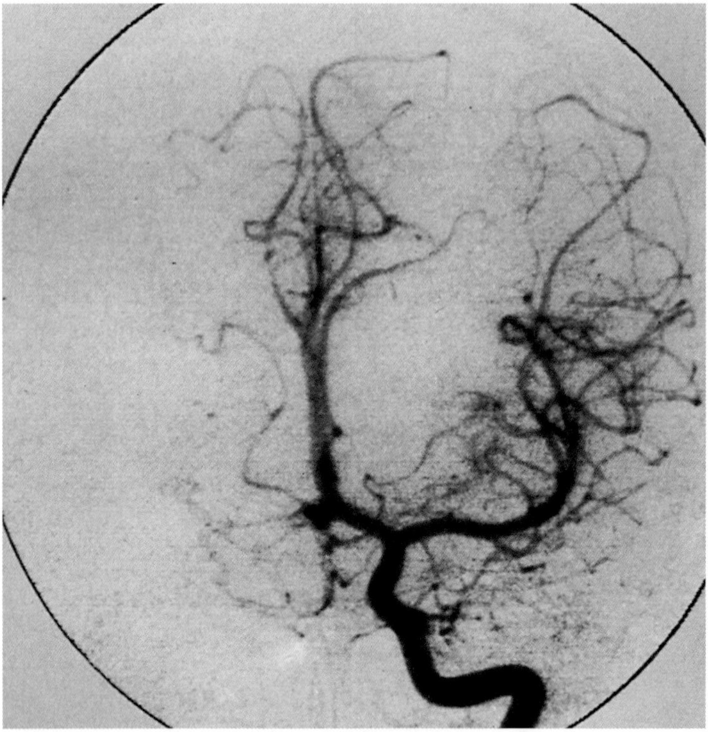

内頸動脈造影　正面（前後）　動脈相　281

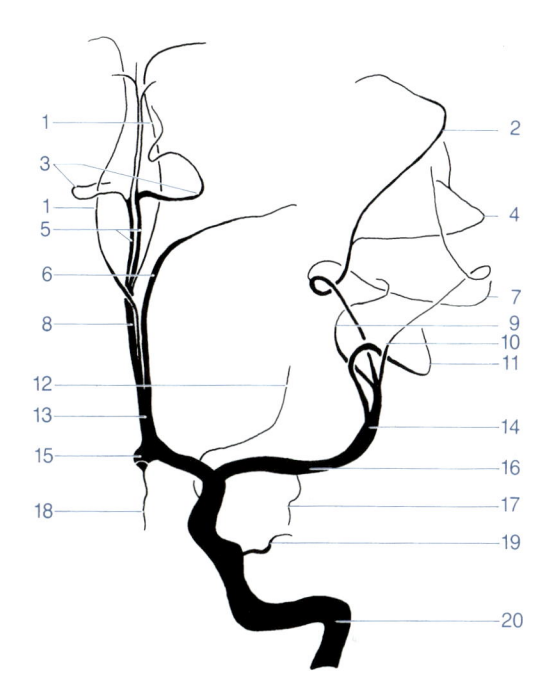

1. 脳梁辺縁動脈　Callosomarginal artery
2. 前頭頂動脈　Anterior parietal artery
3. 脳梁周囲動脈　Pericallosal artery
   口ひげ様に見える
4. 後頭頂動脈　Posterior parietal artery
5. 脳梁周囲動脈　Pericallosal artery
   A4部脳梁より上方
6. 前頭極動脈　Frontopolar artery
7. 前中心溝動脈　Prerolandic artery
8. 前大脳動脈A3部　Third segment of the anterior cerebral artery
   脳梁周囲動脈　Pericallosal artery
9. 角回動脈　Artery of the angular gyrus
10. 後側頭動脈　Posterior temporal artery
11. 前前頭動脈　Prefrontal arteries
12. 前脈絡叢動脈　Anterior choroidal artery
13. 前大脳動脈A2部　Second segment of the anterior cerebral artery
   （脳梁周囲動脈　Pericallosal artery）
14. 中大脳動脈M2部（島部）　Second segment of the middle cerebral artery
15. 前交通動脈　Anterior communicating artery of the cerebrum
   静脈弓により見えない
16. 中大脳動脈M1部　First segment of the middle cerebral artery（蝶形骨部 Sphenoid part）
17. 側頭極動脈　Temporal polar artery
18. 前眼動脈　Fronto orbital artery
19. 眼動脈　Ophthalmic artery
20. 内頸動脈　Internal carotid artery

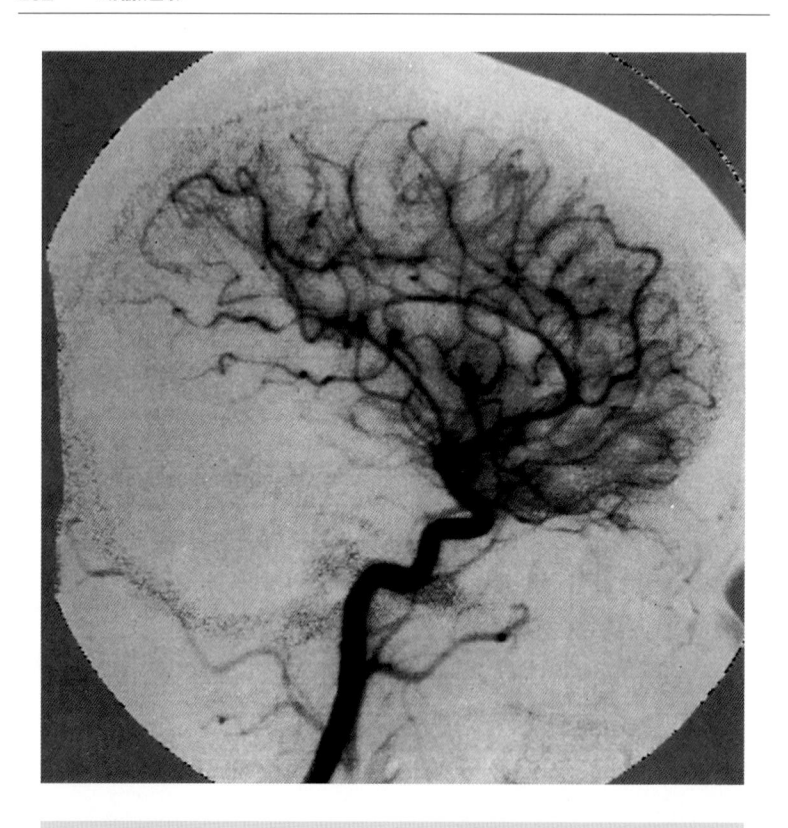

1	内側後前頭動脈 Posterior internal frontal artery	6	内側上頭頂動脈 Superior internal parietal artery
2	前頭頂動脈 Anterior parietal artery	7	内側中前頭動脈 Medial internal frontal artery
3	傍中心動脈 Paracentral artery		
4	後頭頂動脈 Posterior parietal artery	8	内側下頭頂動脈 Inferior internal parietal artery
5	内側前前頭動脈 Anterior internal frontal artery	9	前頭極動脈 Frontal polar artery

内頸動脈造影　側面　動脈相

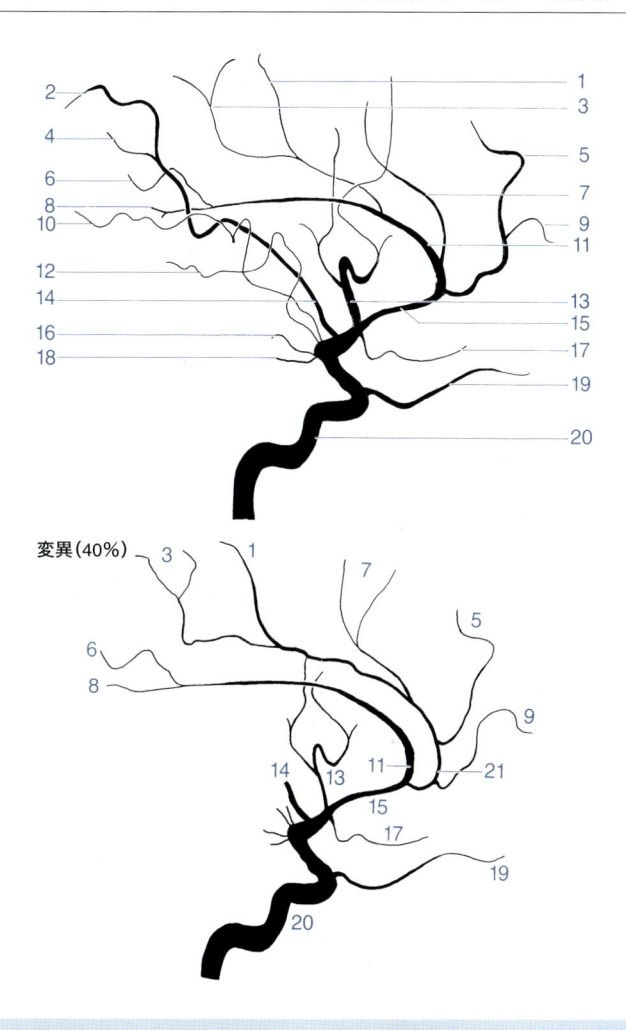

変異(40%)

10	角回動脈 Artery of the angular gyrus
11	脳梁周囲動脈 Pericallosal artery
12	後側頭動脈 Posterior temporal artery
13	前前頭動脈 Prefrontal arteries
14	中大脳動脈M2部 Second segment of the middle cerebral artery
15	前大脳動脈A2部 Second segment of the anterior cerebral artery
16	前脈絡叢動脈 Anterior choroidal artery
17	前眼動脈 Fronto-orbital artery
18	後交通動脈 Posterior communicating artery
19	眼動脈 Ophthalmic artery
20	内頸動脈 Internal carotid artery
21	脳梁辺縁動脈 Callosomarginal artery

動脈造影

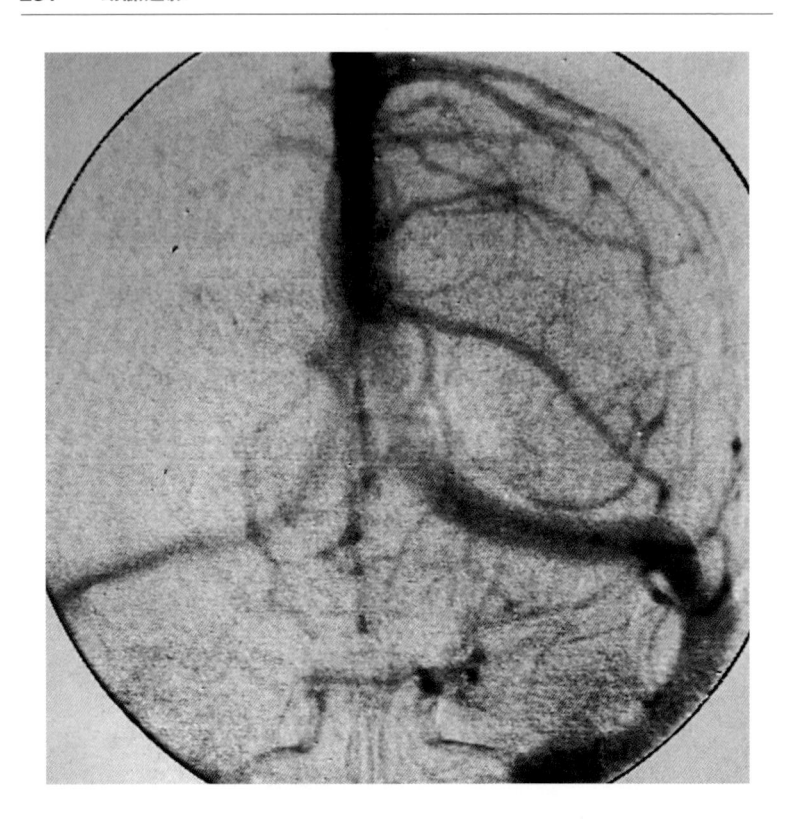

内頸動脈造影　正面（前後）　静脈相　285

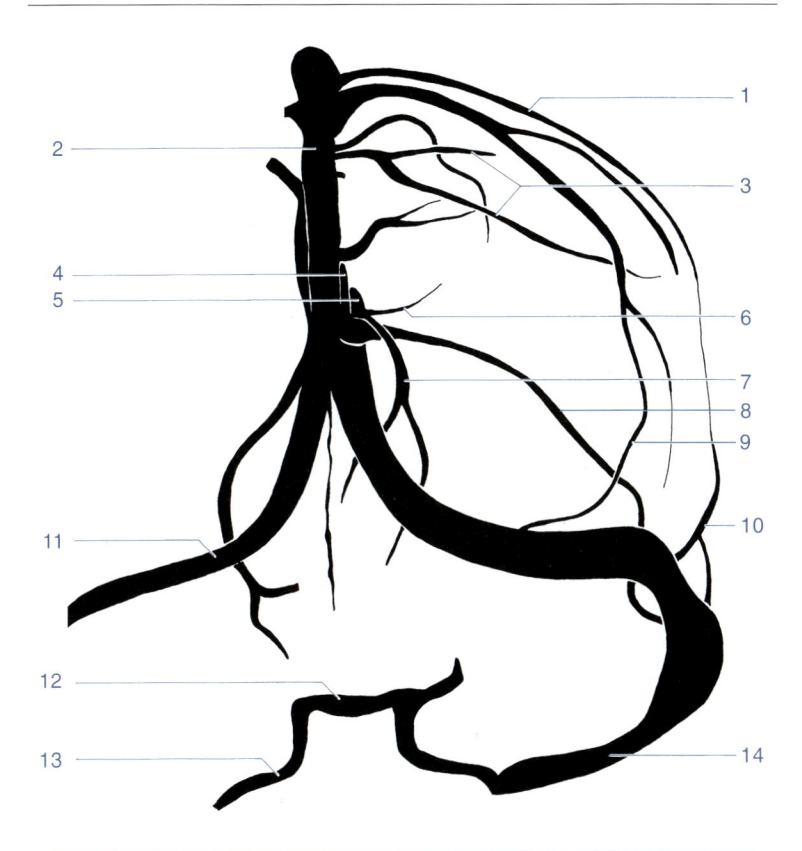

1 頭頂静脈 Parietal vein
2 上矢状静脈洞 Superior sagittal sinus
3 上吻合静脈 Superior anastomotic vein
 （**Trolard静脈** Vein of Trolard）*
4 Galen 大静脈 Great cerebral vein of Galen
5 内大脳静脈 Internal cerebral vein
6 上視床線条体静脈 Superior thalamostriate vein
7 **Rosenthal 脳底静脈** Basal vein of Rosenthal
8 前頭静脈 Frontal vein
9 シルビウス静脈 Veins of the fossa of Sylvius
10 蝶形頭頂静脈洞 Sphenoparietal sinus
11 横静脈洞 Transverse sinus
12 海綿間静脈洞 Intercavernous sinus
13 下錐体静脈洞 Inferior petrosal sinus
14 S状静脈洞 Sigmoid sinus

*訳注
通常はもっと下方まで走行し，側頭葉表面の静脈と吻合する．

動脈造影

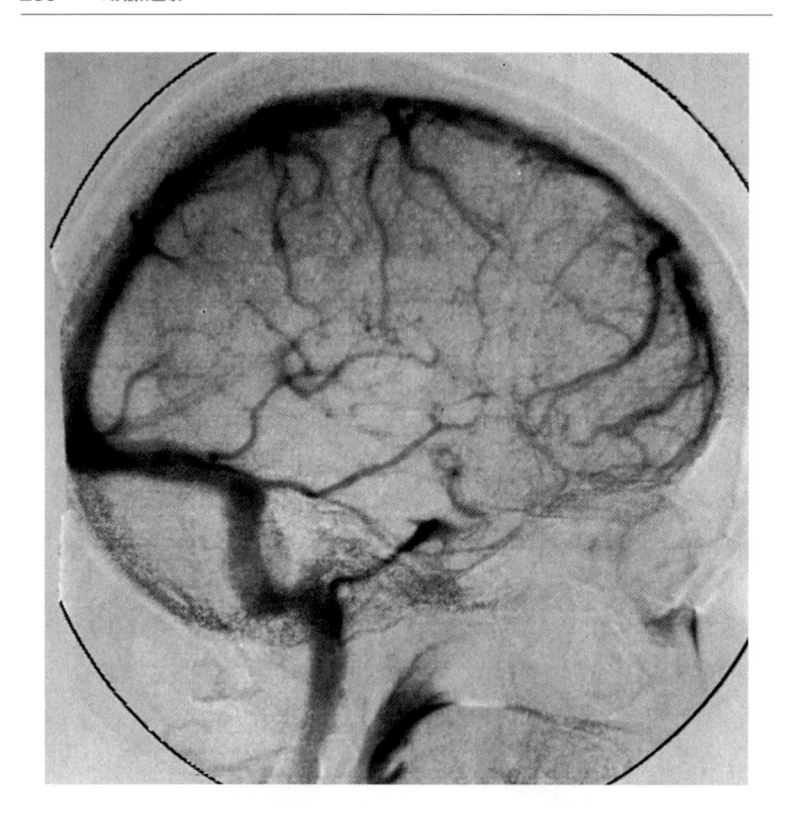

内頸動脈造影 側面 静脈相

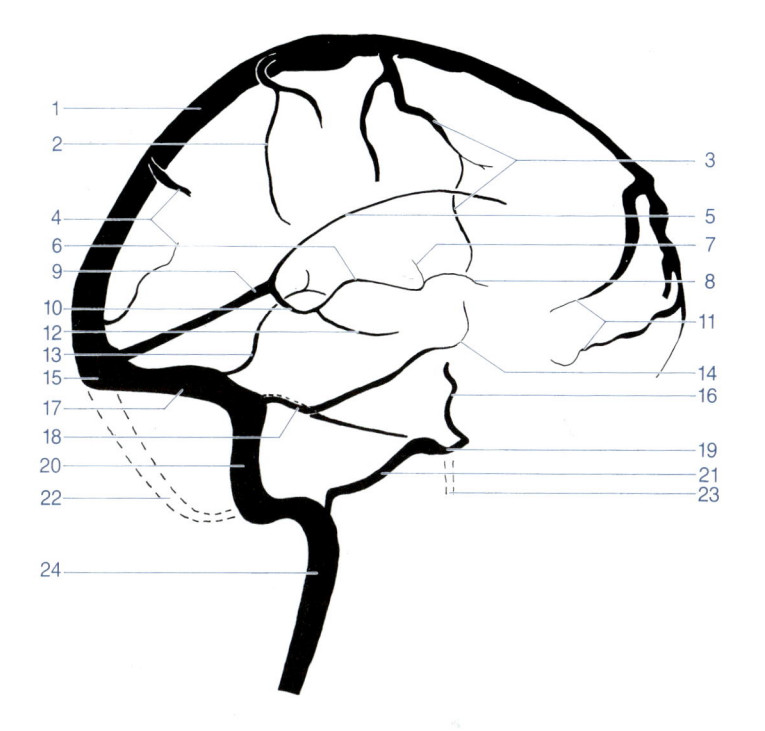

1 上矢状静脈洞 Superior sagittal sinus	13 下吻合静脈 Inferior anastomotic vein (**Labbé**静脈 Vein of Labbé)
2 頭頂静脈 Parietal vein	
3 上吻合静脈 Superior anastomotic vein (**Trolard**静脈 Vein of Trolard)	14 シルビウス静脈 Veins of the fossa of Sylvius
4 後頭静脈 Occipital veins	15 静脈洞交会 Cofluence of sinuses
5 下矢状静脈洞 Inferior sagittal sinus	16 海綿静脈洞 Cavernous sinus
6 内大脳静脈 Internal cerebral vein	前方を還流
7 上視床線条体静脈 Superior thalamostriate veins	17 横静脈洞 Transverse sinus
	18 上錐体静脈洞 Superior petrosal sinus
8 透明中隔静脈 Vein of the septum pellucidum	19 海綿静脈洞 Cavernous sinus
	後方を還流
9 直静脈洞 Straight sinus	20 S状静脈洞 Sigmoid sinus
10 Galen大静脈 Great cerebral vein of Galen	21 下錐体静脈洞 Inferior petrosal sinus
11 上行前頭静脈 Ascending frontal veins	22 後頭静脈洞 Occipital sinus
12 Rosenthal脳底静脈 Basal vein of Rosenthal	23 翼突筋静脈叢 Pterygoid plexus
	24 内頸静脈 Internal jugular vein

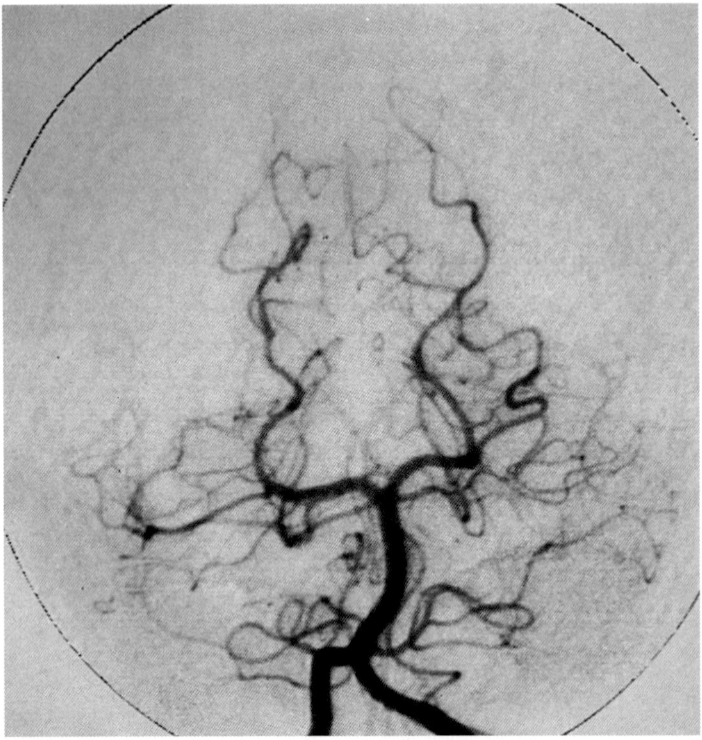

椎骨動脈造影　正面（前後）　動脈相　289

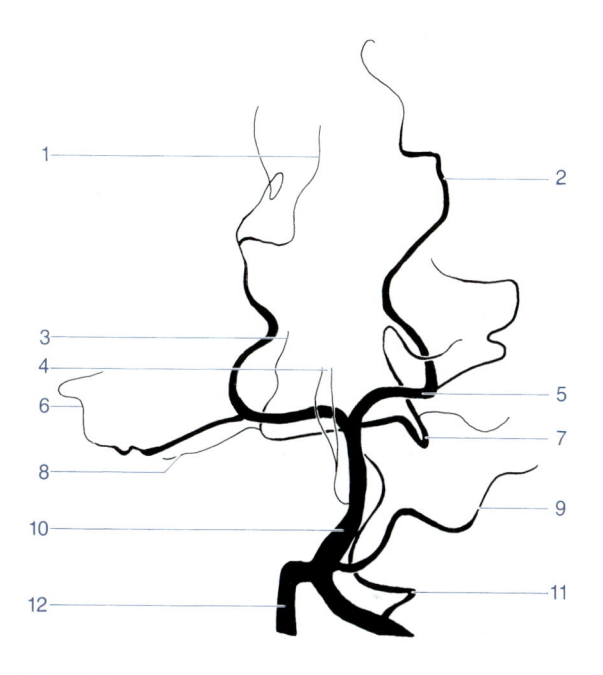

1　内側後頭動脈の鳥距動脈 Calcarine branch of the medial occipital artery	8　辺縁動脈 Marginal artery
2　頭頂後頭動脈 Parieto-occipital artery	9　前下小脳動脈 Anterior inferior cerebellar artery
3　虫部枝 Vermian branch	10　脳底動脈 Basilar artery
4　視床穿通動脈 Thalmoperforate arteries	11　後下小脳動脈 Posterior inferior cerebellar artery
5　後大脳動脈 Posterior cerebral artery	12　椎骨動脈 Vertebral artery
6　側頭後頭動脈 Temporo-occipital artery	
7　上小脳動脈 Superior cerebellar artery	

動脈造影

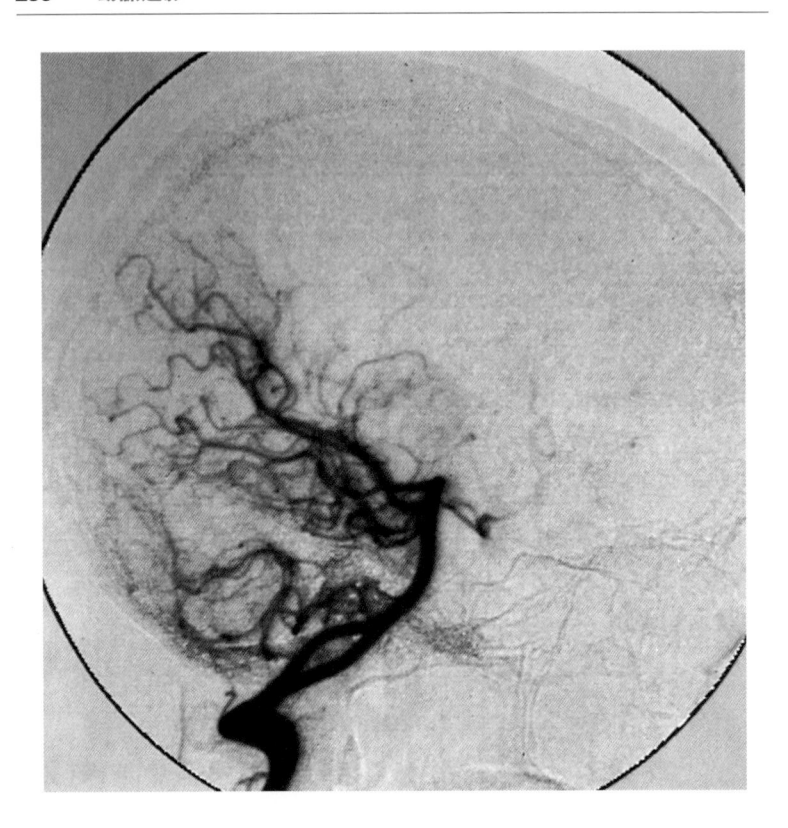

椎骨動脈造影　側面　動脈相

1　頭頂後頭動脈 Parieto-occipital artery	8　後交通動脈 Posterior communicating artery
2　後脳梁枝 Posterior corpus callosal branch	9　上小脳動脈 Superior cerebellar artery
3　内側後頭動脈の鳥距動脈 Calcarine branch of the medical occipital artery	10　脳底動脈 Basilar artery
4　後, 内側, 外側, 脈絡叢動脈 Choroidal arteries (posterior, medial, and lateral)	11　前下小脳動脈 Anterior inferior cerebellar artery
5　側頭後頭動脈 Temporo-occipital artery	12　後下小脳動脈 Posterior inferior cerebellar artery
6　後大脳動脈 Posterior cerebral artery	13　椎骨動脈 Vertebral arteries
7　後大脳動脈視床枝 Branches of the posterior cerebral artery to the thalamus	

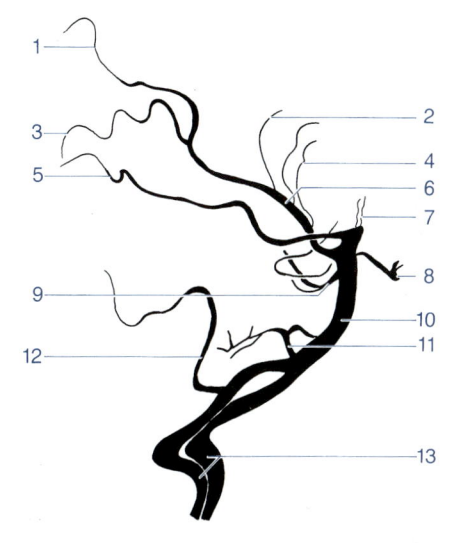

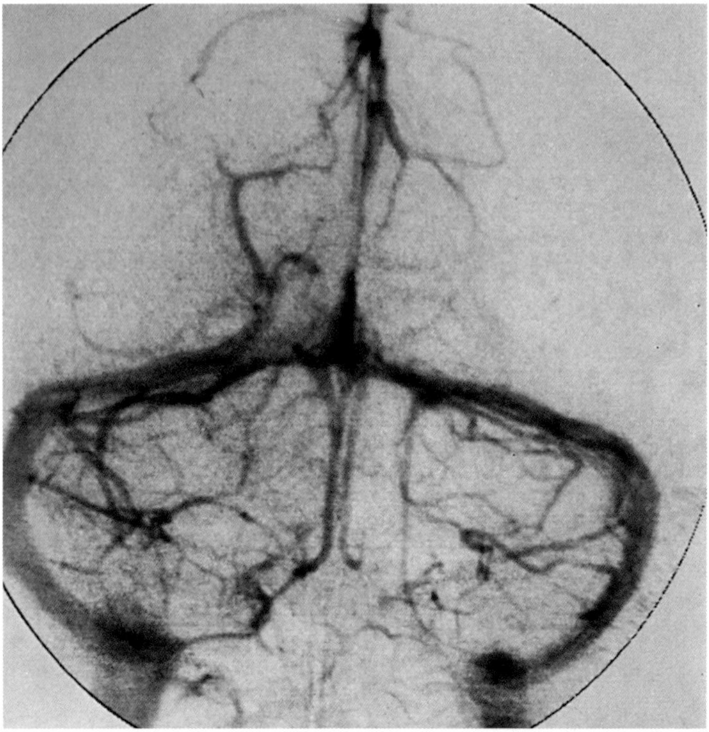

椎骨動脈造影　正面（前後）　静脈相　293

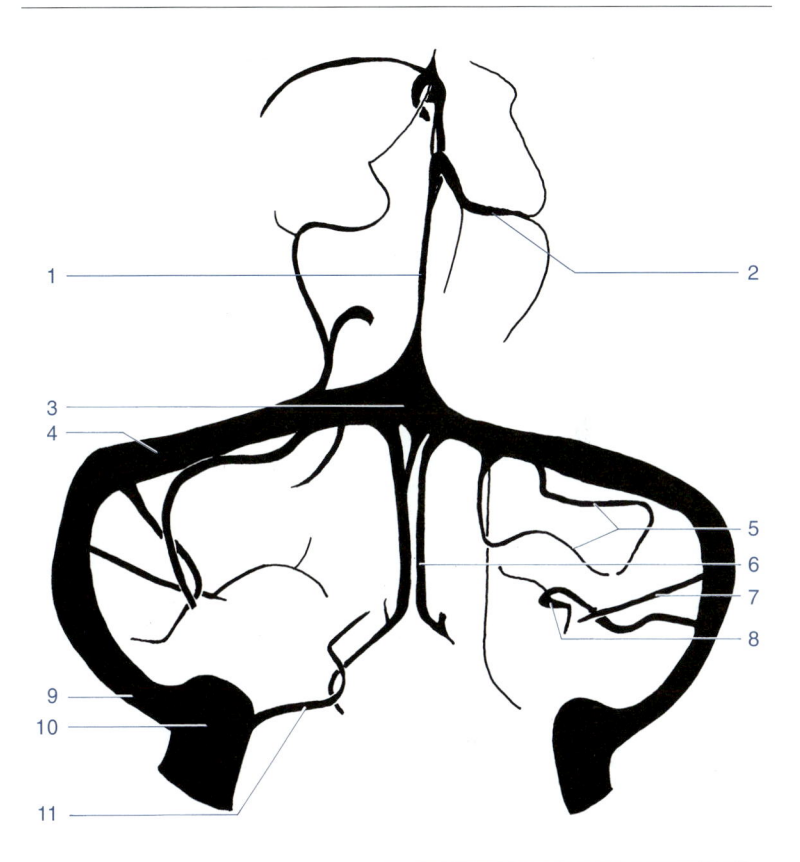

1	直静脈洞 Straight sinus
2	上大脳静脈 Superior cerebral veins
3	静脈洞交会 Confluence of sinuses
4	横静脈洞 Transverse sinus
5	小脳半球静脈 Veins of the cerebellar hemisphere
6	下虫部静脈 Inferior vein of the vermis
7	下小脳半球静脈 Inferior vein of the cerebellar hemisphere
8	錐体静脈 Petrosal vein 上錐体静脈洞に合流
9	S状静脈洞 Sigmoid sinus
10	頸静脈球 Bulb of the jugular vein
11	下錐体静脈洞 Inferior petrosal sinus

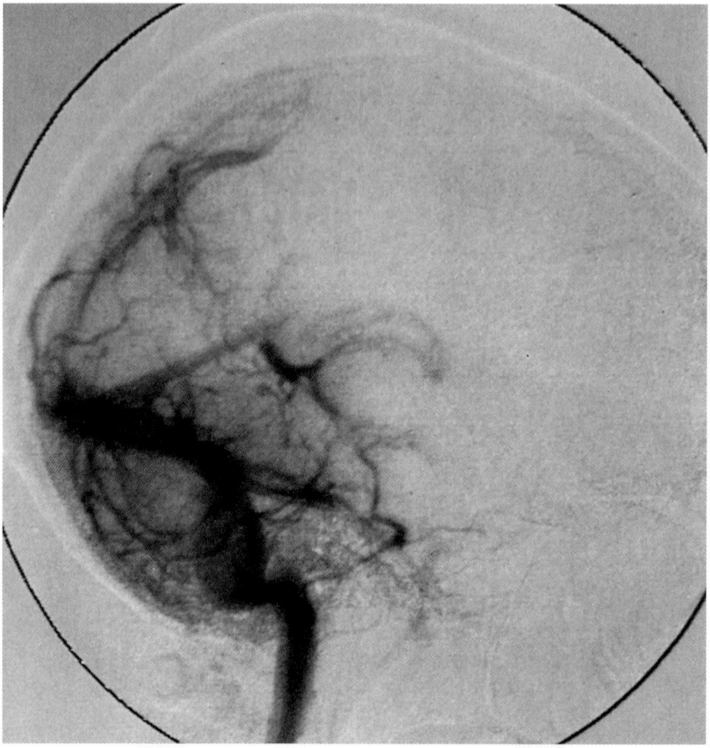

椎骨動脈造影　側面　静脈相　**295**

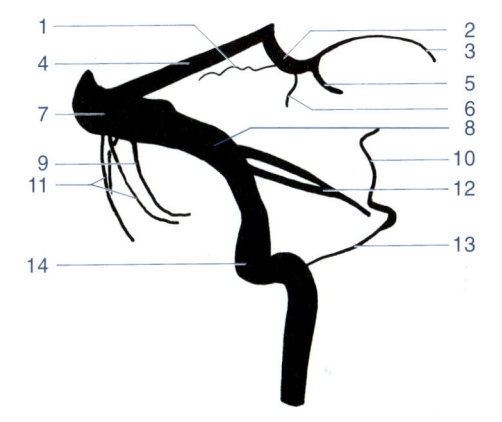

1　上小脳半球静脈 Superior veins of the cerebellar hemisphere	9　下小脳半球静脈 Inferior veins of the cerebellar hemisphere
2　Galen大静脈 Great cerebral vein of Galen	10　海綿静脈洞 Cavernous sinus
3　内大脳静脈 Internal cerebral vein	11　下小脳半球静脈 Inferior veins of the cerebellar hemisphere
4　直静脈洞 Straight sinus	12　上錐体静脈洞 Superior petrosal sinus
5　Rosenthal脳底静脈 Basal vein of Rosenthal	13　下錐体静脈洞 Inferior petrosal sinus
6　前中心小脳静脈 Precentral cerebellar vein	14　S状静脈洞 Sigmoid sinus
7　静脈洞交会 Confluence of sinuses	
8　横静脈洞 Transverse sinus	

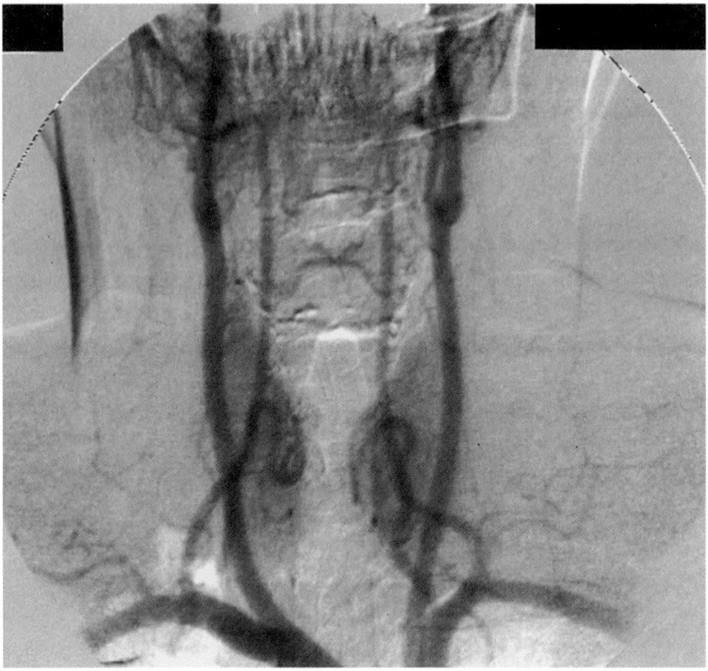

頸部動脈造影　正面(前後)

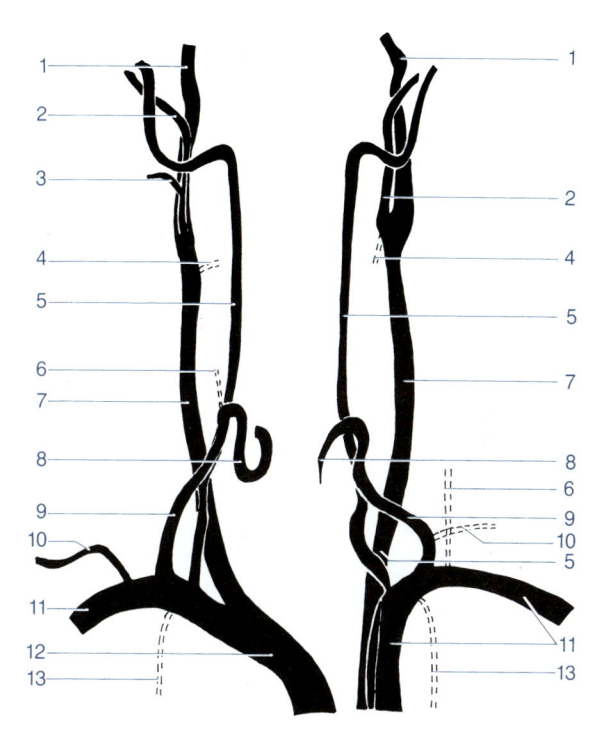

1　内頸動脈 Internal carotid artery	8　下甲状腺動脈 Inferior thyroid artery
2　外頸動脈 External carotid artery	9　甲状頸動脈 Thyrocervical trunk
3　顔面動脈 Facial artery	10　肩甲上動脈 Suprascapular artery
4　上甲状腺動脈 Superior thyroid artery	11　鎖骨下動脈 Subclavian artery
5　椎骨動脈 Vertebral artery	12　腕頭動脈 Brachiocephalic trunk
6　上行頸動脈 Ascending cervical artery	13　内胸動脈 Internal thoracic artery
7　総頸動脈 Common carotid artery	

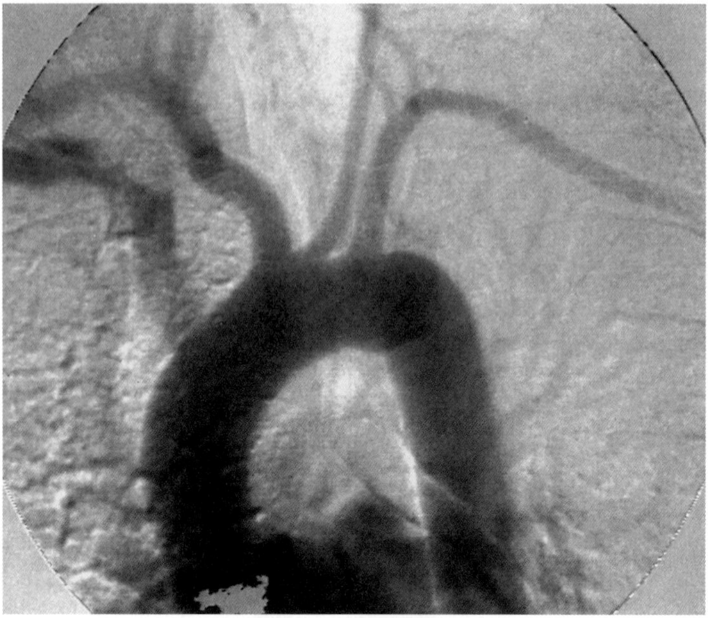

大動脈造影　正面（前後） **299**

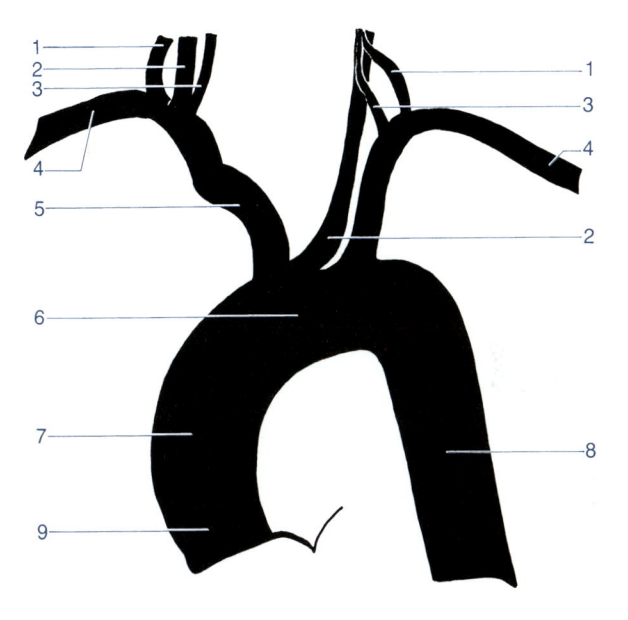

1	甲状頸動脈 Thyrocervical trunk	6	大動脈弓 Aortic arch
2	総頸動脈 Common carotid artery	7	上行大動脈 Ascending aorta
3	椎骨動脈 Vertebral artery	8	下行大動脈 Descending aorta
4	鎖骨下動脈 Subclavian artery	9	大動脈根部 Aortic root
5	腕頭動脈 Brachiocephalic trunk		

動脈造影

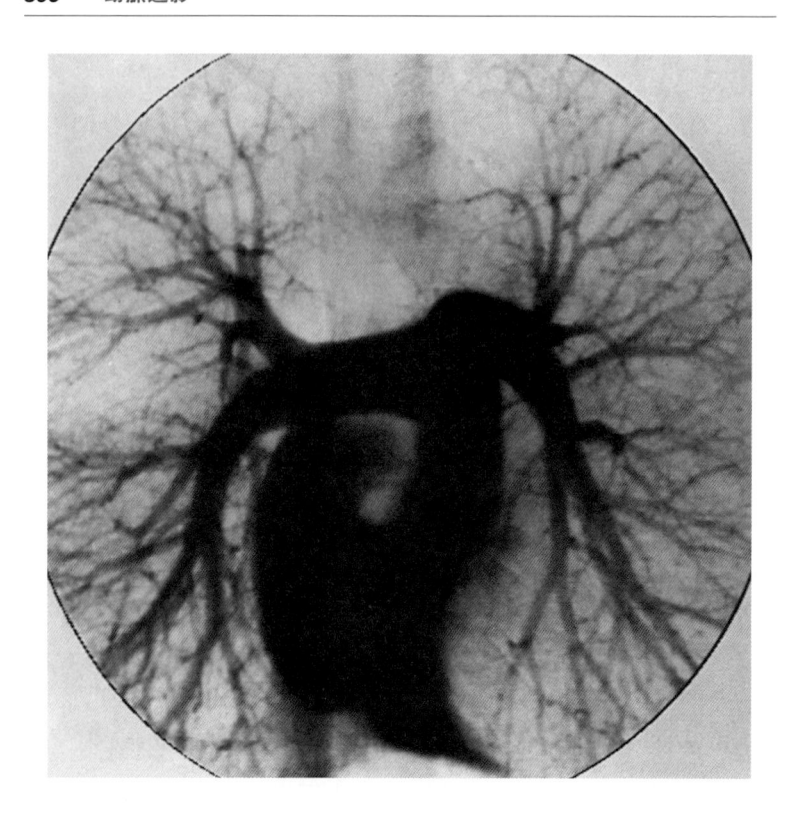

肺動脈造影　動脈相

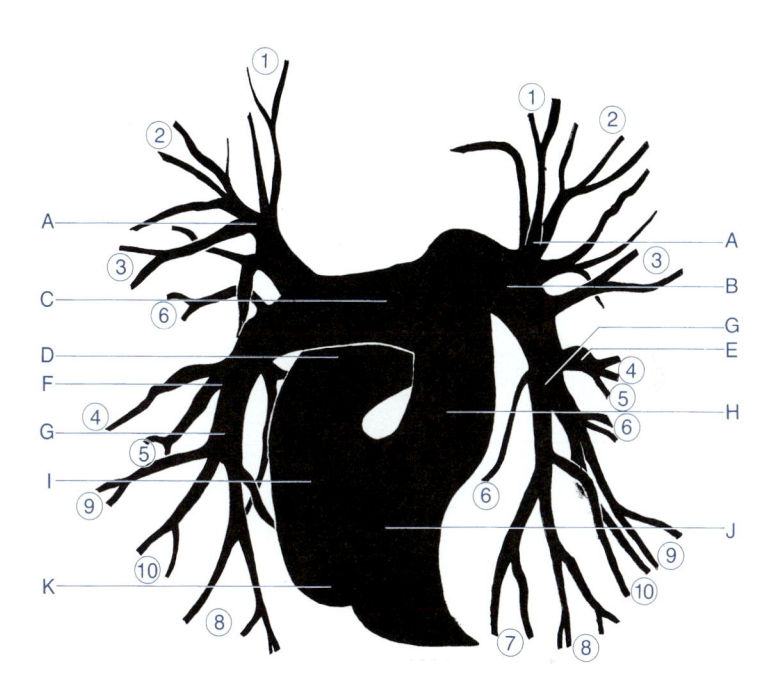

○＝区域動脈1〜10

- A　肺尖枝　Apical branch
- B　左肺動脈　Left pulmonary artery
- C　右肺動脈　Right pulmonary artery
- D　上大静脈　Superior vena cava
- E　肺舌動脈　Lingular artery
- F　肺動脈中葉枝　Middle lobe branch of the pulmonary artery
- G　肺動脈下葉枝　Inferior lober branch of the pulmonary artery
- H　肺動脈幹　Pulmonary trunk
- I　右心房　Right atrium
- J　右心室　Right ventricle
- K　下大静脈　Inferior vena cava

302 動脈造影

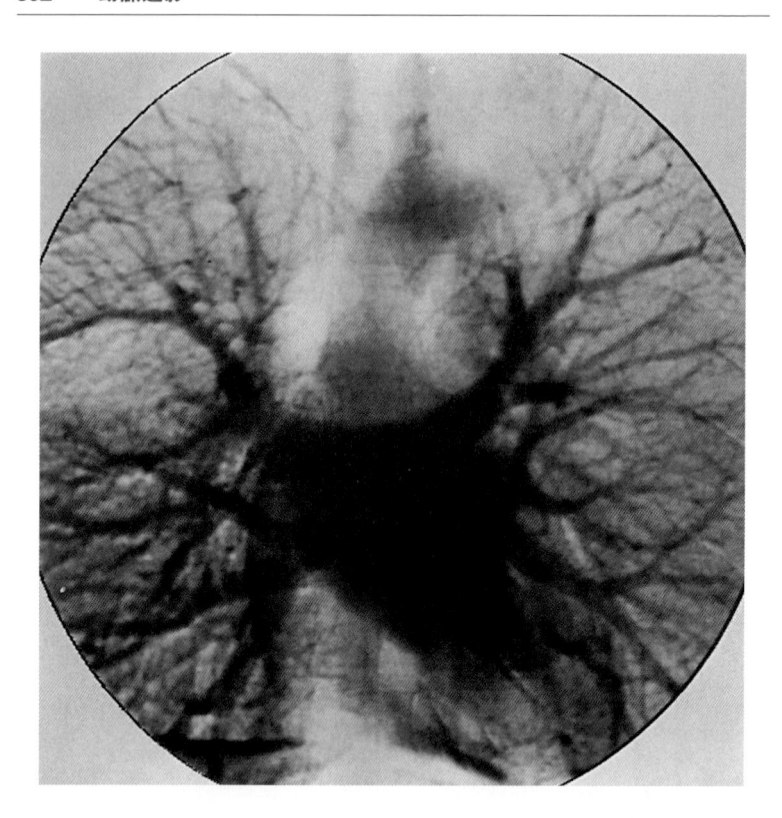

肺動脈造影　正面（前後）　静脈相

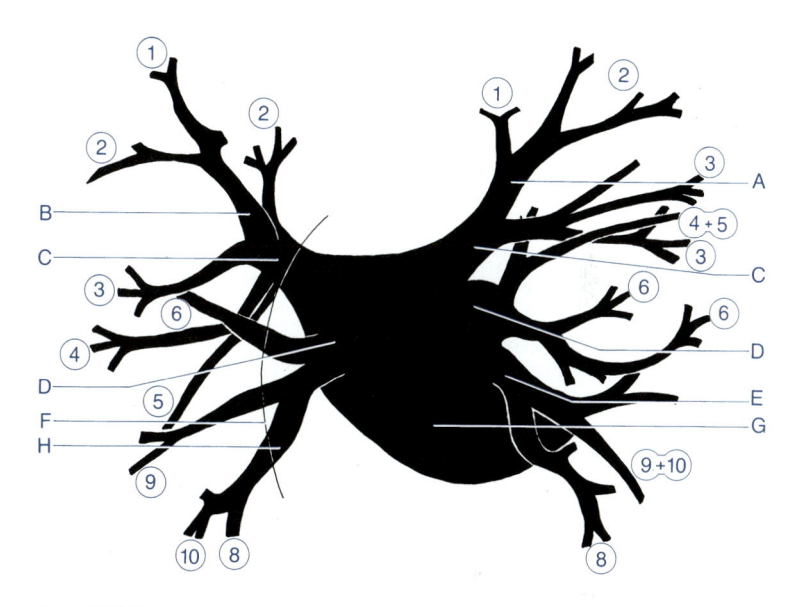

○＝区域動脈1〜10

A　左肺静脈の肺尖後枝 Apicoposterior branch of left superior pulmonary vein	D　下肺静脈 Inferior pulmonary veins
B　右上肺静脈の肺尖枝 Apical branch of right superior pulmonary vein	E　左下葉静脈 Left lower lobe vein
	F　右心房 Right atrium
C　上肺静脈 Superior pulmonary veins	G　左心房 Left atrium
	H　右下葉静脈 Right lower lobe vein

304　動脈造影

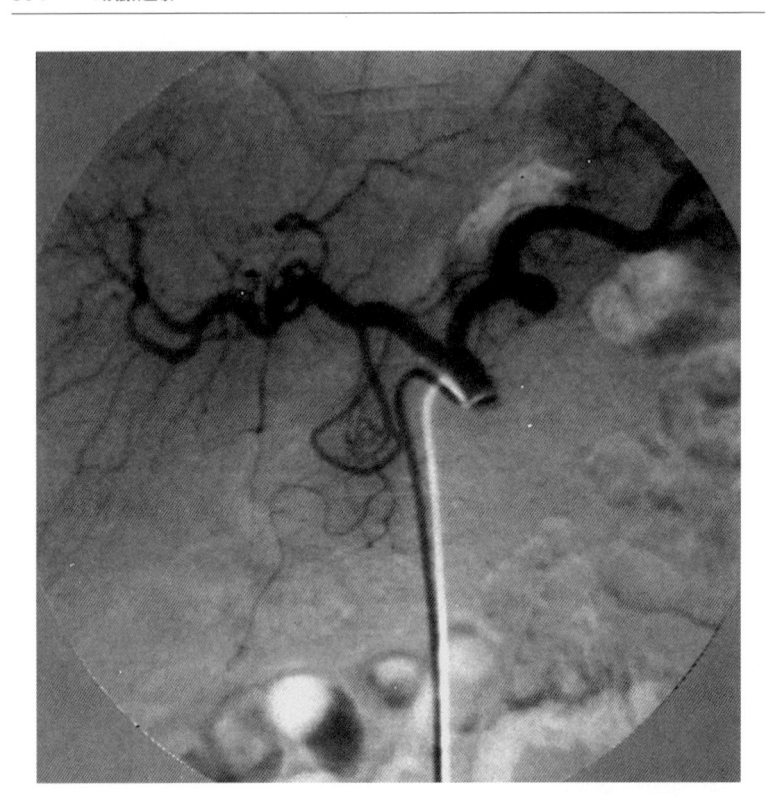

腹腔動脈幹造影　動脈相　305

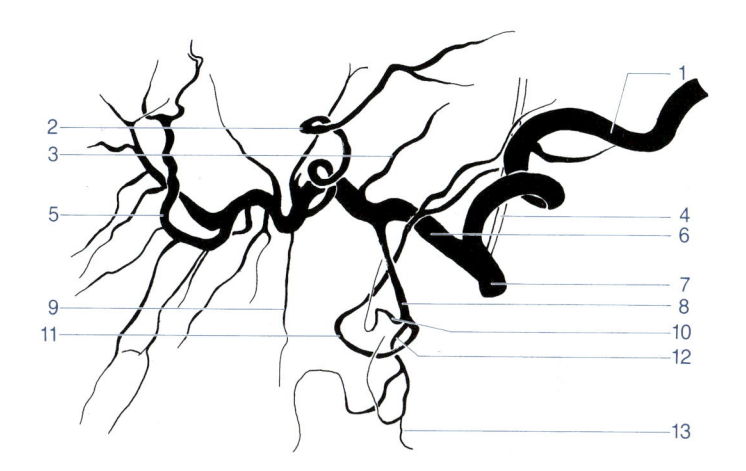

1 脾動脈 Splenic artery
2 左肝動脈 Left branch of the proper hepatic artery
3 右胃動脈 Right gastric artery
4 左胃動脈 Left gastric artery
5 右肝動脈 Right branch of the proper hepatic artery
6 総肝動脈 Common hepatic artery
7 腹腔動脈 Celiac trunk
8 胃十二指腸動脈 Gastroduodenal artery
9 胆嚢動脈 Cystic artery
10 上十二指腸上動脈 Superior supraduodenal artery
11 右胃大網動脈 Right gastroepiploic artery
12 上膵十二指腸動脈 Superior pancreaticoduodenal artery
13 下膵十二指腸動脈 Inferior pancreaticoduodenal artery
　　上腸間膜動脈と交通

動脈造影

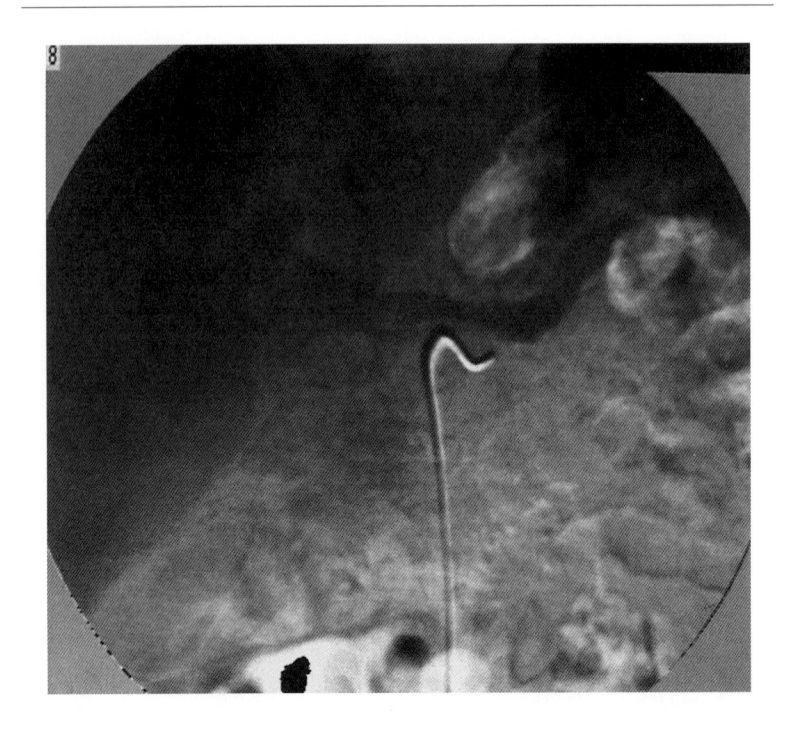

腹腔動脈幹造影 静脈相 **307**

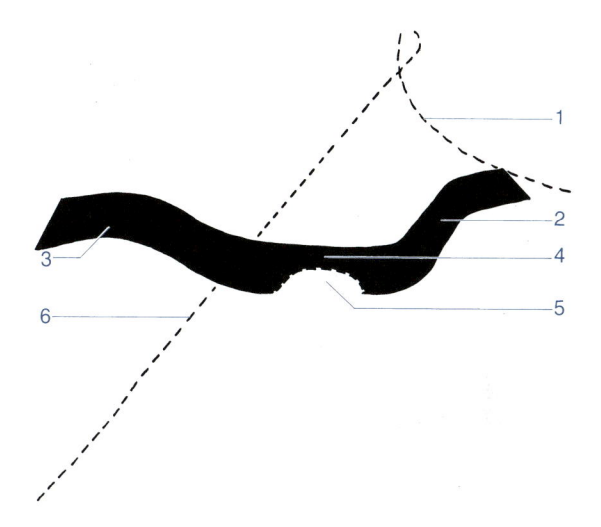

1 脾臓 Spleen
2 脾静脈 Splenic vein
3 門脈 Portal vein
4 合流部 Confluence
5 腸間膜静脈合流部の洗い流し
 Wash-out at the junction of the mesenteric vein
6 肝臓 Liver

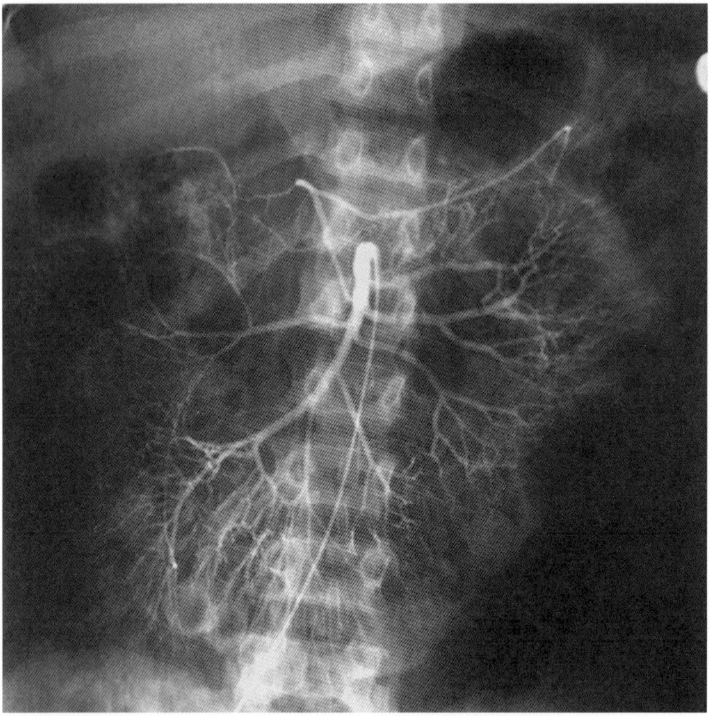

上腸間膜動脈造影　動脈相

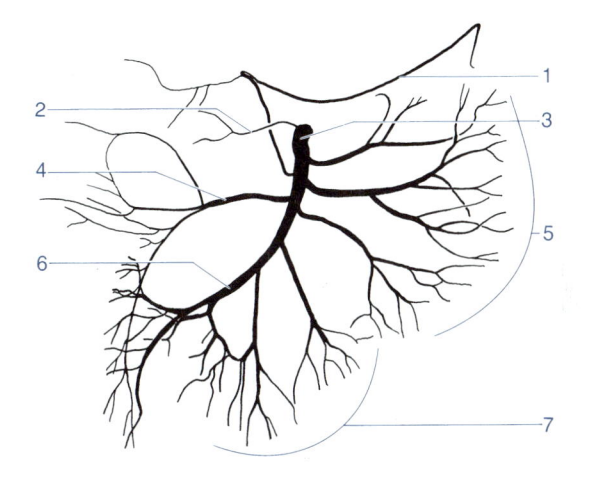

1　中結腸動脈　Middle colic artery
2　下膵十二指腸動脈　Inferior pancreaticoduodenal artery
3　上腸間膜動脈　Superior mesenteric artery
4　右結腸動脈　Right colic artery
5　空腸動脈　Jejunal arteries
6　回結腸動脈　Ileocolic artery
7　回腸動脈　Ileal arteries

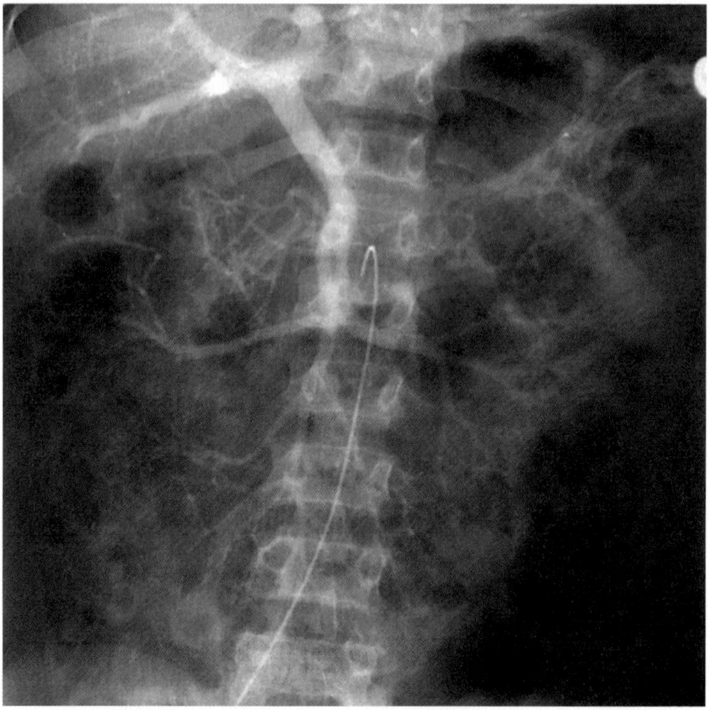

上腸間膜動脈造影　静脈相　*311*

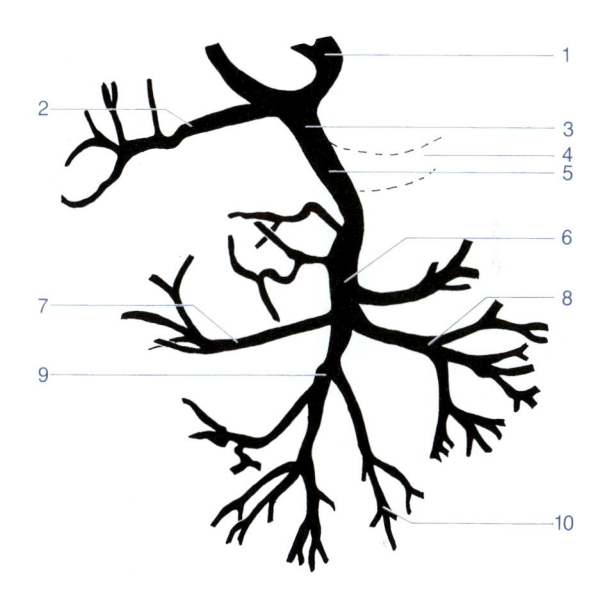

1　門脈左枝 Left branch of the portal vein	6　上腸間膜静脈 Superior mesenteric vein
2　門脈右枝 Right branch of the portal vein	7　右結腸静脈 Right colic vein
3　門脈 Portal vein	8　空腸静脈 Jejunal veins
4　脾静脈 Splenic vein	9　回結腸静脈 Ileocolic vein
5　合流部 Confluence	10　回腸静脈 Ileal veins

312　動脈造影

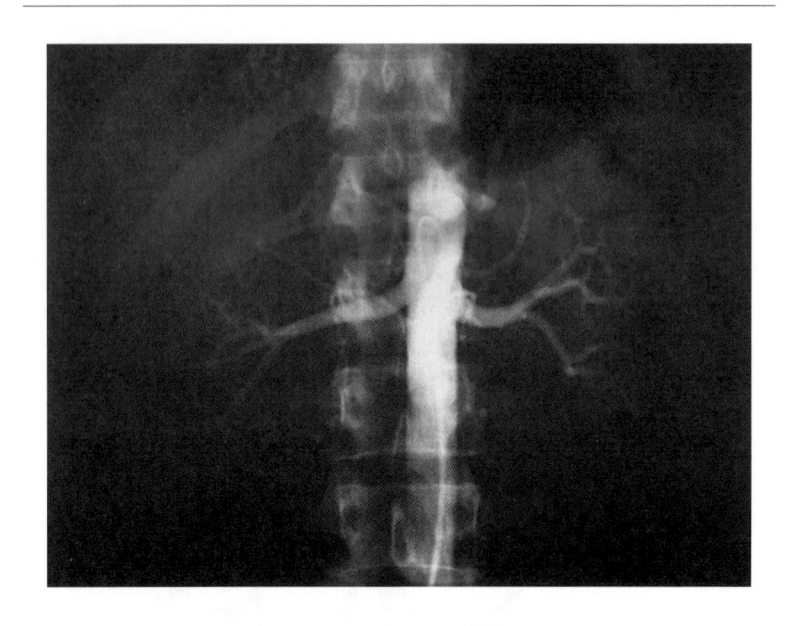

腎動脈造影　動脈相

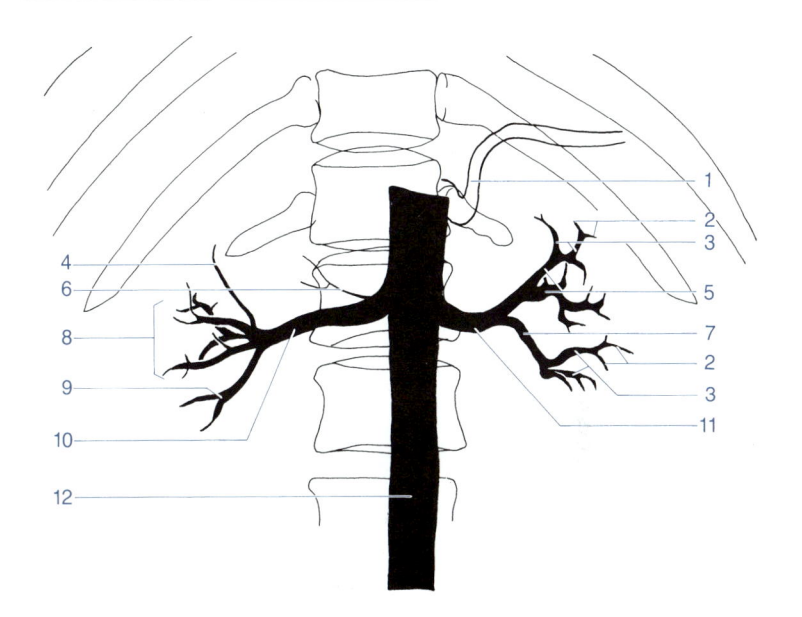

1	脾動脈 Splenic artery	7	区域動脈 Segmental arteries (後枝 Posterior branch)
2	弓状動脈 Arcuate arteries	8	中区動脈 Middle segmental artery
3	葉間動脈 Interlobular arteries	9	下区動脈 Inferior segmental artery
4	上区動脈 Superior segmental artery	10	右腎動脈 Right renal artery
5	区域動脈 Segmental arteries (前枝 Anterior branch)	11	左腎動脈 Left renal artery
6	下副腎動脈 Inferior adrenal artery	12	腹大動脈 Abdominal aorta

314 動脈造影

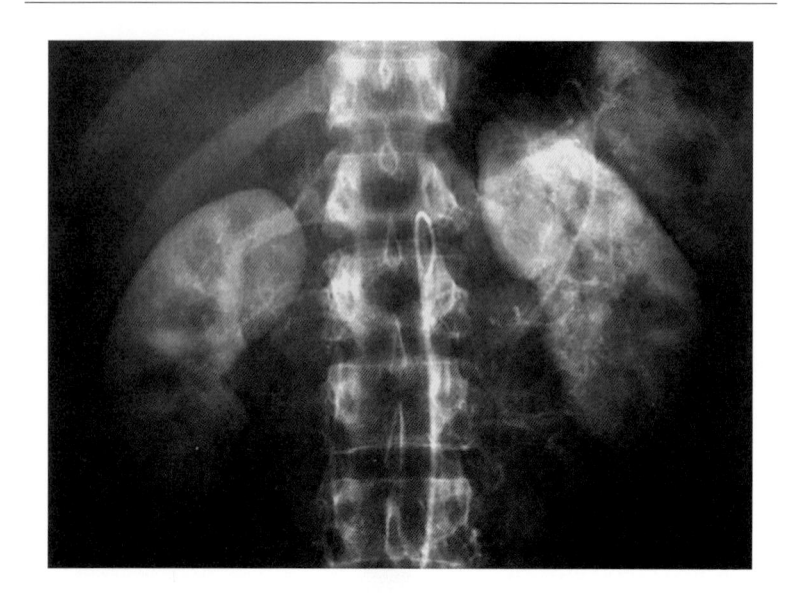

腎動脈造影　静脈相

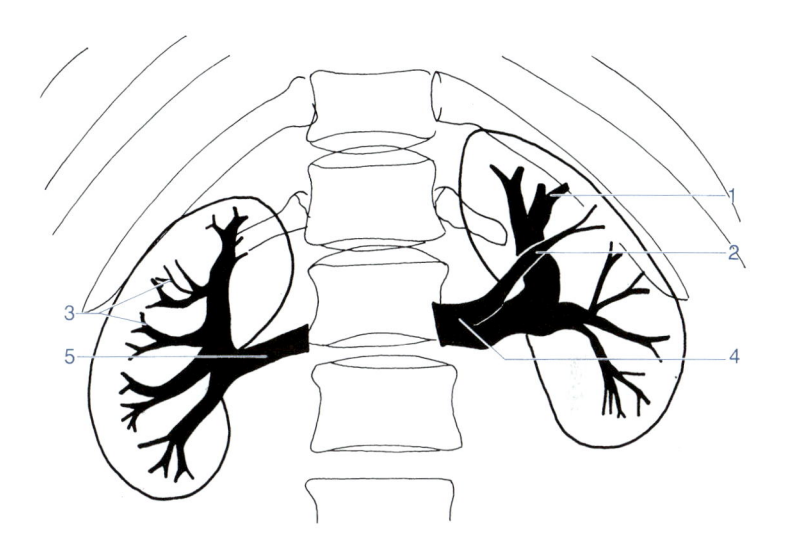

1　葉間静脈 Interlobular vein	3　弓状静脈 Arcuate vein
2　腎静脈上枝 Superior branch of the renal vein	4　左腎静脈 Left renal vein
	5　右腎静脈 Right renal vein

316　動脈造影

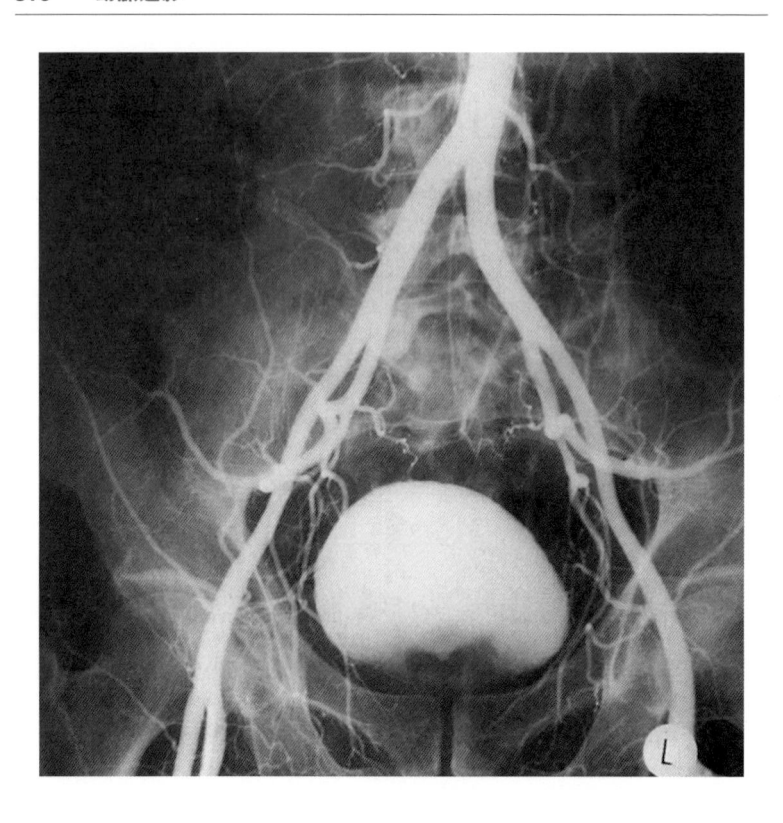

骨盤・下肢動脈造影　骨盤部

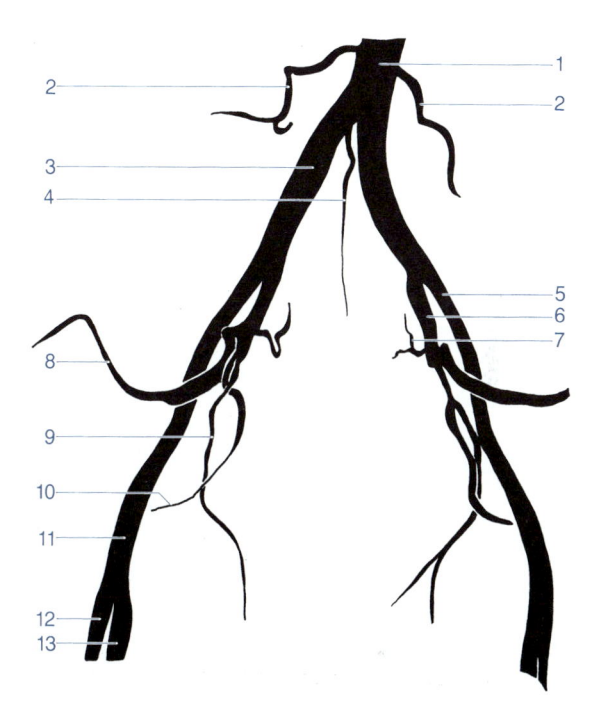

1　腹大動脈 Abdominal aorta	8　上殿動脈 Superior gluteal artery
2　腰動脈 Lumbar artery	9　閉鎖動脈 Obturator artery
3　総腸骨動脈 Common iliac artery	10　下殿動脈 Inferior gluteal artery
4　正中仙骨動脈 Median sacral artery	11　総大腿動脈 Common femoral artery
5　外腸骨動脈 External iliac artery	12　深大腿動脈 Deep femoral artery
6　内腸骨動脈 Internal iliac artery	13　浅大腿動脈 Superficial femoral artery
7　外側仙骨動脈 Lateral sacral artery	

318 動脈造影

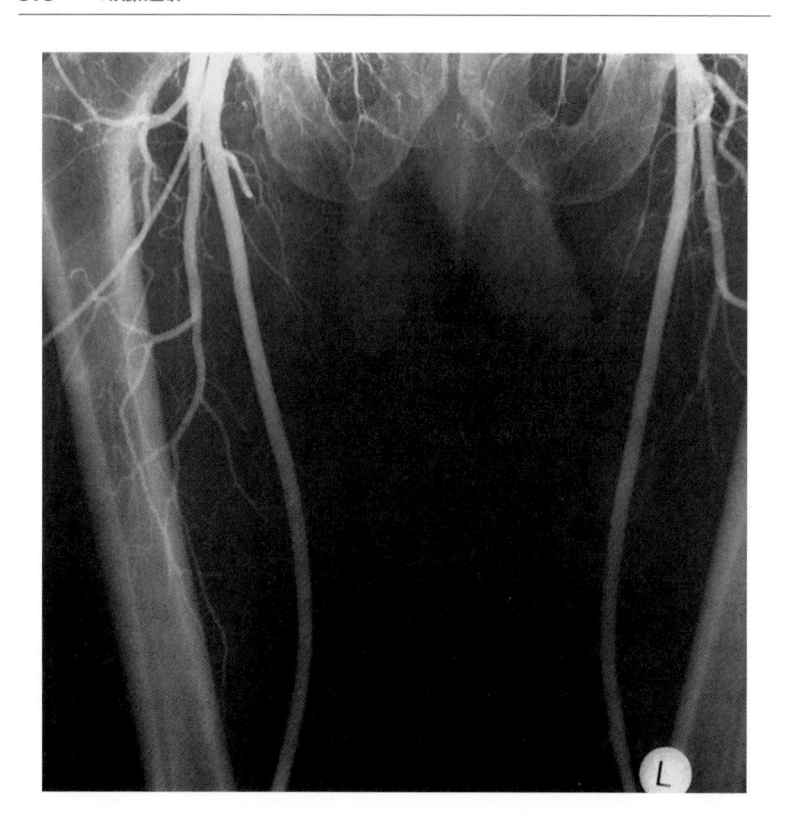

骨盤・下肢動脈造影　大腿部　**319**

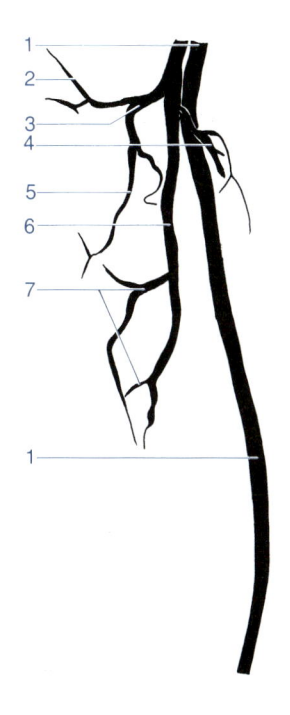

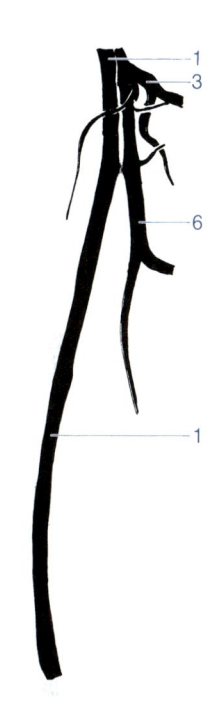

1　浅大腿動脈　Superficial femoral artery
2　外側大腿回旋動脈の上行枝　Ascending branch of the lateral femoral circumflex artery
3　外側大腿回旋動脈　Lateral femoral circumflex artery
4　内側大腿回旋動脈　Medial femoral circumflex artery
5　外側大腿回旋動脈の下行枝　Descending branch of the lateral femoral circumflex artery
6　深大腿動脈　Deep femoral artery
7　貫通動脈　Perforating artery

320 動脈造影

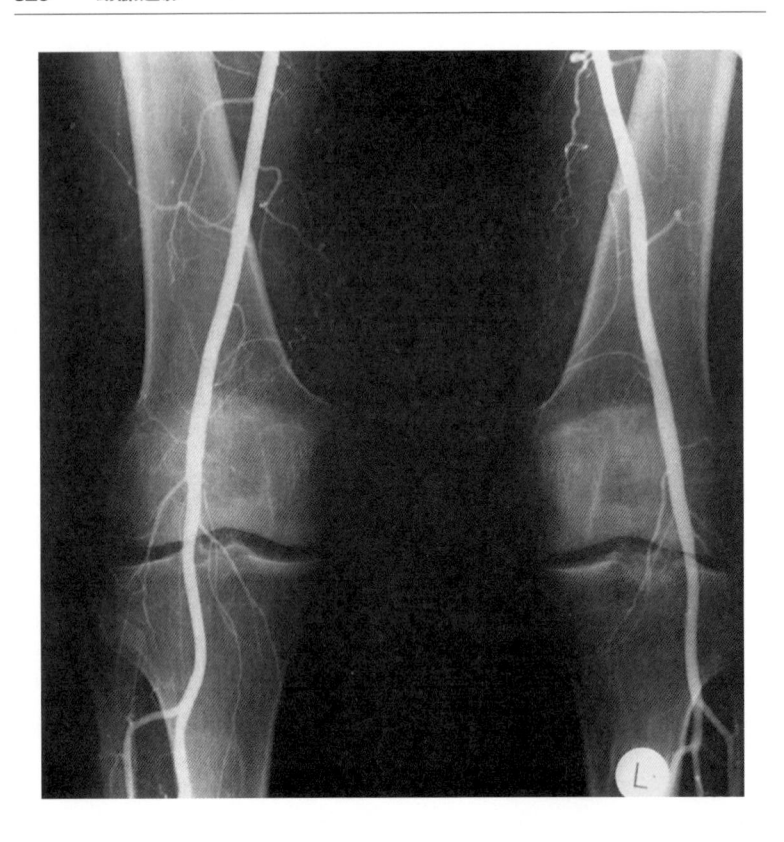

骨盤・下肢動脈造影　膝部

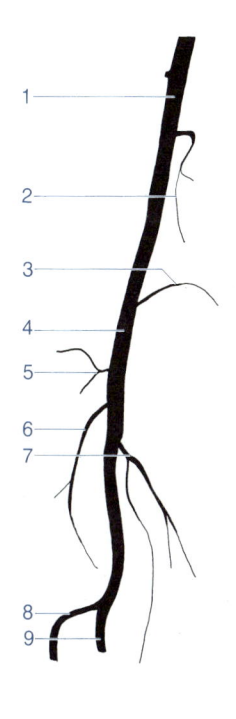

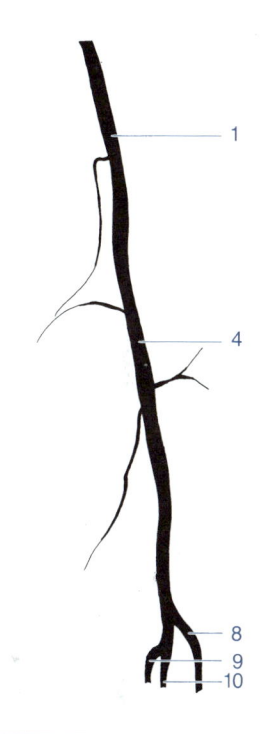

1 浅大腿動脈 Superficial femoral artery
2 下行膝動脈 Descending genicular artery
3 内側上膝動脈 Superior medial genicular artery
4 膝窩動脈 Popliteal artery
5 外側上膝動脈 Superior lateral genicular artery
6 中膝動脈 Middle genicular artery
7 内側下膝動脈 Inferior medial genicular artery
8 前脛骨動脈 Anterior tibial artery
9 後脛骨動脈 Posterior tibial artery
10 腓骨動脈 Peroneal artery

322 動脈造影

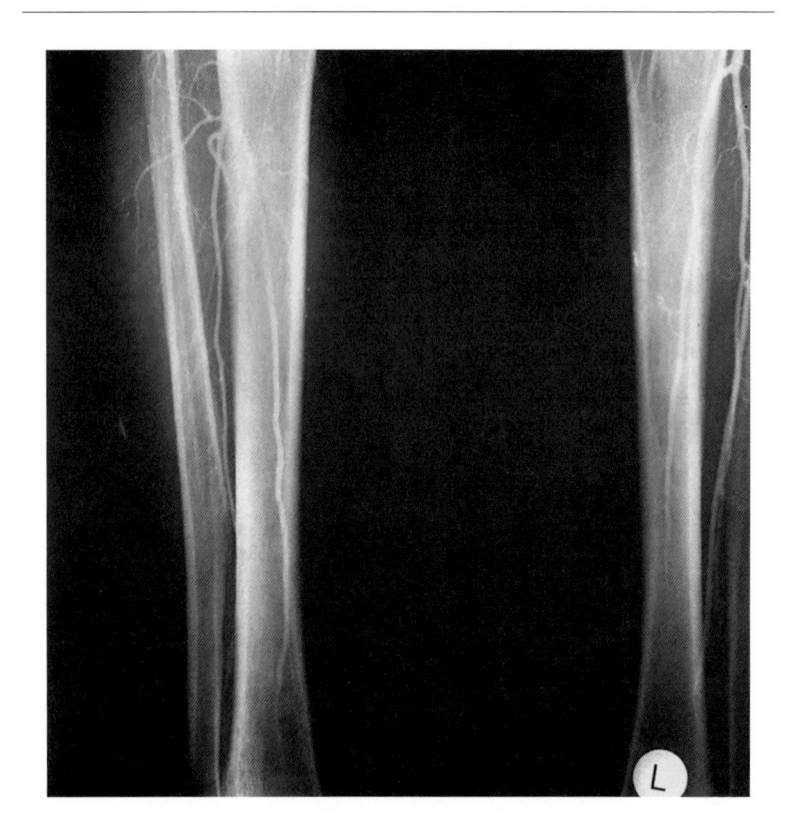

骨盤・下肢動脈造影　下腿部　**323**

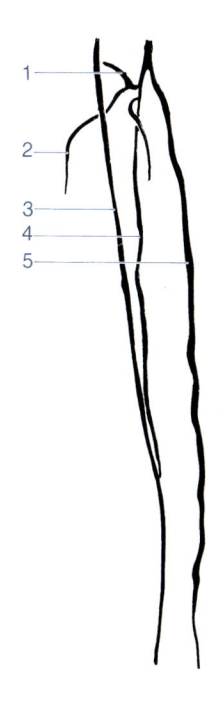

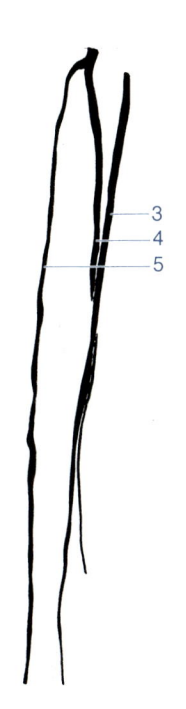

1　(後脛骨動脈の)腓骨回旋枝　Circumflex fibular branch	3　前脛骨動脈　Anterior tibial artery
2　筋枝　Muscular branch	4　腓骨動脈　Peroneal artery
	5　後脛骨動脈　Posterior tibial artery

324 動脈造影

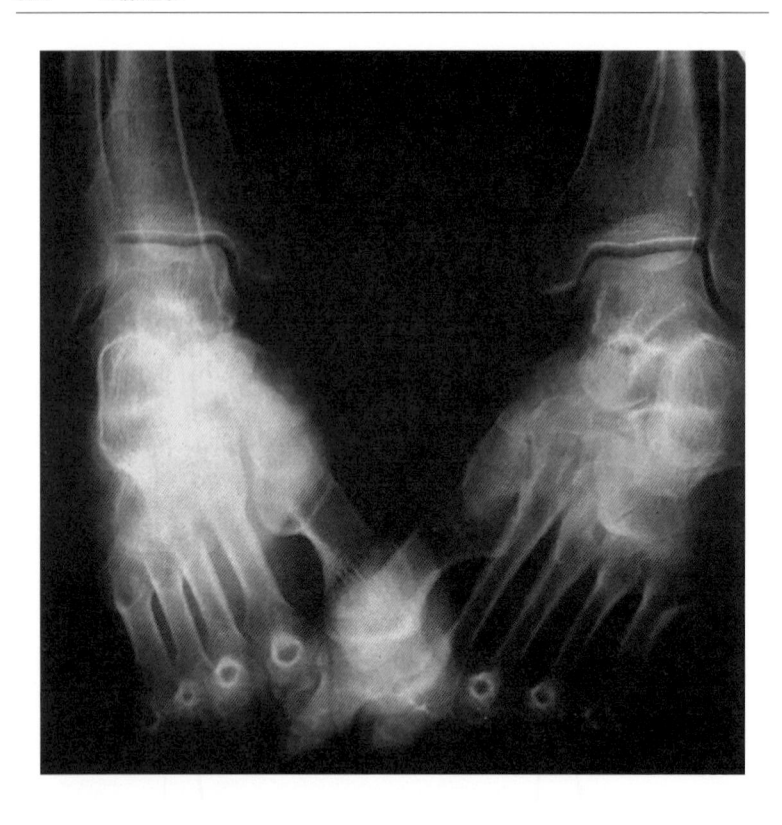

骨盤・下肢動脈造影　足部

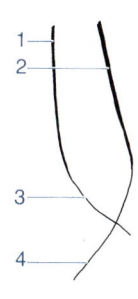

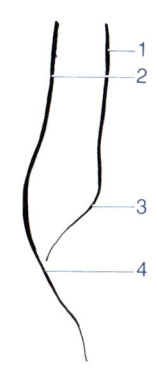

1　前脛骨動脈　Anterior tibial artery
2　後脛骨動脈　Posterior tibial artery
3　足背動脈　Dorsalis pedis artery
4　足底動脈　Plantar artery

326 静脉造影

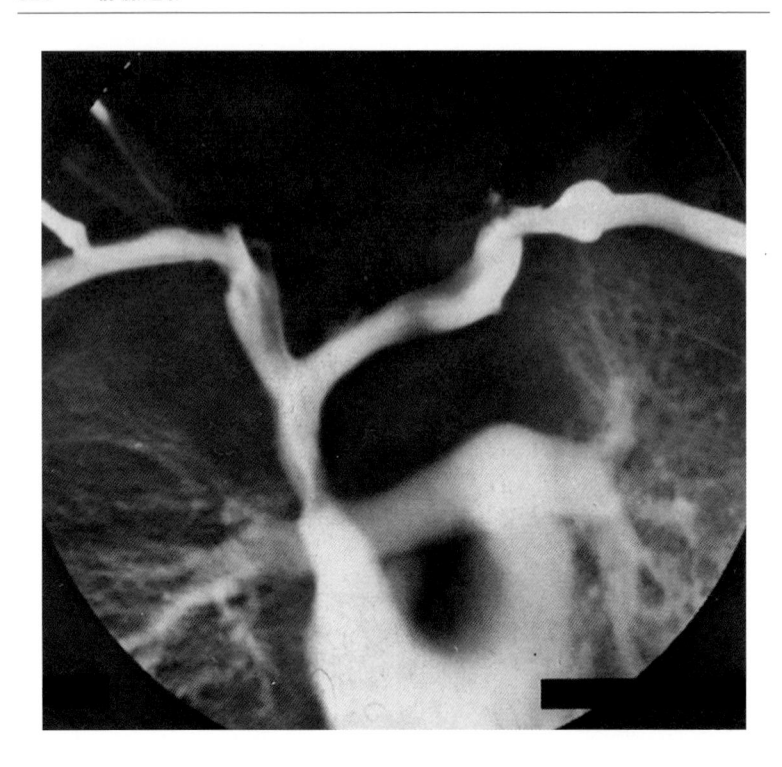

上大静脈　正面（前後） 327

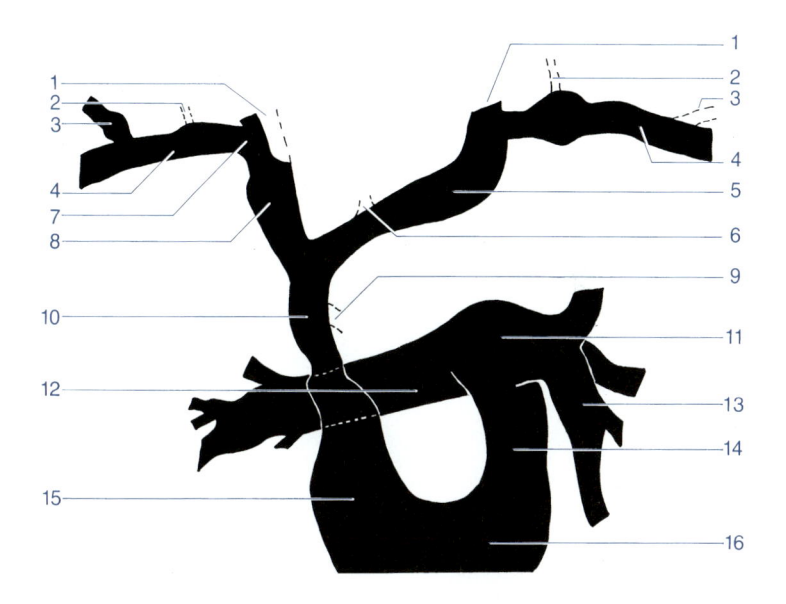

1　内頸静脈　Internal jugular vein	9　奇静脈　Azygos vein
2　外頸静脈　External jugular vein	10　上大静脈　Superior vena cava
3　橈側皮静脈　Cephalic vein	11　肺動脈幹　Pulmonary trunk
4　鎖骨下静脈　Subclavian vein	12　右肺動脈　Right pulmonary artery
5　左腕頭静脈　Left brachiocephalic vein	13　左肺動脈　Left pulmonary artery
6　下甲状腺静脈　Inferior thyroid vein	14　動脈円錐　Infundibulum
7　静脈角　Venous angle	15　右心房　Right atrium
8　右腕頭静脈　Right brachiocephalic vein	16　右心室　Right ventricle

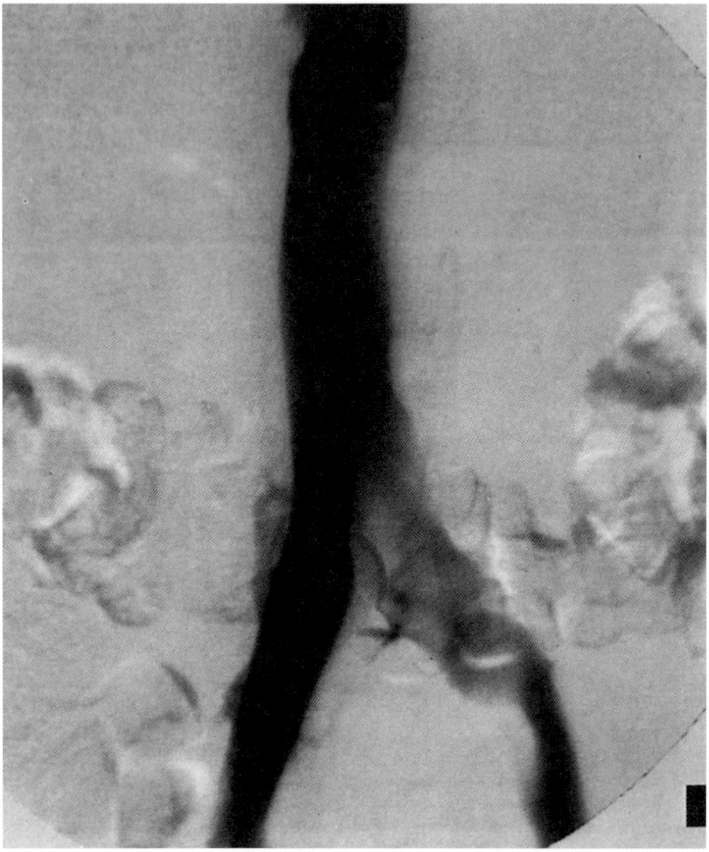

下大静脈　正面（前後）　329

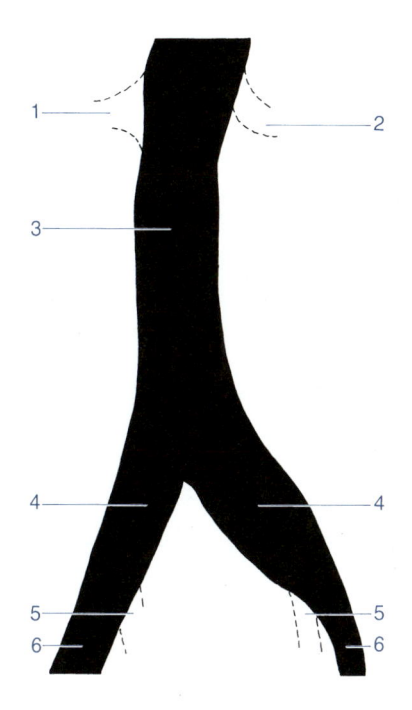

1　右腎静脈 Right renal vein	4　総腸骨静脈 Common iliac vein
2　左腎静脈 Left renal vein	5　内腸骨静脈 Internal iliac vein
3　下大静脈 Inferior vena cava	6　外腸骨静脈 External iliac vein

330　静脉造影

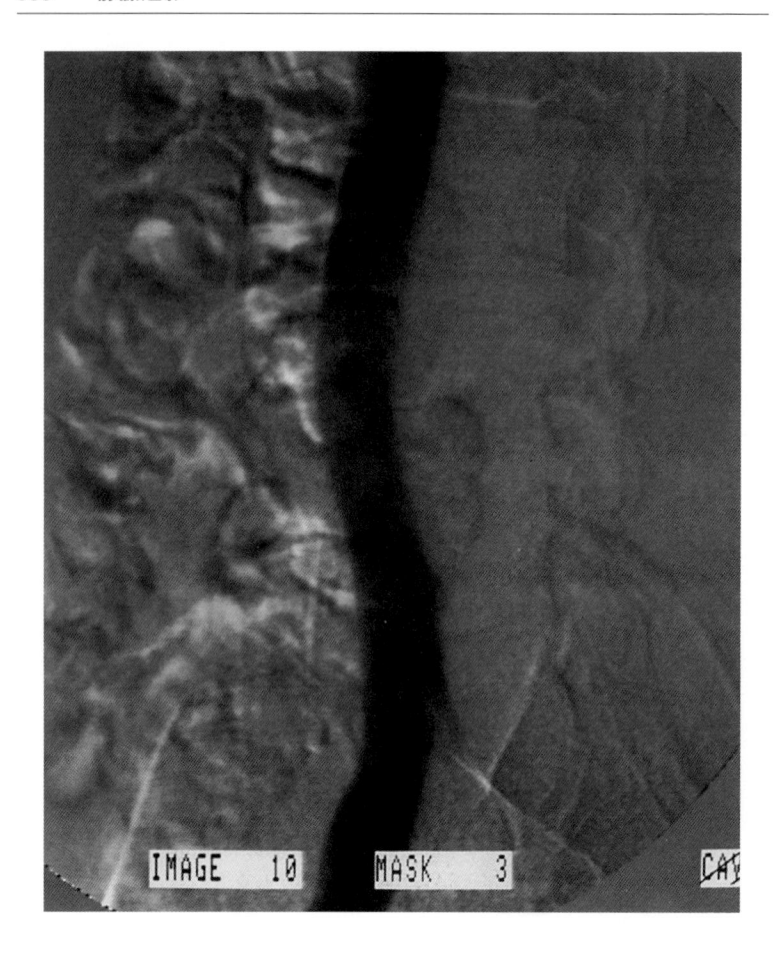

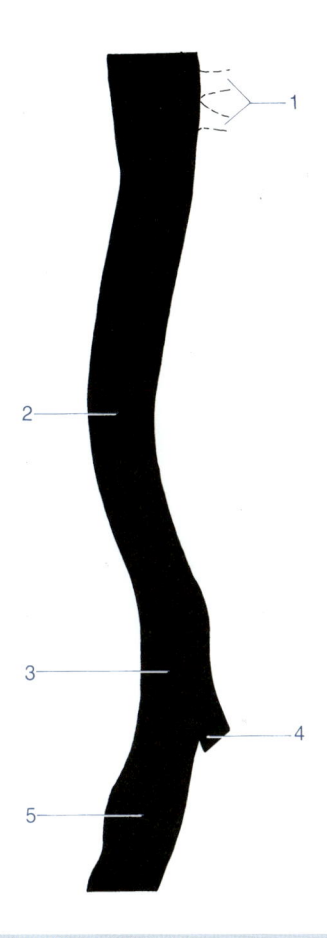

下大静脈　側面　　*331*

1　腎静脈　Renal veins
2　下大静脈　Inferior vena cava
3　総腸骨静脈　Common iliac vein
4　内腸骨静脈　Internal iliac vein
5　外腸骨静脈　External iliac vein

静脉造影

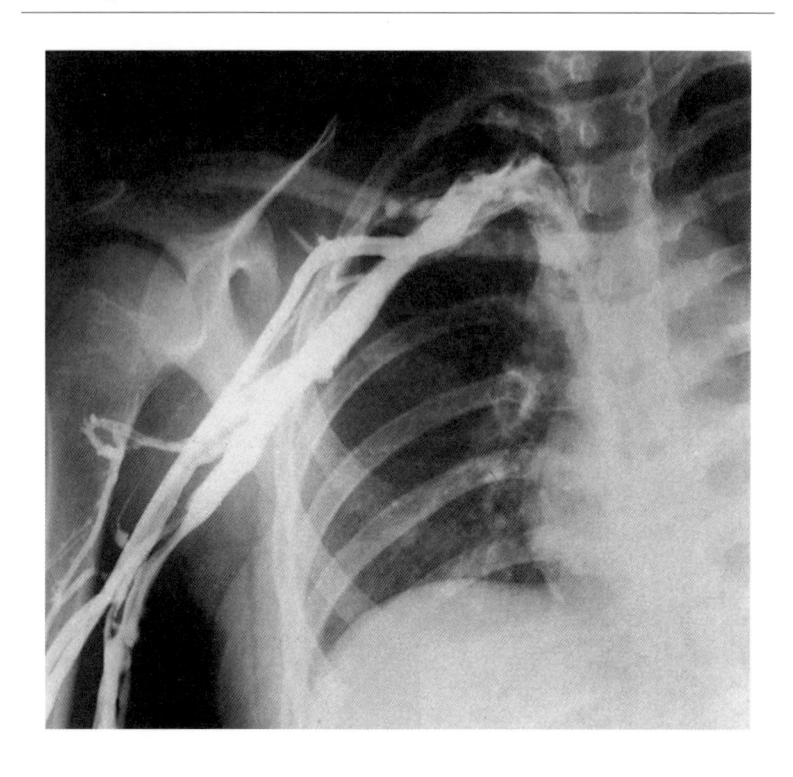

上腕静脈造影　**333**

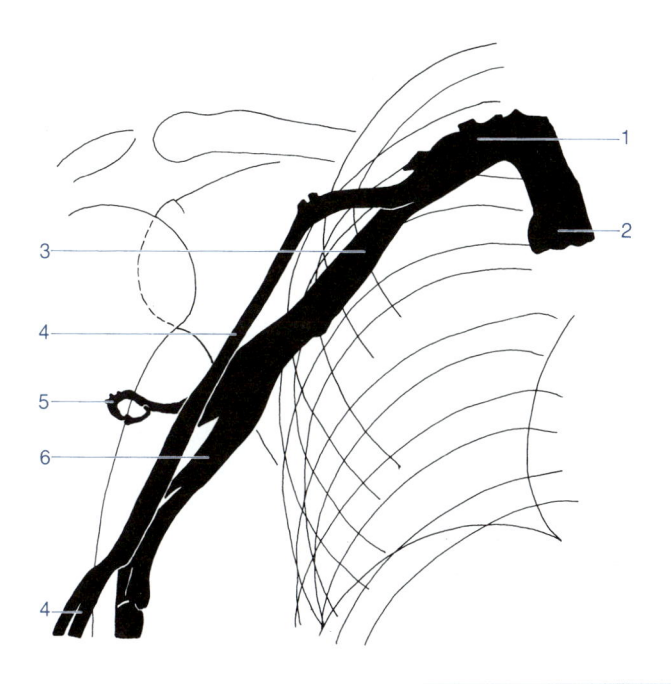

1 鎖骨下静脈 Subclavian vein	4 橈側皮静脈 Cephalic vein
2 上大静脈 Superior vena cava	5 上腕深部静脈 Deep veins of the arm
3 腋窩静脈 Axillary vein	6 上腕静脈 Brachial veins

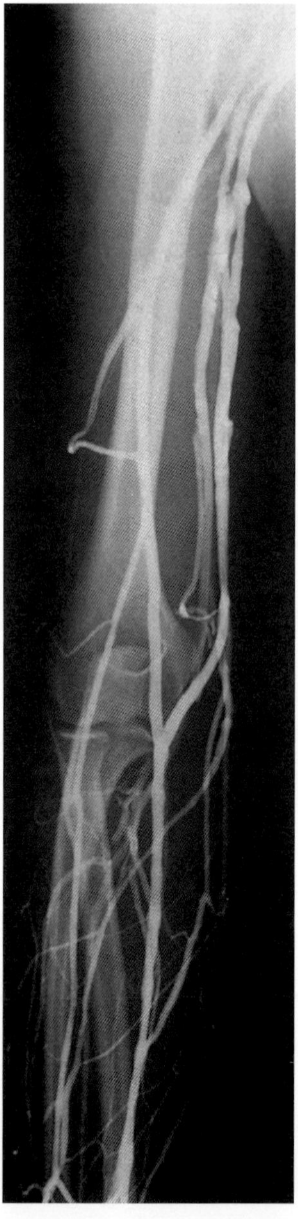

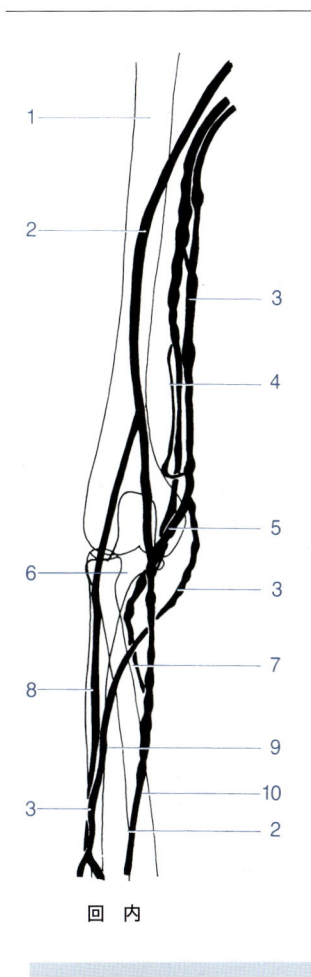

前腕静脈造影

回 内 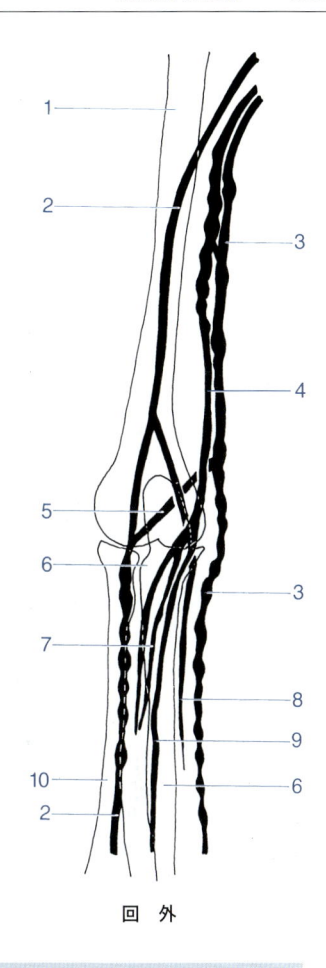 　　　　　　　　　　回 外

1　上腕骨 Humerus	6　尺骨 Ulna
2　橈側皮静脈 Cephalic vein	7　橈骨静脈 Radial veins
3　尺側皮静脈 Basilar vein	8　尺骨静脈 Ulnar veins
4　上腕静脈 Brachial vein	9　前腕正中皮静脈 Median antebrachial vein
5　肘正中皮静脈 Median cubital vein	10　橈骨 Radius

336 静脉造影

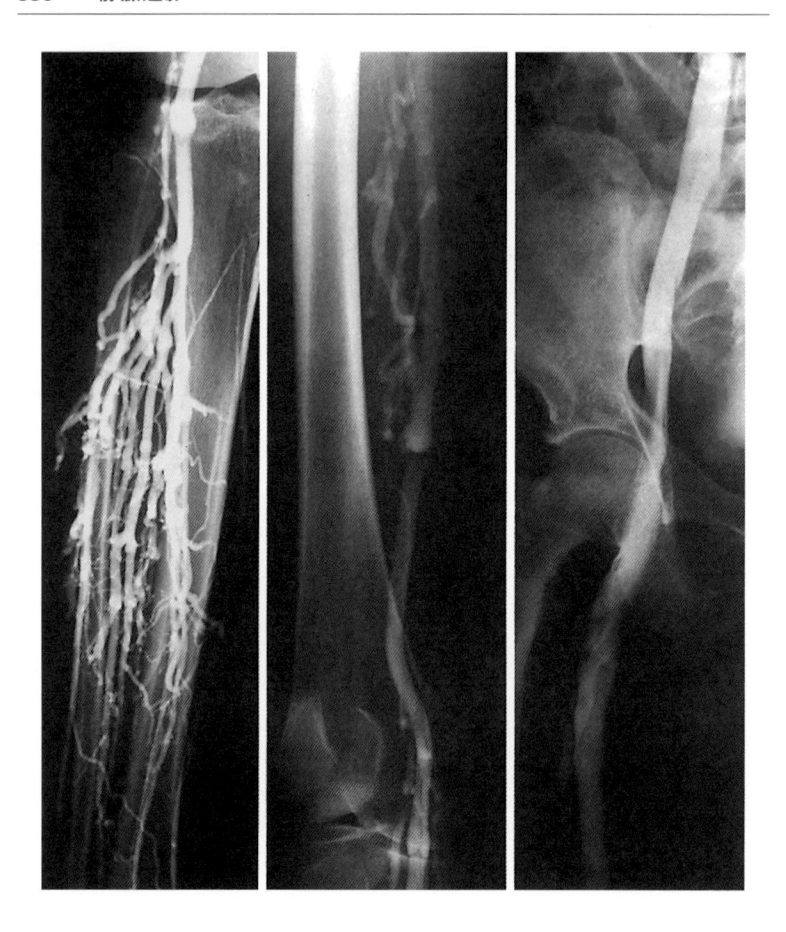

内 旋　　　　　　　　外 旋

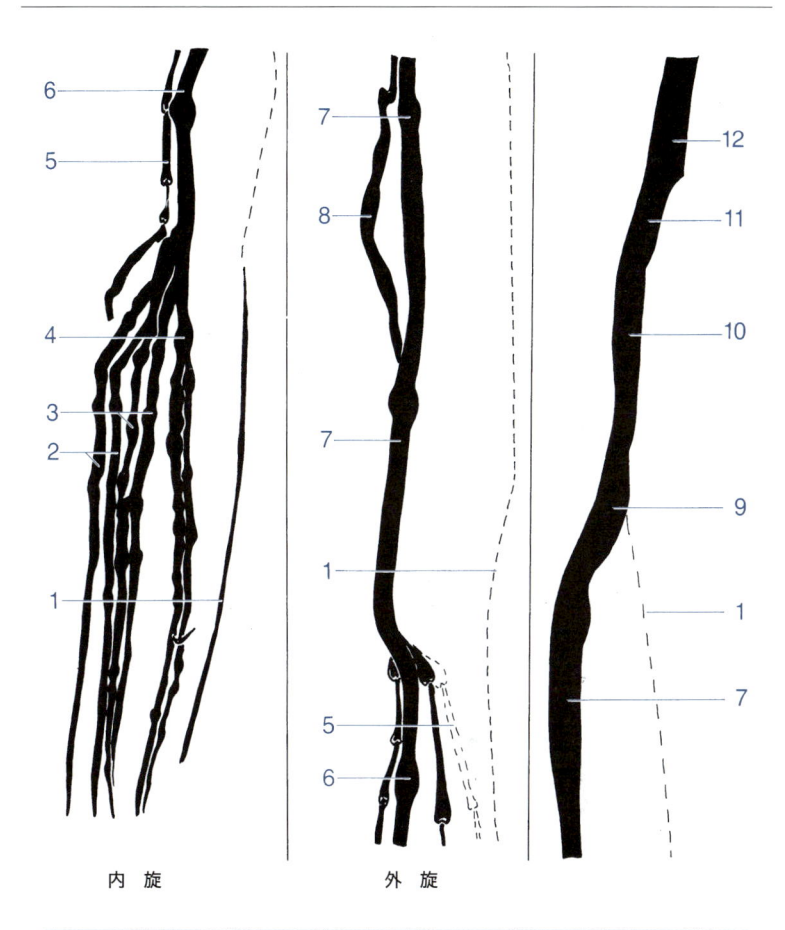

1	大伏在静脈 Greater saphenous vein	7	浅大腿静脈 Superficial femoral vein
2	前脛骨静脈 Anterior tibial veins	8	深大腿静脈 Deep femoral vein
3	腓骨静脈 Peroneal veins	9	大腿静脈 Femoral vein
4	後脛骨静脈 Posterior tibial veins	10	外腸骨静脈 External iliac vein
5	小伏在静脈 Small saphenous vein	11	総腸骨静脈 Common iliac vein
6	膝窩静脈 Popliteal vein	12	下大静脈 Inferior vena cava

特殊な造影検査

特殊な造影検査 340

340　特殊な造影検査

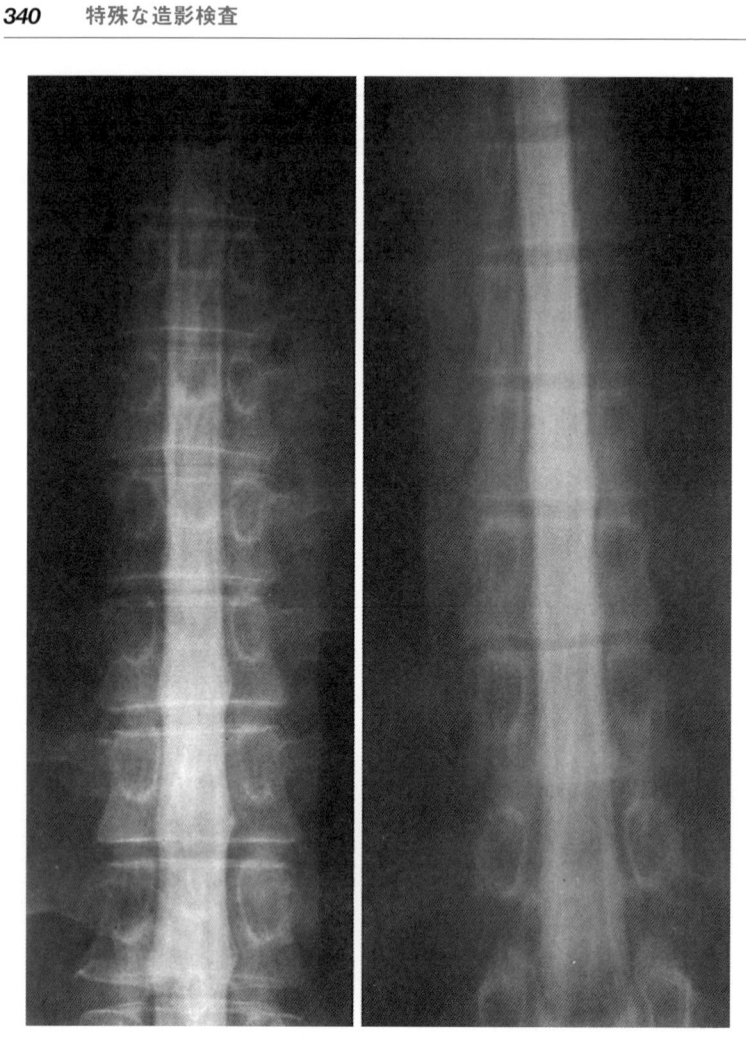

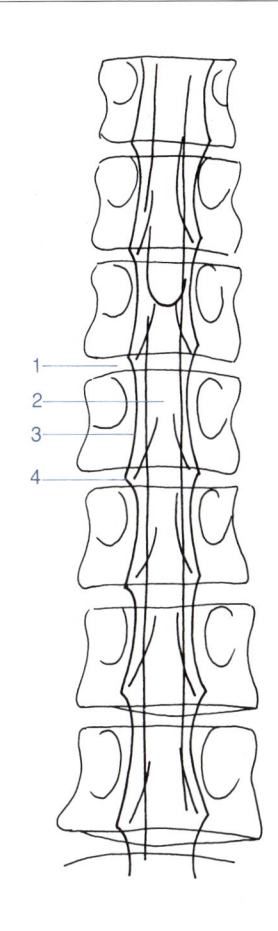

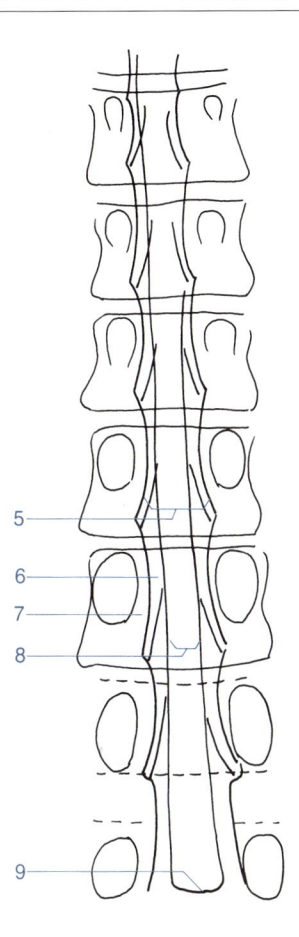

胸部ミエログラフィー　正面（前後） 341

1　椎間板　Intervertebral disk	5　硬膜内腔　Intradural space
2　脊髄　Spinal cord	6　外側クモ膜下腔　Lateral subarachnoid space
3　硬膜嚢外側縁　Lateral margin of the dural sac	7　硬膜外腔　Extradural space
4　神経根袖　Nerve root sleeve	8　髄内部　Intramedullary region
	9　脊髄円錐　Medullary cone

342　特殊な造影検査

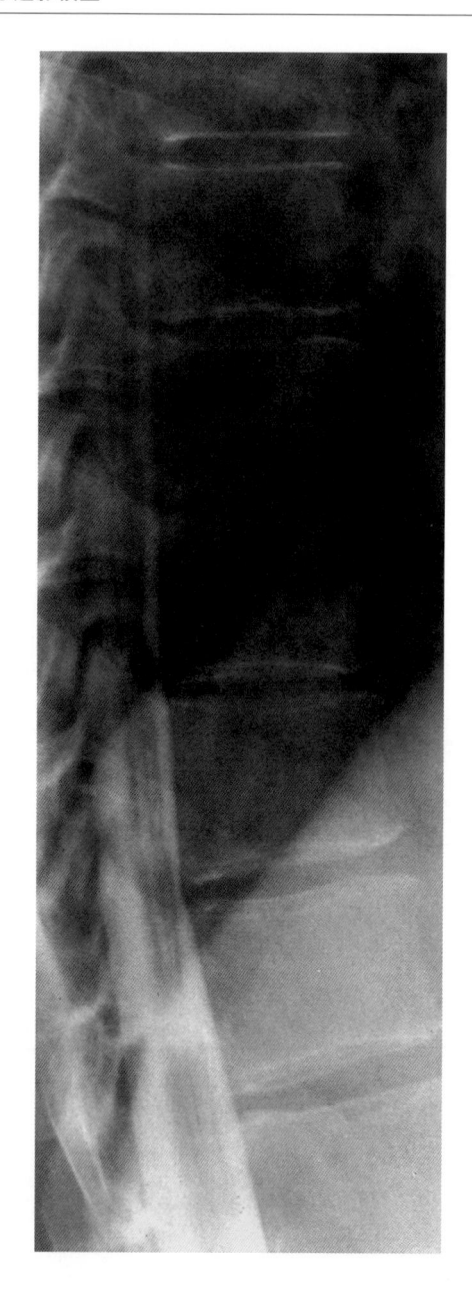

胸部ミエログラフィー 側面

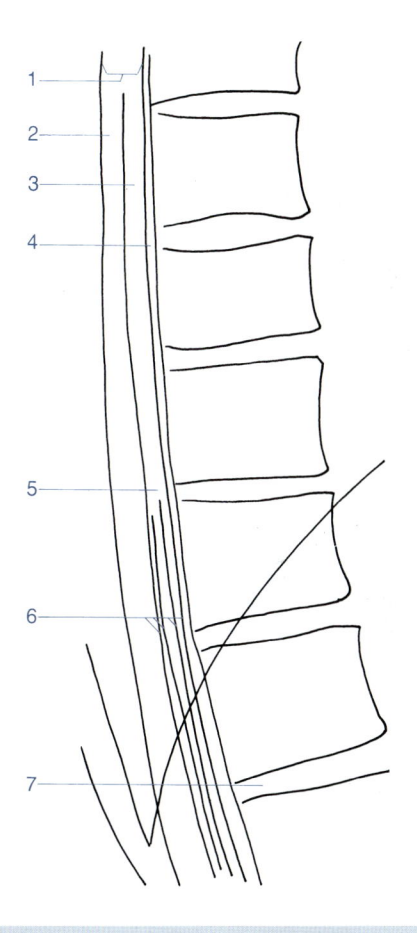

1 硬膜囊 Dural sac
2 後クモ膜下腔 Posterior subarachnoid space
3 脊髄 Spinal cord
4 前クモ膜下腔 Anterior subarachnoid space
5 脊髄円錐 Medullary cone
6 馬尾 Cauda equina
7 椎間板 Intervertebral disk

344 特殊な造影検査

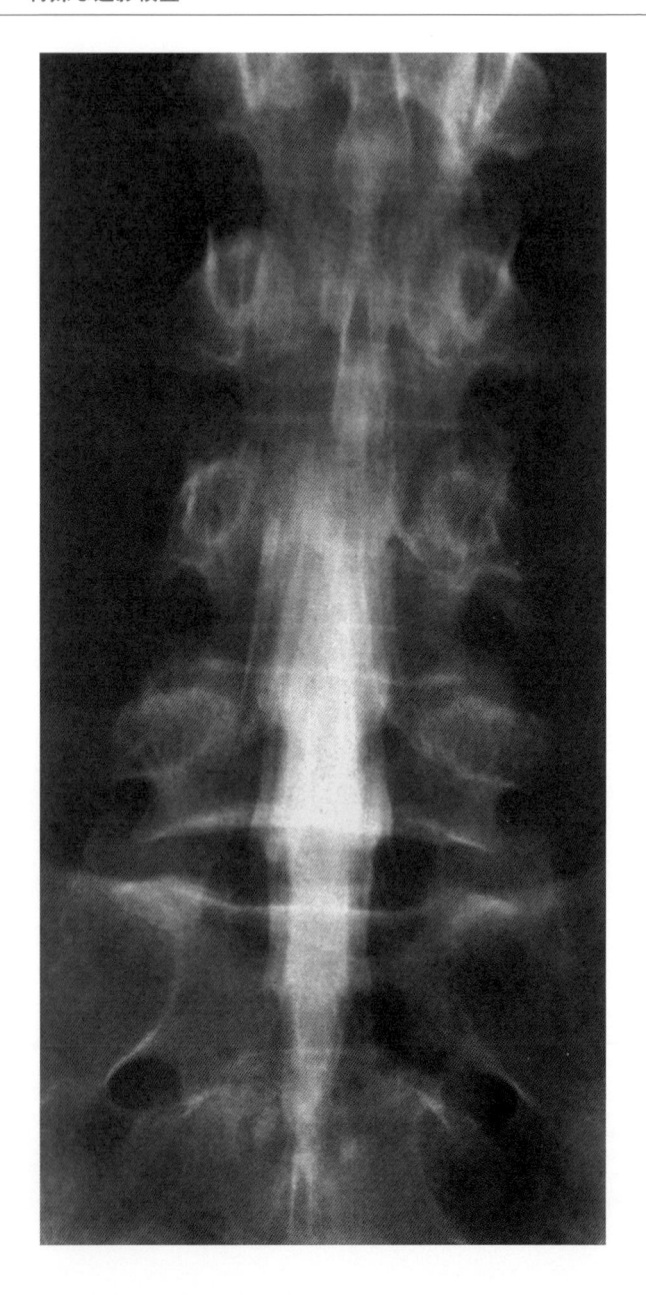

腰部ミエログラフィー　正面（前後） 345

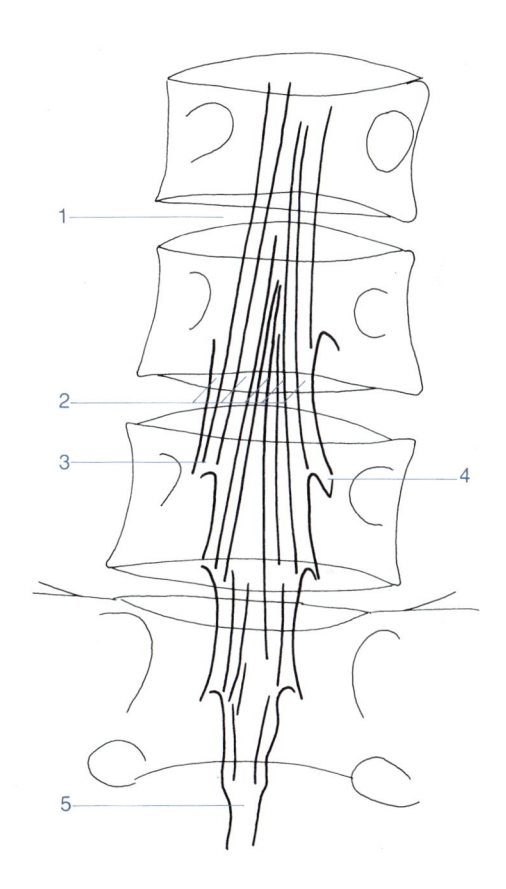

1 椎間板　Intervertebral disk
2 馬尾　Cauda equina
3 クモ膜下腔の脊髄神経根　Spinal nerve root in the subarachnoid space
4 神経根袖　Nerve root sleeve
5 硬膜嚢遠位端　Distal end of the dural sac

346　特殊な造影検査

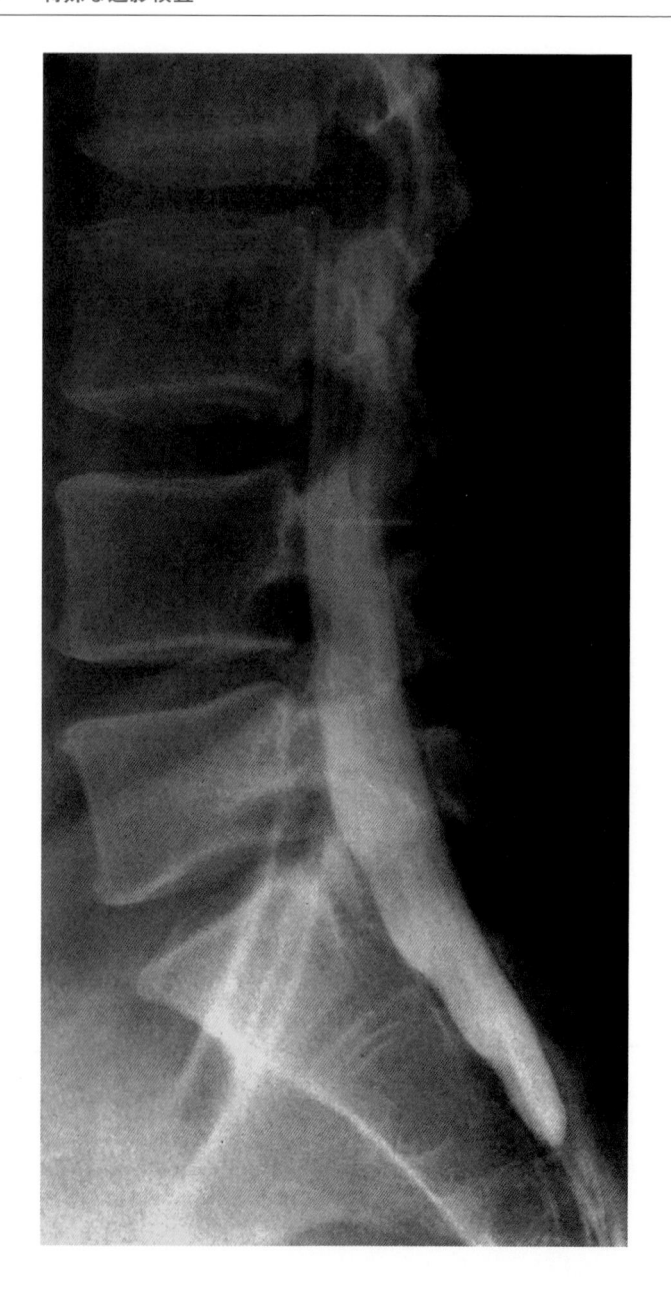

腰部ミエログラフィー 側面 347

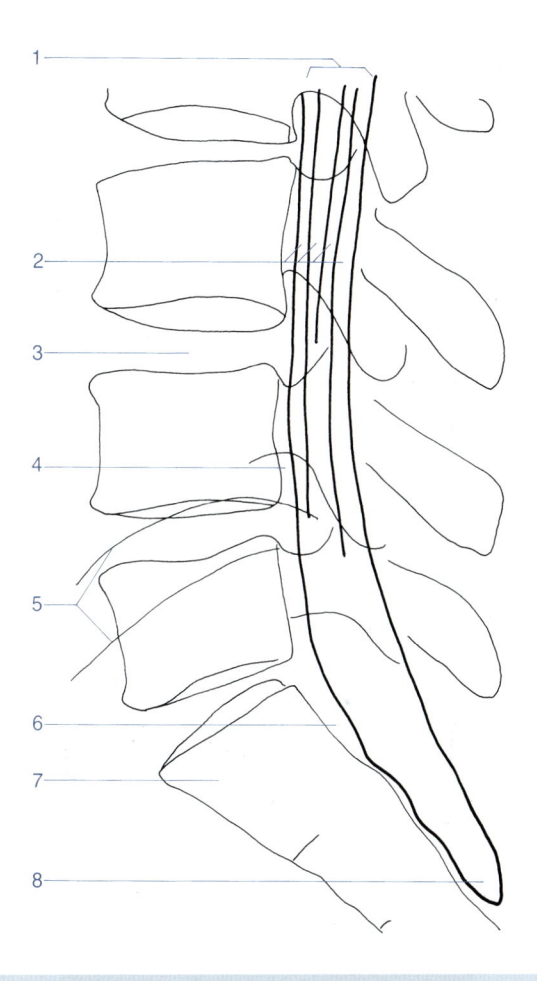

1 硬膜囊　Dural sac
2 馬尾　Cauda equina
3 椎間板　Intervertebral disk
4 椎間孔　Intervertebral foramen
5 腸骨稜　Iliac crest
6 硬膜外脂肪　Epidural fat
7 仙骨　Sacrum
8 硬膜囊遠位端　Distal end of the dural sac

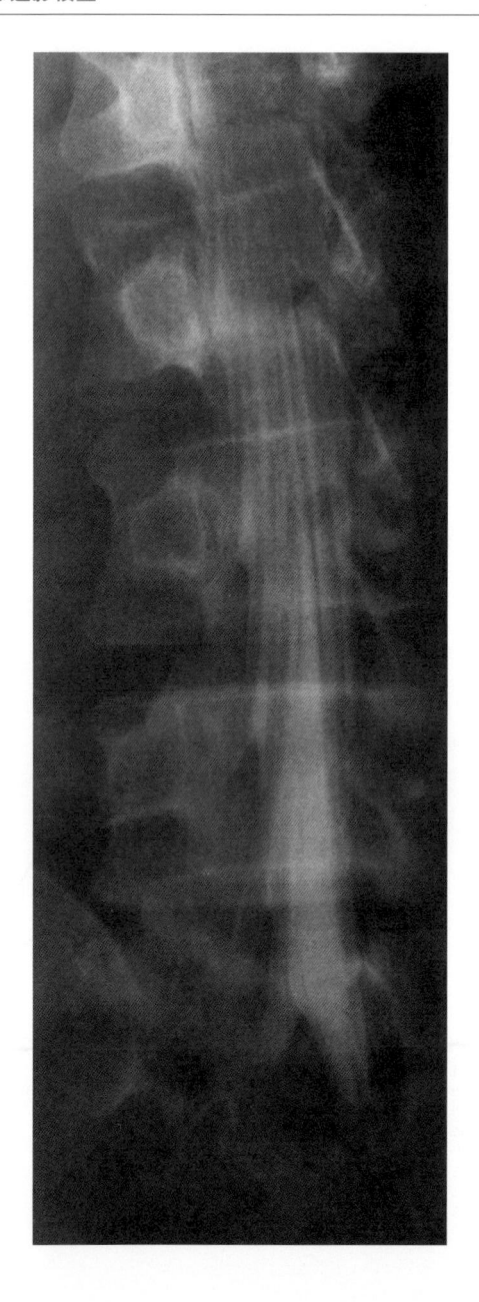

特殊な造影検査

腰部ミエログラフィー　斜位　**349**

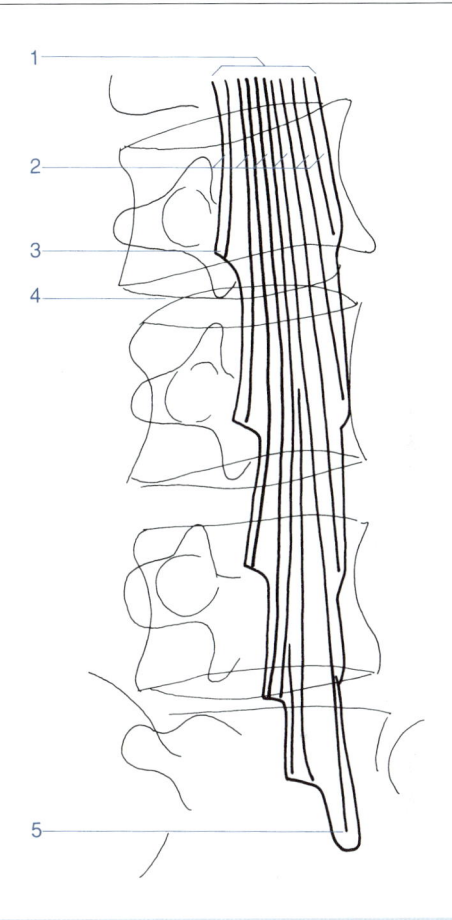

1 硬膜嚢　Dural sac
2 馬尾　Cauda equina
3 神経根鞘（第3腰椎）Nerve root sheath, L3
4 椎間板（L3/L4）Intervertebral disk L3–L4
5 硬膜嚢遠位端（S1あるいはS2レベル）
　Distal end of the dural sac (at level of S1 or S2)

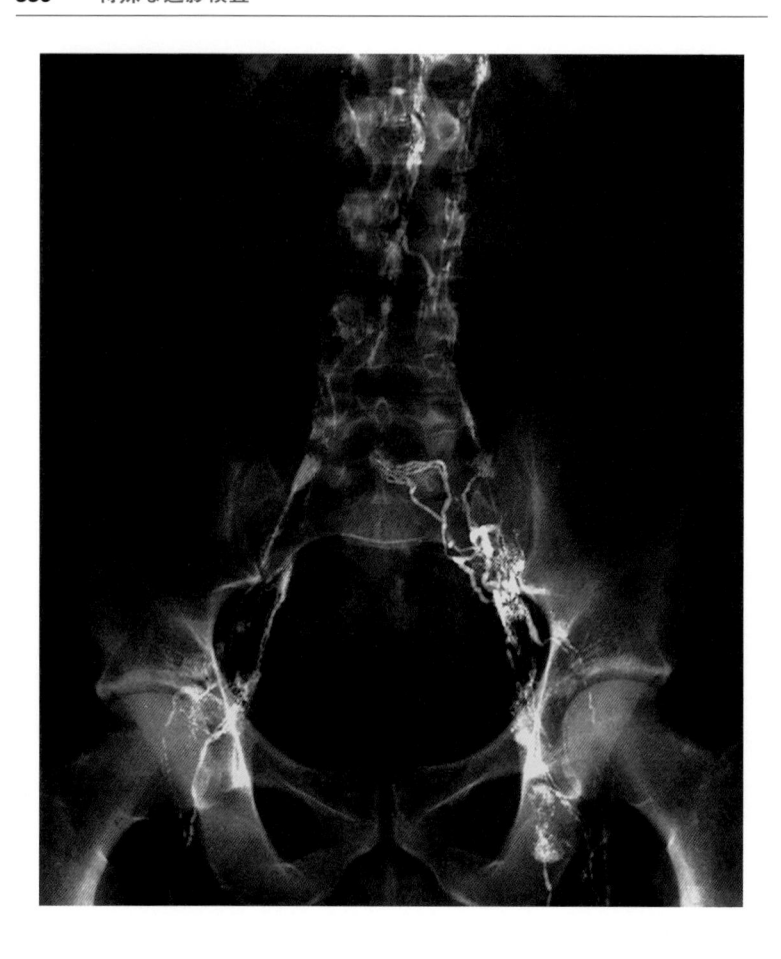

特殊な造影検査

両足リンパ管造影　正面（前後）注入相　　351

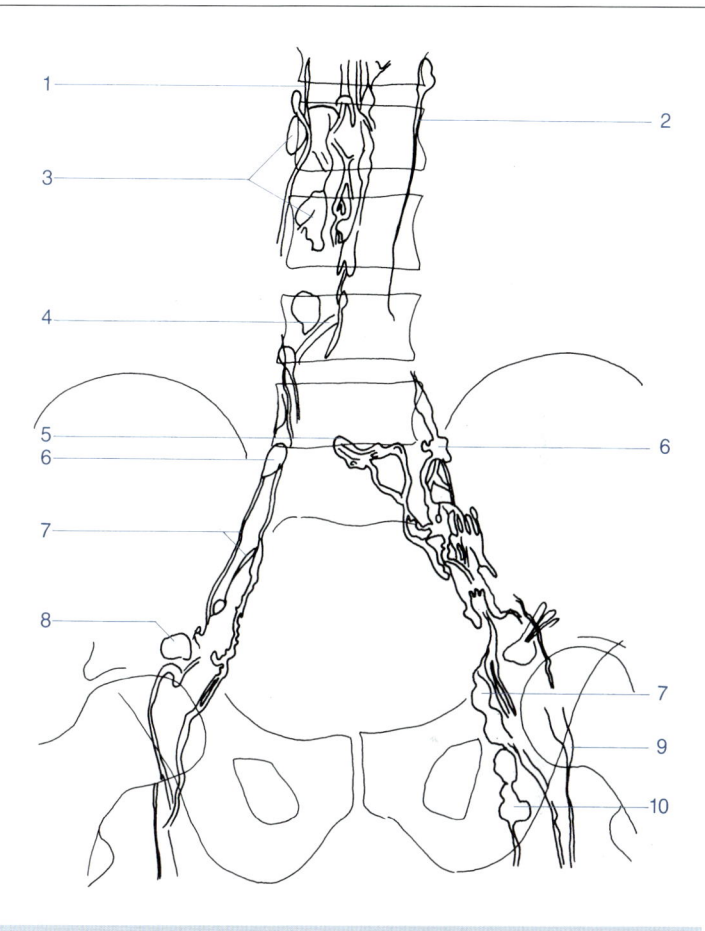

1　右腰リンパ本幹　Right lumbar trunk
2　左腰リンパ本幹　Left lumbar trunk
3　腰リンパ節　Lumbar lymph nodes
4　交通枝　Crossover
5　岬角リンパ節　Promontory lymph nodes
6　総腸骨リンパ節　Common iliac lymph nodes
7　外腸骨リンパ節群のリンパ管　Lymph channels of the external iliac lymph nodes
8　外側裂孔リンパ節　Lateral lacunar lymph nodes
9　浅鼠径リンパ節　Superficial inguinal lymph nodes
10　深鼠径リンパ節　Deep inguinal lymph nodes

352 特殊な造影検査

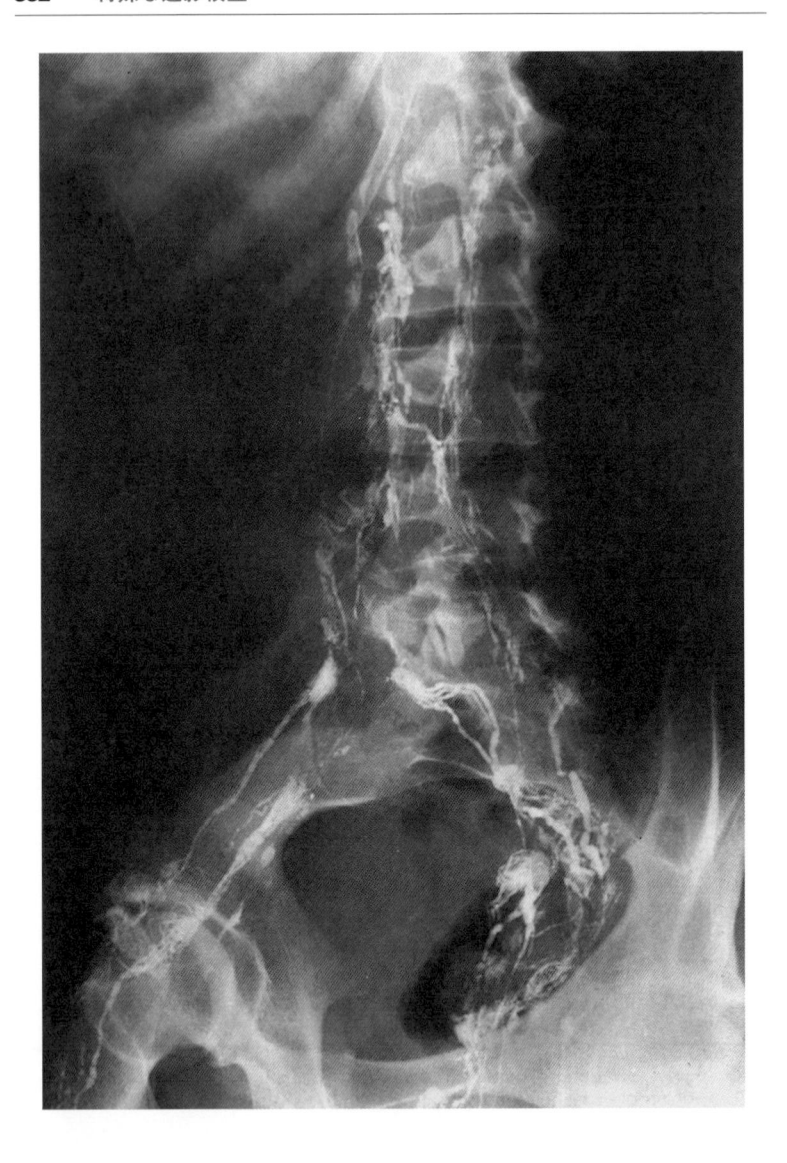

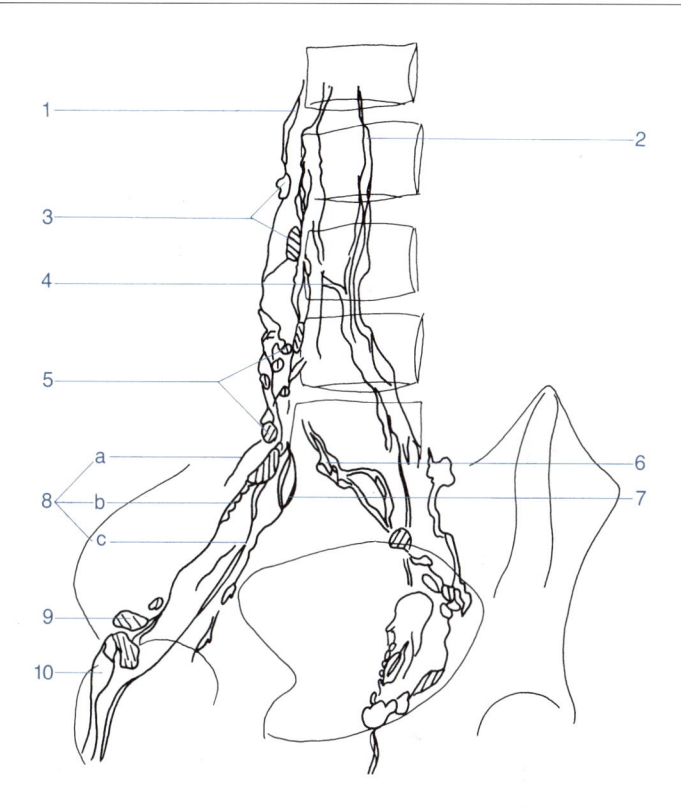

両足リンパ管造影 斜位 注入相

1 右腰リンパ本幹 Right lumbar trunk
2 左腰リンパ本幹 Left lumbar trunk
3 腰リンパ節 Lumbar lymph nodes
4 交通枝 Crossover
5 総腸骨リンパ節 Common iliac lymph nodes
6 岬角リンパ節 Promontory lymph nodes
7 内腸骨リンパ節と外腸骨・総腸骨リンパ節を結ぶリンパ管 Lymph channels connecting the internal iliac lymph nodes with the external and common illiac lymph nodes
8 外腸骨・結腸骨リンパ節 External and common iliac lymph nodes:
 a 外鎖 External chain
 b 中鎖 Middle chain
 c 内鎖 Internal chain
9 裂孔リンパ節 Lacunar lymph node
10 浅鼠径リンパ節 Superficial inguinal lymph nodes

354 特殊な造影検査

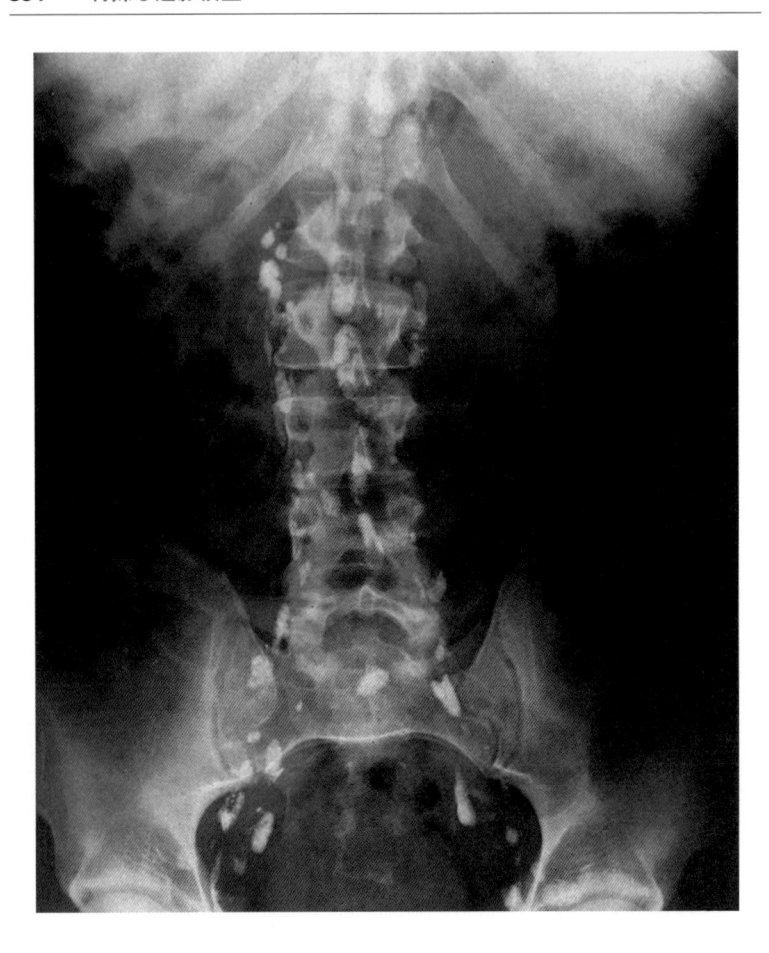

両足リンパ管造影　正面(前後)　貯留相

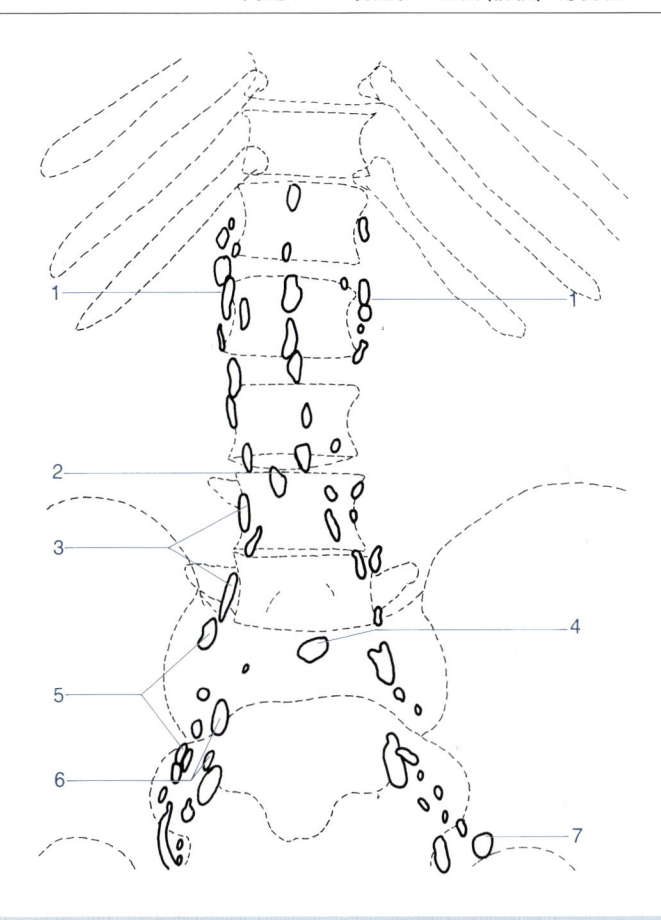

1　傍大動脈リンパ節(外側大動脈, 前大動脈, 後大動脈) Para-aortic lymph nodes (lateral aortic, preaortic, and retroaortic)
2　交通枝 Crossover
3　総腸骨リンパ節 Common iliac lymph nodes
4　岬角リンパ節 Promontory lymph nodes
5　外腸骨リンパ節 External iliac lymph nodes
6　内腸骨リンパ節 Internal iliac lymph nodes
7　裂孔リンパ節 Lacunar lymph node

356 特殊な造影検査

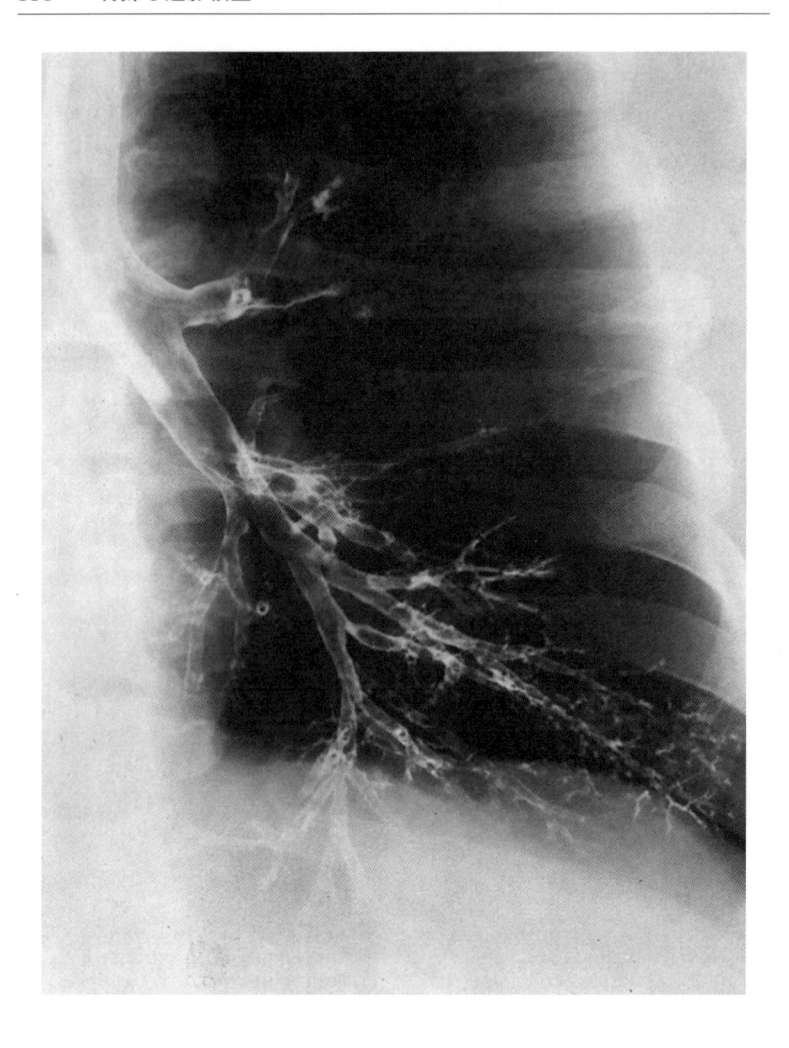

左気管支造影　正面（前後）

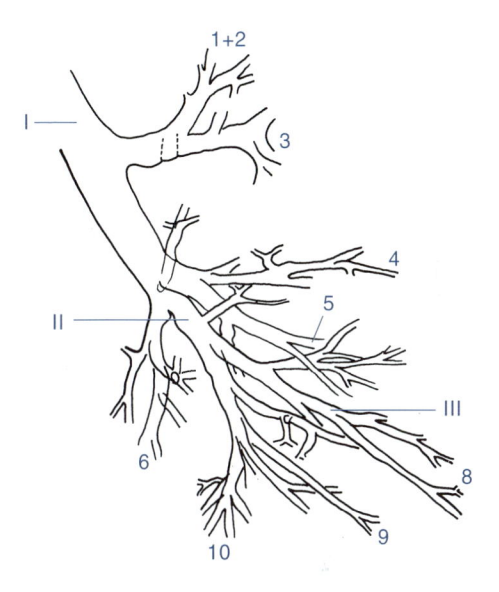

1+2　上葉の肺尖後枝 Apical-posterior segment of the upper lobe	8　下葉の前肺底枝 Anterior-media basal segment of lower lobe
3　上葉の前上葉枝 Anterior segment of the upper lobe	9　下葉の外側肺底枝 Lateral basal segment of the lower lobe
4　上葉の上舌枝 Lingula of the superior segment of the upper lobe	10　下葉の後肺底枝 Posterior basal segment of the lower lobe
5　上葉の下舌枝 Lingula of the inferior segment of the upper lobe	
6　上下葉枝 Superior segment of the lower lobe　左肺には B^7 はない	I　主気管支 Main bronchus
	II　葉気管支 Lobar bronchus
	III　区域気管支 Segmental bronchus

358　特殊な造影検査

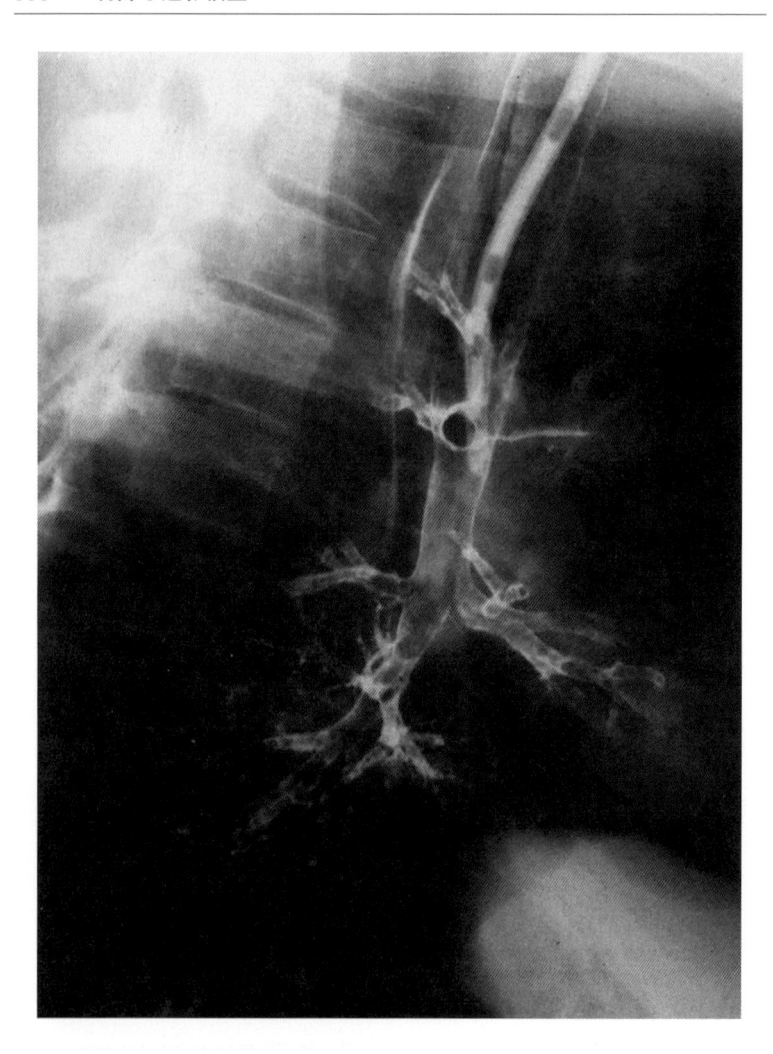

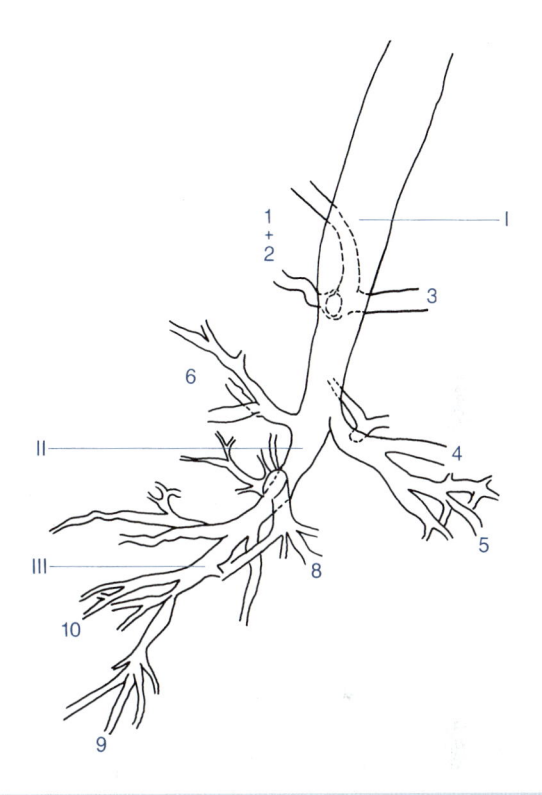

左気管支造影　側面

1+2	上葉の肺尖後枝 Apical-posterior segment of the upper lobe
3	上葉の前上葉枝 Anterior segment of the upper lobe
4	上舌枝 Lingula of the superior segment of the upper lobe
5	下舌枝 Lingula of the inferior segment of the upper lobe
6	上下葉枝 Superior segment of the lower lobe 左肺には B^7 はない
8	下葉の前肺底枝 Anteriormedial basal segment of the lower lobe
9	下葉の外側肺底枝 Lateral basal segment of the lower lobe
10	下葉の後肺底枝 Posteriorbasal segment of the lower lobe
I	主気管支 Main bronchus
II	葉気管支 Lobar bronchus
III	区域気管支 Segmental bronchus

360 特殊な造影検査

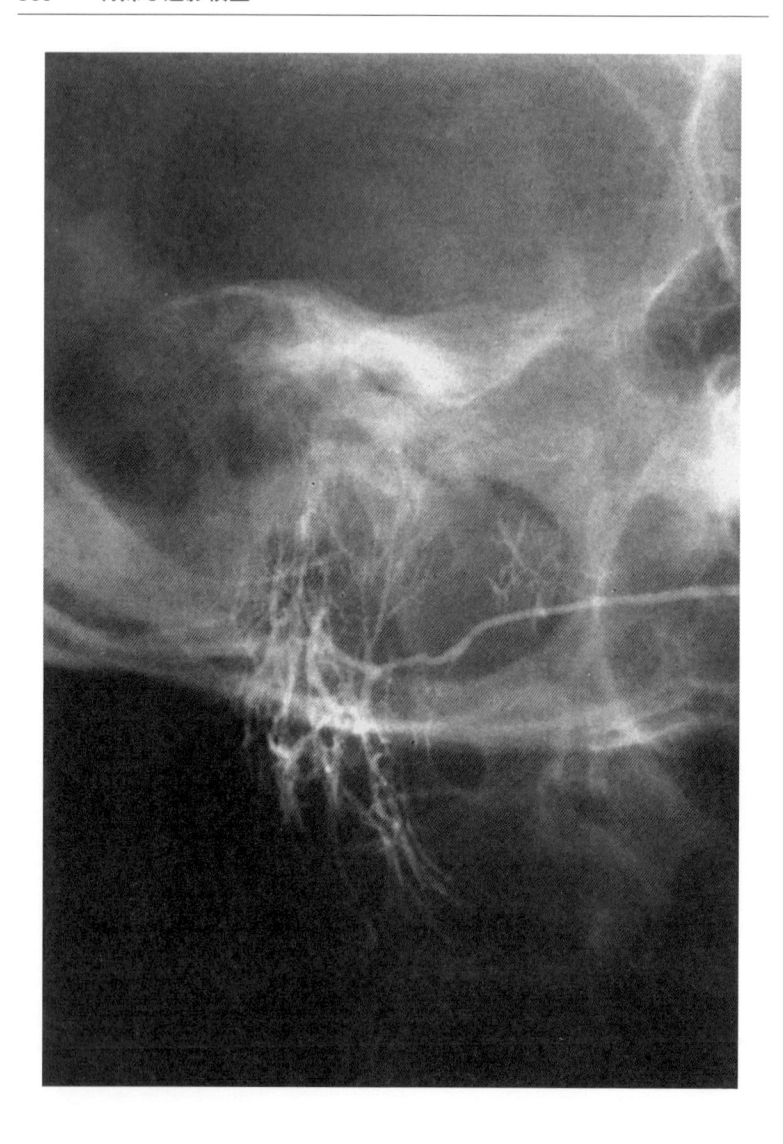

耳下腺造影 側面

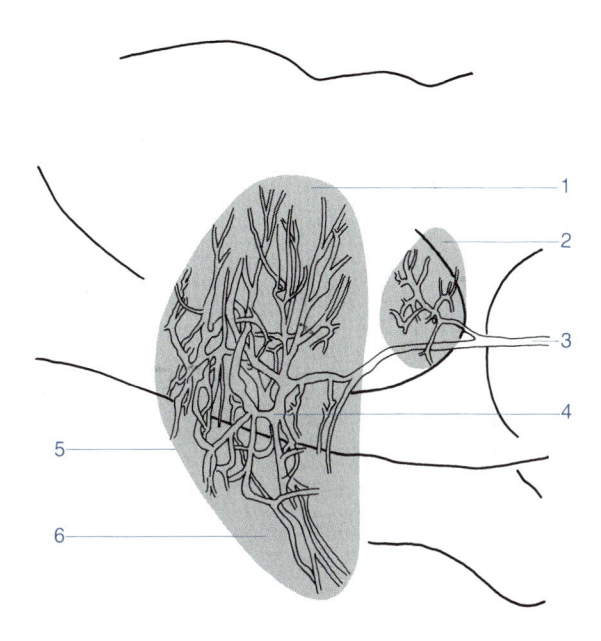

1. 耳下腺浅葉 Superficial lobe of the parotid gland
2. 副耳下腺 Accessory parotid gland
3. 耳下腺管 Parotid duct (**Stensen**管 Stensen's duct)
4. 葉間耳下腺管 Intralobular ductal system
5. 耳下腺 Parotid gland
6. 耳下腺深葉 Deep lobe of the parotid gland　顔面神経より深層

362 特殊な造影検査

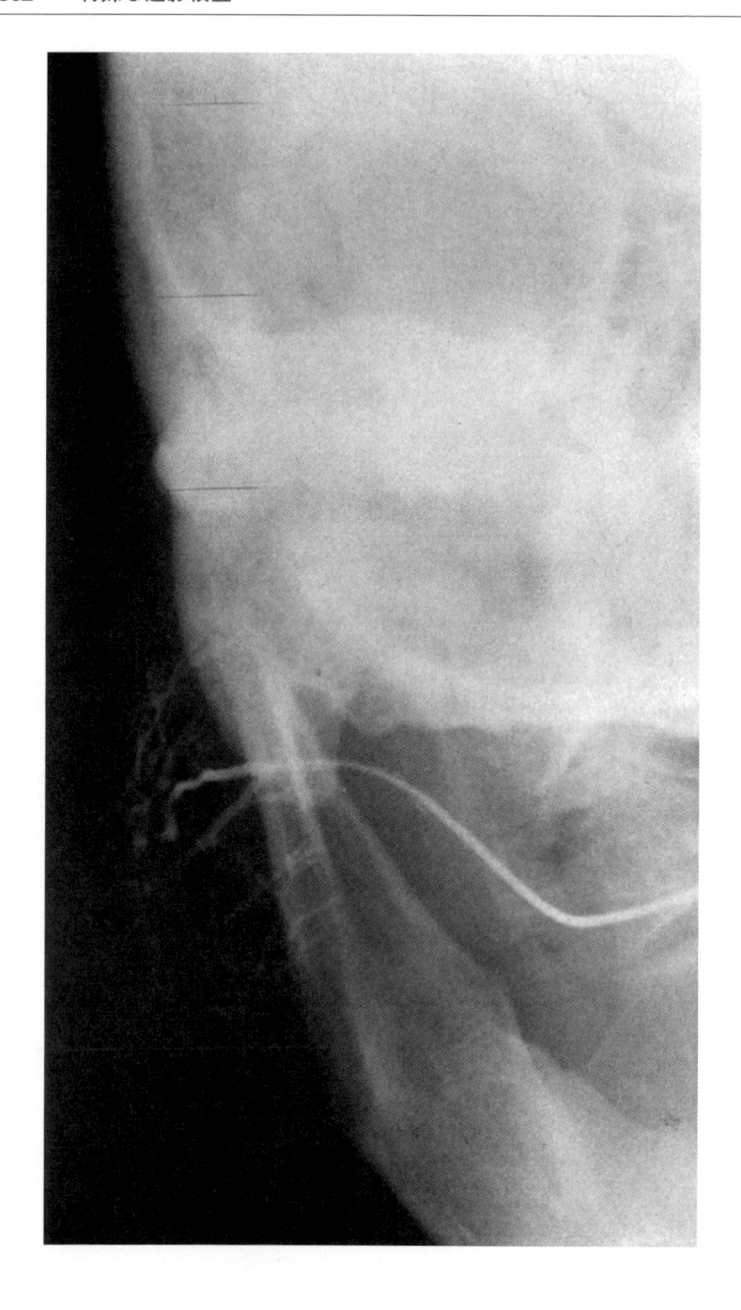

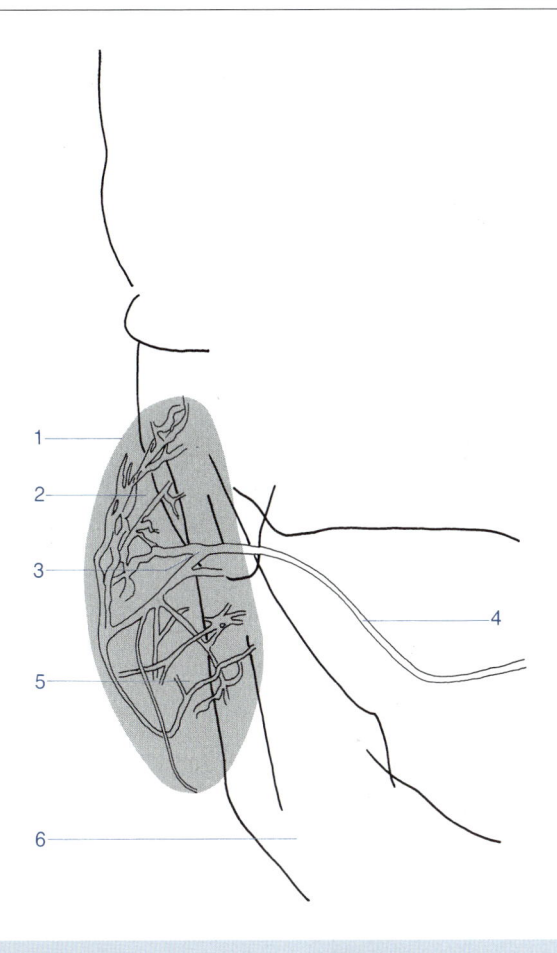

耳下腺造影　正面（前後）

1 耳下腺 Parotid gland
2 耳下腺浅葉 Superficial lobe of the parotid gland　顔面神経より表層
3 葉間耳下腺管 Intralobular parotid ductal system
4 耳下腺管 Parotid duct (Stensen管 Stensen's duct)
5 耳下腺深葉 Deep lobe of the parotid gland　顔面神経より深層
6 下顎骨 Mandible

364　特殊な造影検査

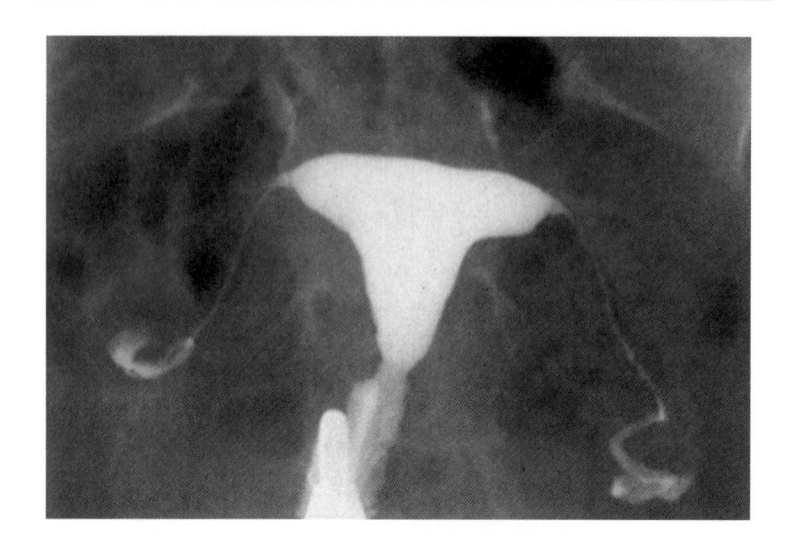

子宮卵管造影

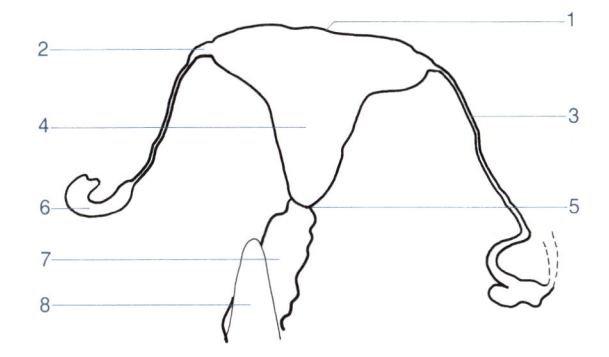

1 子宮底 Fundus of the uterus
2 卵管子宮開口部 Uterine ostium of the fallopian
3 卵管 Fallopian tube
4 子宮腔 Uterine cavity
5 峽部頸管 Cervical canal
6 卵管采 Fimbriae of the fallopian tube
7 腟 Vagina
8 支持鈎 Instrument

366 特殊な造影検査

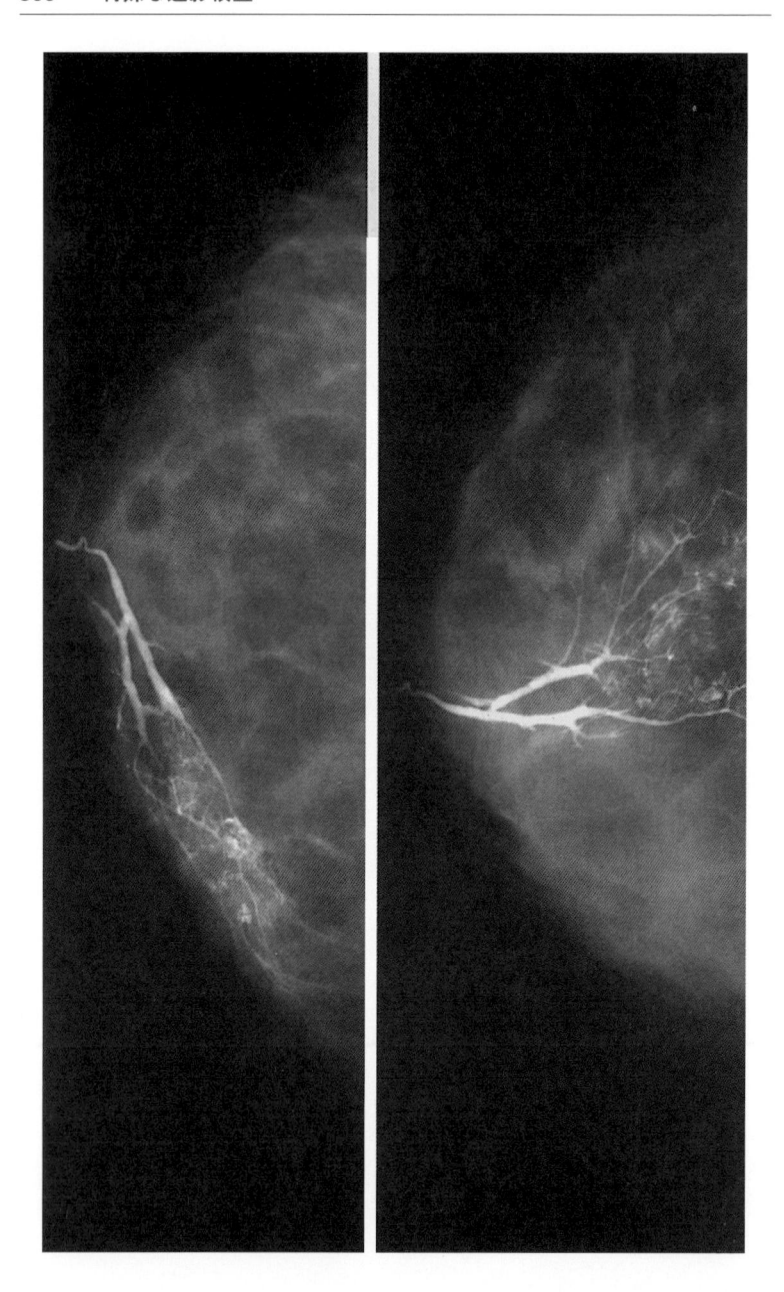

乳管造影　**367**

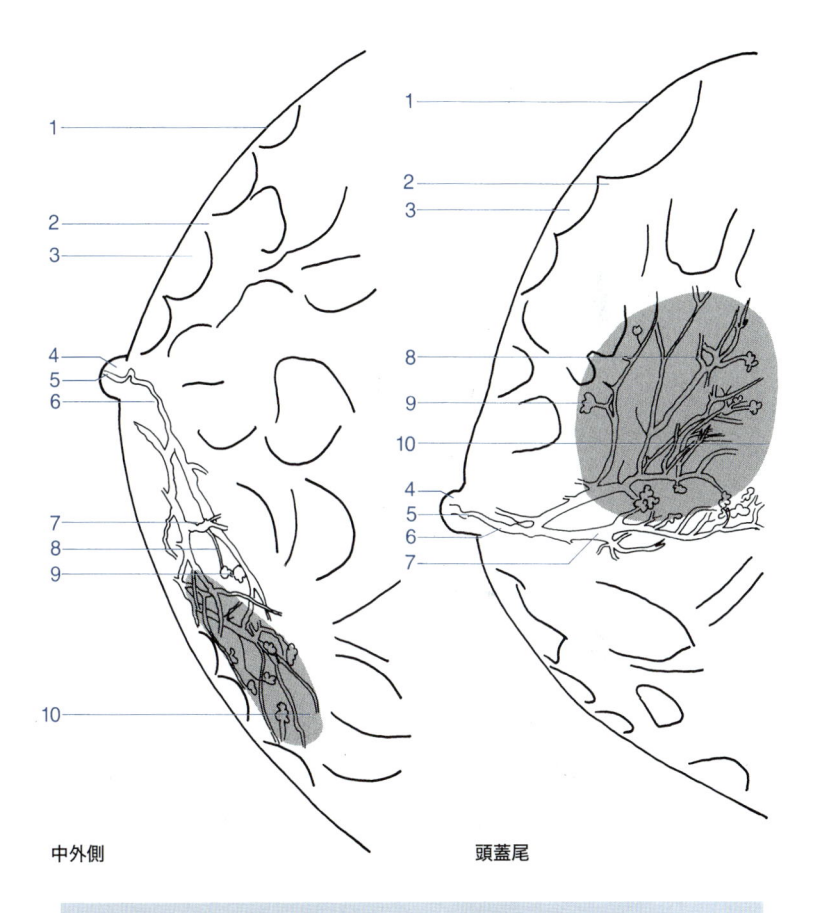

中外側

頭蓋尾

1	皮膚 Skin, 皮下組織 Subcutaneous tissue
2	Cooper 靱帯 Cooper's ligament
3	皮下脂肪組織 Subcutaneous fatty tissue
4	乳頭 Nipple
5	乳頭後方の主乳管 Main lactiferous duct posterior to the nipple
6	乳管洞 Lactiferous sinus
7	乳管 Lactiferous duct
8	乳管 Mammary ductule
9	乳腺小葉 Lobules of the mammary gland
10	乳腺腺葉 Lobe of the mammary gland

368 特殊な造影検査

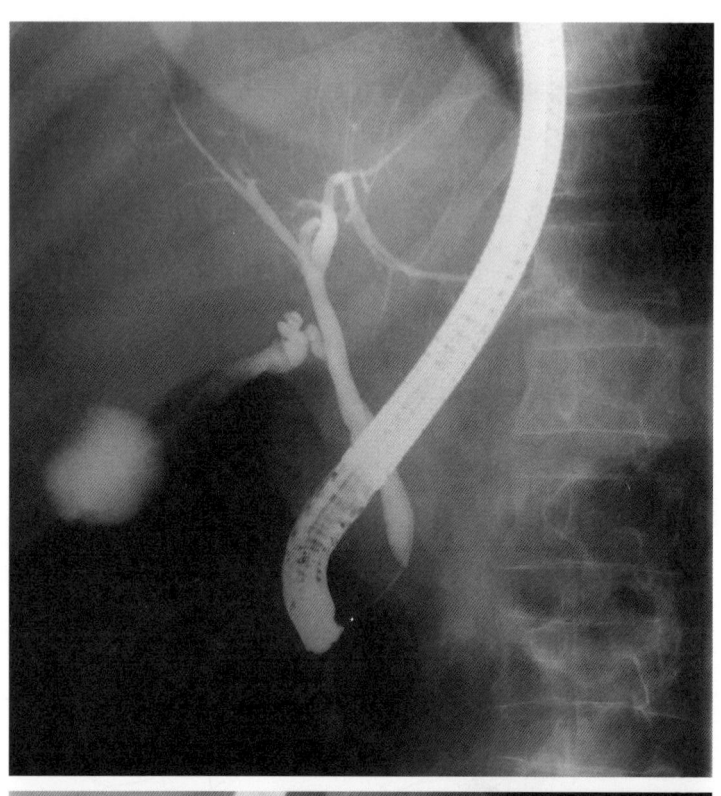

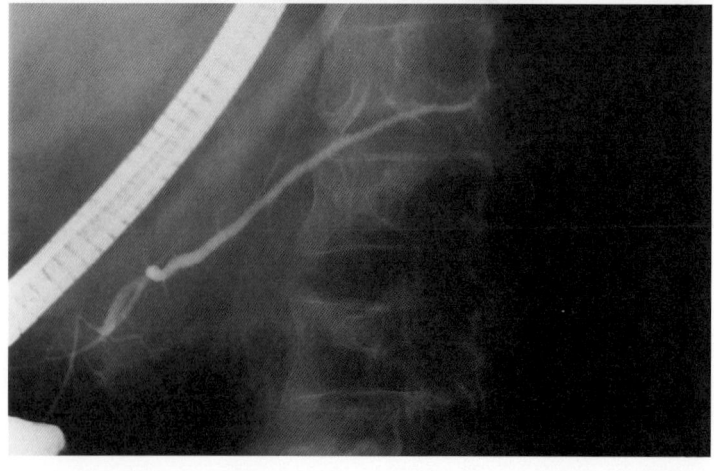

ERCP(内視鏡的膵胆管造影法)

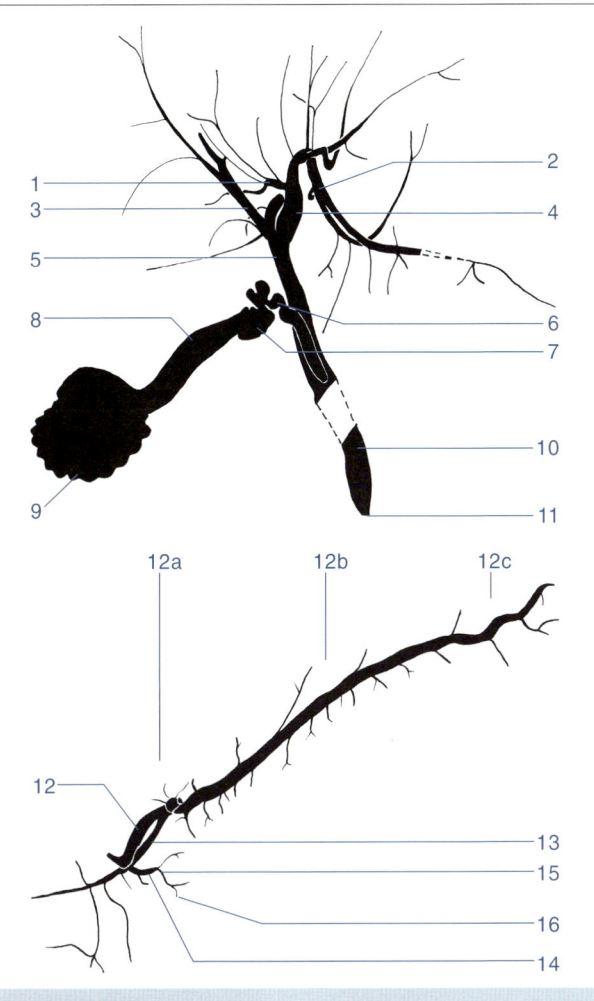

1 (左肝管の)内側枝 Medial branch of the left hepatic duct	12 膵管 Pancreatic duct (Wirsung管 Wirsung's duct)
2 外側枝 Lateral branch	a 頭部 Head region
3 右肝管 Right hepatic duct	b 体部 Body region
4 左肝管 Left hepatic duct	c 尾部 tail region
5 総肝管 Common hepatic duct	13 副膵管 Accessory pancreatic duct (Santorini管 Santorini's duct)
6 胆囊管 Cystic duct	14 一次分枝膵管 Primary lateral duct
7 胆囊頸部 Neck of the gallbladder	15 二次分枝膵管 Secondary lateral duct
8 胆囊体部 Body of the gallbladder	16 三次分枝膵管 Tertiary lateral duct
9 胆囊底部 Fundus of the gallbladder	
10 総胆管 Common bile duct	
11 Vater乳頭 Papilla of Vater (十二指腸乳頭 Duodenal papilla)	

和文索引

あ

アキレス腱　181,191
鞍結節　39
鞍背　31,39

い

胃　249,253
胃十二指腸動脈　305
胃食道角　247
胃底　249
胃泡　209,213,217～221
咽頭　241
咽頭後隙　231

う

ヴェサリウス骨　187
右胃大網動脈　305
右胃動脈　305
右下肺静脈　217
右下肺動脈　217
右下葉気管支　233
右肝動脈　305
右気管傍線　209
右結腸静脈　311
右結腸動脈　309
右主気管支　209,219,233
右上肺静脈　303
右上葉気管支　212,233
右心室　211～213,219,301,327
右心房　211,217～219,301～303,327
右腎　223,265
右腎静脈　315,329
右腎動脈　313
右肺　217～219
右肺静脈　219
右肺動脈　211,219,233～235,301,327
右腕頭静脈　211,327
烏口突起　83,89～111,115,273～275

え

エナメル質　22
腋窩　215,273,333
腋窩陥凹　273～275
腋窩静脈　333
遠位指節間関節　128～131,145,186,201～205

お

オトガイ孔　19～22
オトガイ隆起　3,19～21
横隔膜　51～53,209,213～214,217～219,221,245
横隔膜下腔　221
横行結腸　221,259
横静脈洞　285～287,293～295
横足根関節　186,203
横洞溝　7
横突起　45～59,75,79,83,237

か

下顎角　3,17～22
下顎管　3,19～22
下顎孔　19
下顎骨　3～5,9,47～49,229～231,243,363
　　関節突起　3
　　筋突起　5
下顎枝　17～21
下顎頭　7～9,19～22,29～37
下陥凹　277
下関節突起　47～59,237
下区動脈　313
下甲状腺静脈　327
下甲状腺動脈　297
下行結腸　259
下行膝動脈　321
下行大動脈　209,212,217～219,233,299
下後腸骨棘　61,65,75,237
下矢状静脈洞　287
下小脳半球静脈　293～295
下垂体窩　5,39～41

下膵十二指腸動脈　305,309
下錐体静脈洞　285〜287,293〜295
下前腸骨棘　67〜69,149〜153,157
下腿　146,177
下大静脈　211〜213,217〜219,301,329〜331,337
下虫部静脈　293
下殿動脈　317
下橈尺関節　124,129,133
下肺　214,303
下肺静脈　303
下鼻甲介　3,13
下部腎杯　265
下副腎動脈　313
下吻合静脈　287
下葉気管支　213,235
仮声帯　229
蝸牛　29〜31,35
顆間窩　161,167〜173
顆間隆起　146,161,165,169〜171,177
回結腸静脈　311
回結腸動脈　309
回腸　253〜257
　末端部　257
回腸静脈　311
回腸動脈　309
回盲弁　257〜259
海綿静脈洞　285〜287,295
解剖頸（上腕骨）　103,113
外脛骨　187
外頸静脈　327
外頸動脈　297
外後頭隆起　7
外耳　33
外耳孔　5
外耳道　33,37
外側顆間結節　159,163,167,175
外側クモ膜下腔　341
外側上顆（上腕骨）　113,117〜124
外側上顆（大腿骨）　159,163,167
外側上膝動脈　321
外側楔状骨　183,186〜189,197〜203
外側舌喉頭蓋ヒダ　241,245
外側仙骨動脈　317
外側仙骨稜　75,79〜81
外側大腿回旋動脈　319
外側中葉区　215
外側半規管　31,35
外側脈絡叢動脈　291
外側裂孔リンパ節　351
外腸骨リンパ節　353〜355
外腸管静脈　329〜331,337

外腸管動脈　317
角回動脈　281〜283
角切痕　249
顎関節　7,19〜21,33
滑車（上腕骨）　113〜117,121〜124
肝管　369
肝臓　221〜223,307
冠状縫合　5
貫通動脈　319
寛骨臼蓋　61〜63,69〜71,149〜157
寛骨涙痕　61
関節窩　89〜91,95,101〜103,107,111,115
関節結節　33
関節腔　169〜171,279
関節唇　103
関節突起　7〜9,19〜22,29〜37,45
関節突起間部　59
関節面　97,173
環軸関節　11,45
環椎　7,29,47〜49
　後弓　7,47
　前弓　29,47
眼窩　3〜5,9〜17,22,31,39
眼窩下孔　9
眼窩底　13,17,22
眼窩板　13,41
眼動脈　281〜283
顔面動脈　297

き

気管　45〜47,51,209,212,217〜219,229〜235,243
気管支　217,245
気管分岐部　209,219,233
奇静脈　211,233,327
奇静脈食道線　209
基節骨　128〜135,143〜145,186,189,201〜205
弓下窩　35
弓状静脈　315
弓状線　73
弓状動脈　313
弓状隆起　7,31,35
臼蓋　61〜63,69〜73,149,153〜155
臼蓋傾斜角　63
臼蓋嘴　61〜63,149
臼底　69〜71,149〜151,155
距骨　146,175〜199,279
　外側突起　181,191
　滑車　146,179〜181
　後突起　181,189〜191
距骨下関節　179,183〜185,191,199
距舟関節　181

距踵関節　183〜185
距踵舟関節　189,199,201〜203
距腿関節　183〜185,195
峡部頸管　365
胸郭　43
胸骨　219
　角　85〜87,212
　体　85〜87,212
　柄　85〜87,93
胸骨後腔　87,212
胸鎖関節　85,93
胸壁　214
頬骨　4〜5,9〜11,29,37
頬骨陥凹　27
頬骨弓　3,13〜15,22,27,31
頬骨前頭突起　13
頬骨突起　5
棘孔　29
棘上窩　101
棘突起　45〜59,75,237
近位指節間関節　128〜131,145,186,201〜205
近位手根列　124〜126
筋突起(下顎骨)　17〜22,27,29

く

クモ膜下腔脊髄神経根　345
クモ膜顆粒　3
区域気管支　357〜359
空回腸移行部　255
空腸　253〜255
空腸静脈　311
空腸動脈　309

け

外科頸(上腕骨)　103〜105,111〜113
茎状突起　22,33
脛骨　146,161,163〜171,175〜185,189,195,279
　外側顆　146,159,163,169〜171,175〜177
　内果　146,175〜186,195〜199,279
　内側顆　146,159,163,169〜171,175,177
脛骨高原　165〜167
脛骨粗面　165〜167,175〜177
脛腓関節　161,169,279
頸静脈球　293
頸静脈孔　7,29
頸切痕　85
頸椎　29,89
鶏冠　11
結節間腱鞘　273〜275

結腸　221,253,257
　肝弯曲部　259
　脾弯曲部　221,259
月状骨　124〜126,129〜143
犬歯　21〜22
肩関節　107
肩甲上動脈　297
肩甲上腕関節　107
肩甲切痕　105
肩甲下滑液包　273〜275
肩甲棘　89〜91,97〜105
肩甲頸　107
肩甲骨　53,89〜91,97〜107,113,212
　下角　83,97,101
　外側角(頸)　89,97,113
　　関節唇　273〜275
　　上角　89〜91,97〜107
肩鎖関節　89〜111,115
肩峰　83,89〜115,273〜275
剣状突起　85〜87

こ

股関節　43,67,75〜77,146
鼓室　31,35〜37
鼓室蓋　35
後気管腔　231
後クモ膜下腔　343
後交通動脈　283,291
後縦隔　214
後心腔　213
口蓋垂　243〜245
口腔　231
甲状頸動脈　297〜299
甲状軟骨　229〜231
肛門管　263
肛門直腸接合部　261
岬角　57,67,77,237
岬角リンパ節　351〜355
後咽頭腔　231
後下小脳動脈　289〜291
後篩骨洞　9
後床突起　5,39
後接合線　209
後側頭動脈　281〜283
後大脳動脈　289〜291
　視床枝　283
後柱　69〜71,149〜151
後直腸腔　261
後頭骨　4〜7,45
後頭静脈洞　287
後頭頂動脈　281〜282

後頭稜 7
後脈絡叢動脈 291
鉤状突起 45,115〜119,123〜126
鉤椎関節 45
鉤突窩 115,119,126
喉頭 243
喉頭蓋 231,241,245
喉頭蓋谷 229〜231,241〜243
喉頭室 229〜231,243
喉頭前庭 229〜231
硬口蓋 5,13,22
硬膜外腔 341
硬膜外脂肪 347
硬膜囊 341〜349
骨間膜 124〜126,167,175
骨幹端 105
骨髄腔 159,175〜177
骨端板 163
骨皮質 105,115,159,161〜163,175〜177
骨迷路 37

さ

左胃動脈 305
左下肺静脈 217
左下葉気管支 233
左肝動脈 305
左主気管支 209,219,233
左上葉気管支 212,233
左上葉肺動脈 217
左心室 211〜213,217〜219
左心房 211〜213,217,303
左腎 223,265
左腎静脈 315,329
左腎動脈 313
左肺 217〜219
左肺静脈 219,303
左肺動脈 211,217〜219,301,327
左腕頭静脈 327
鎖骨 51,83〜97,99〜115,209,273〜275
鎖骨円錐靱帯結節 91,95
鎖骨下静脈 327,333
鎖骨下動脈 211,297〜299
坐骨 61〜71,75〜77,81,146,149〜157
坐骨棘 61,65〜69,75〜77,81,149〜155
坐骨結節 61,65〜67,71,146,149〜153,157
載距突起 191〜193
三角筋粗面 113
三角骨 124〜126,129〜143,191
三角線維軟骨 269
三尖弁 211〜213

し

シルビウス静脈 285〜287
子宮 365
矢状縫合 3
指節骨 186
指腹 145
視床穿通動脈 289
視神経管 15
歯根 22
歯根管 19〜22
歯根尖孔 19〜22
歯髄腔 19〜22
歯突起 3,7,11,29,43〜49,231
篩骨神経溝 25
篩骨洞 3,5,13〜15,41
篩板 5
耳下腺 361〜363
　深葉 361〜363
　浅葉 361〜363
耳下腺管 361〜363
軸椎 3,7,11,29,43〜49,231
　歯突起 3,29,43〜45
舌 9,22
膝窩 161
膝窩陥凹 277
膝窩静脈 337
膝窩動脈 321
膝蓋下脂肪体 165
膝蓋骨 146,159〜173
膝蓋靱帯 165
膝蓋大腿関節 161,173
膝関節 146,169,171,177
斜台 5,29,39
尺骨 113〜133,139,271,335
　茎状突起 124〜126,129〜141,271
尺骨陥凹 269〜271
尺骨静脈 335
尺骨神経溝 121
尺側皮静脈 335
手根骨 124〜126
手根中手関節 133,143
主気管支 209,219,233,357〜359
種子骨 128〜131,143,186〜205
舟状骨 124〜126,129〜143,179〜191,197〜203
十二指腸 249〜253
　下行部 249〜253
　球部 249〜253
　上行部 253
　水平部 253

十二指腸空腸移行部　253
十二指腸乳頭　251
小臼歯　21〜22
小坐骨切痕　77
小腸　221
小転子　61,71,149〜157
小殿筋　61,149
小頭　115〜117,121〜124
小脳半球静脈　293
小伏在静脈　337
小菱形骨　129〜143
小弯(胃)　249
掌側陥凹　269〜271
踵骨　179〜199,279
踵骨隆起　181,189〜193
踵立方関節　189,201
上顎骨　3,17,21,25
上顎洞　3〜5,9〜17,21〜22,27〜31,41
　歯槽陥凹　9,22
上陥凹　277
上関節突起　47〜59,75
上眼窩裂　13〜15
上距骨骨　187
上区動脈　313
上甲状腺動脈　297
上行頸動脈　297
上行結腸　257〜259
上行前頭静脈　287
上行大動脈　212,217〜219,299
上後腸骨棘　61,65,75,237
上矢状静脈洞　285〜287
上視床線条体静脈　285〜287
上十二指腸上動脈　305
上小脳動脈　289〜291
上小脳半球静脈　295
上踵骨陥凹　279
上膝十二指腸動脈　305
上錐体静脈洞　287,295
上舌枝　359
上前腸骨棘　61,65〜69,149〜155
上大静脈　211,233,301,327,333
上大脳静脈　293
上腸間膜静脈　311
上腸間膜動脈　305,309
上殿動脈　317
上橈尺関節　117,123〜124
上肺静脈　303
上半規管　31,35
上吻合静脈　285〜287
上腕骨　83,89〜126,335
　解剖頸　103,113
　外側上顆　113,117〜124

上腕骨(続き)
　滑車　126
　外科頸　103〜105,111〜113
　三角筋粗面　113
　小結節　89,93〜95,103,107〜115
　小頭　115〜117,121〜124
　大結節　89,93〜95,103,107〜113
　頭　83,89〜115
　内側上顆　113,117〜124
上腕静脈　333〜335
上腕深部静脈　333
上腕二頭筋　273〜275
　長頭腱鞘　273〜275
静脈角　327
静脈洞交会　287,293〜295
食道　231,241〜247
食道裂孔　247
神経根袖　341,345
神経根鞘　349
深鼠径リンパ節　351
深大腿静脈　337
深大腿動脈　317〜319
腎盂　265
腎臓　265
腎静脈　315,331
腎動脈　313
腎杯　265

す

膵管　369
錐体　3,7〜13,31〜39
錐体静脈　293

せ

正円孔　9,13
正中仙骨動脈　317
正中仙骨稜　75〜81
成長板　159,163,167,175,179〜181
声帯　229
声門下腔　229〜231
声門裂　229
脊髄　341〜343
脊髄円錐　341〜343
切歯　21〜22
楔舟関節　189,199
舌　22,231,243
舌根　243
仙骨　43,55〜57,61,65〜69,73〜81,149,221〜
　223,237,261,237,347
　外側部　73

仙骨（続き）
　岬角　57,67,77,237
仙骨角　75〜81
仙骨管　77,81
仙骨孔　55,73〜79,237
仙骨翼　65,75,237
仙骨裂孔　75,79
仙腸関節　43,55,61,69〜75,149〜155,237
浅鼠径リンパ節　351〜353
浅大腿静脈　337
浅大腿動脈　317〜321
前大脳動脈A2部　281〜283
前大脳動脈A3部　281
腺組織　225〜227
前下小脳動脈　289〜291
前眼動脈　281〜283
前弓　49
前クモ膜下腔　343
前脛骨静脈　337
前脛骨動脈　321〜325
前交通動脈　281
前篩骨洞　9〜11
前縦隔　214
前床突起　5,39
前前頭動脈　281〜283
前中心溝動脈　281
前中心小脳静脈　295
前柱　69〜71,149〜153
前庭　31,35
　ひだ　229
前頭蓋底　39
前頭頬骨縫合　3
前頭極動脈　281〜282
前頭骨　4
前頭静脈　285
前頭頂動脈　281〜282
前頭洞　3,5,9〜15,31,41
前頭鼻骨縫合　25
前半規管　31,35
前鼻棘　17,25
前脈絡叢動脈　281〜283
前腕　124〜126
前腕正中皮静脈　335

そ

僧帽弁　211〜213
総肝管　267〜369
総肝動脈　305
総頸動脈　297〜299
総大腿動脈　317
総胆管　267〜369

総腸骨静脈　329〜331,337
総腸骨動脈　317
総腸骨リンパ節　351〜353,355
象牙質　22
足関節　146,179〜185,189,195
足根間関節　201〜203
足根中足関節　186,189,199,201〜205
足根洞　181,191,199
足底腱膜　191
足底動脈　325
足背動脈　325
側頭下顎関節　21
側頭窩　27
側頭頬骨縫合　27
側頭極動脈　281
側頭後頭動脈　289〜291
側頭骨　4,5,15,21,27,33
　岩様部　5,15
　頬骨突起　27,33

た

大臼歯　21〜22
大結節稜　109
大後頭孔　5〜7,29〜31,45
大坐骨切痕　67,75〜77,81
大腿骨　61〜67,146〜167
　内側顆　146,159〜163,167〜177
　内側上顆　159,163,167
　外側顆　146,159,161〜177
　外側上顆　159,163,167
　頸　61,71,149〜157
　頭　65〜71,75,146,149〜157,261
　体　159,169〜171
大腿骨頭窩　149
大腿静脈　337
大転子　61,69,146,149〜157
大動脈弓　211〜212,217〜219,233,245,299
大動脈根部　299
大動脈肺動脈窓　212
大動脈弁　211〜213
大動脈傍線　209
大伏在静脈　337
大腰筋　55
大翼（蝶形骨）　5,9,13,29,39
大菱形骨　129〜143
大弯（胃）　249
第1胸椎横突起　45
第1頸椎外側塊　45
第1中足骨　205
第1腰椎　43
第1肋骨　45,51

第 1 肋骨（続き）
　肋骨結節　51
第 2 胸椎　43
第 2 頸椎　49,243
　椎体　49
第 2 立方骨　187
第 3～第 5 中手骨　143
第 3 腰椎　43,349
　椎弓根　43
第 5 中手骨　133,143
第 5 中足骨　181,186,189～191,195～203
第 5 腰椎　73～77,237
　横突起　73
　関節突起　75
　椎弓根　75
　椎体　73
第 6 腰椎棘突起　43
第 7 頸椎　43,231
第 12 胸椎　43
第 12 肋骨　265
胆嚢　267,369
胆嚢管　267,369
胆嚢動脈　305

ち

恥骨　63,69～71,146,149～157
　下枝　61,65～67,71,151
　上枝　61,65～67,75,79,149～151
恥骨結合　61,65～67,79
恥骨直腸筋　263
腟　365
中咽頭　243
中間気管支　209,233～235
中間楔状骨　183,186～189,197～203
中区動脈　313
中結腸動脈　309
中硬膜動脈溝　5
中膝動脈　321
中手骨　128～131,135,139～145
中手指節関節　128～131,143～145
中縦隔　214
中節骨　128,145,186～189,201～205
中足骨　183,186～189,197～203
中足骨間骨　187
中足指節関節　186～205
中大脳動脈　281～283
　M1 部　281
　M2 部　281～283

中頭蓋窩　29
中頭蓋窩前壁　29
中葉　214
中葉気管支　233～235
虫垂　255,259
虫部枝　289
肘正中皮静脈　335
肘頭　113～126
肘頭窩　113～119,123～126
肘部管　121
長腓骨筋腱溝　193
腸間膜静脈合流部　307
腸骨　43,63,73,153～155,221～223,237
腸骨坐骨線　149
腸骨恥骨線　65,71
腸骨翼　61,65,69,73～75
腸骨稜　57,61,65,67～69,77,81,221～223,347
腸腰筋　221～223,265
蝶形骨　3～4,11～15,39～41
　小翼　13～15
　大翼　5,9,13,29,39
蝶形骨洞　5,9,15,29,39
蝶形骨頂静脈洞　285
蝶錐体裂　35
蝶鱗縫合　35
直静脈洞　287,293～295
直腸　81,259～263
　膨大部　261～263
直腸 S 状結腸移行部　261
直腸横ヒダ　261

つ

椎間関節　47～49,53～55
椎間関節柱　47
椎間孔　49,53,57～59,347
椎間板　341～349
椎間板腔　45～47,53～59
椎弓　45
椎弓根　45,49～51,55,59,237
椎弓板　47,59,237
椎骨動脈　289～291,297～299
椎骨傍線　51
椎体　47,51～59

て

転子間稜　61,149,153～155

と

トルコ鞍底 41
豆状骨 124〜126,129,133〜143
島部 281
透明中隔静脈 287
頭蓋底 17,47,231
頭頂後頭動脈 289〜291
頭頂骨 4,5
頭頂静脈 285〜287
橈骨 113〜135,139〜143,271,335
　茎状突起 124,129〜135,139,143
　頸 117,123〜126
　頭 113〜126
橈骨手根関節 124〜126,133,143
橈骨静脈 335
橈骨粗面 119,123〜124
橈側皮静脈 327,333〜335
同側の横突起 59
動脈円錐 327

な

内胸動脈 297
内頸静脈 287,327
内頸動脈 281〜283,297
内後頭隆起 7,35
内後頭稜 35
内耳道 3,7,11,29〜35
内側下膝動脈 321
内側顆間結節 159,163,167,175
内側後前頭動脈 282
内側後頭動脈の鳥距動脈 289〜291
内側上顆（上腕骨） 113,119〜123
内側上顆（大腿骨） 159,163,167
内側上膝動脈 321
内側上頭頂動脈 282
内側楔状骨 181〜183,186,189,197〜203
内側前前頭動脈 282
内側大腿回旋動脈 319
内側中前頭動脈 282
内側中葉区 215
内側脈絡叢動脈 291
内大脳静脈 285〜287,295
内腸骨静脈 329〜331
内腸骨動脈 317
内腸骨リンパ節 353,355
内閉鎖筋 61,223
軟口蓋 5,22
軟骨 277

に

二頭筋溝 93〜95,103,107〜113
乳管 225〜227,367
乳管洞 367
乳腺 367
乳頭 225〜227,367
乳突洞 31〜37
乳突洞口 37
乳突蜂巣 7,29〜31
乳様突起 3,33,37
尿管 265

の

脳底動脈 289〜291
脳梁周囲動脈 281〜283
脳梁辺縁動脈 281〜283
囊状陥凹 269

は

ハウストラ 257,259
パキオニ顆粒 3
破裂孔 29
馬尾 343〜349
背側陥凹 269〜271,279
肺区域 215
肺静脈 211〜213
肺舌動脈 301
肺尖 209
肺動脈 211,217,235,301
　下葉枝 301
　中葉枝 235,301
　肺尖枝 235,301
肺動脈幹 211〜212,217,301,327
肺動脈弁 211〜212
肺門部 214
半規管 7,29
半月圧痕 269
半月板 277
板間層 5

ひ

披裂間切痕 229
披裂軟骨 229
脾静脈 307,311
脾臓 223,307
脾臓下縁 221
脾動脈 305,313

和文索引

腓骨　146,161〜163,175〜185,189,195,279
　外果　146,175〜186,191〜199,279
　頸　165〜167,175
　体　169〜171
　頭　159〜171,175〜177
腓骨筋骨　187
腓骨静脈　337
腓骨動脈　321〜323
尾骨　61,65〜67,75〜81,261
尾骨角　75,79
鼻咽頭　5
鼻腔　11,21〜22,31
鼻甲介　41
鼻骨　5,9,25
鼻骨上顎縫合　25
鼻前庭　25
鼻中隔　3,9〜13,17,29〜31,41
鼻軟骨　25
左胃動脈　305
左下肺静脈　217
左下葉気管支　233
左肝動脈　305
左主気管支　209,219,233
左上葉気管支　212,233
左上葉肺動脈　217
左腎　223,265
左腎静脈　315,329
左腎動脈　313
左肺　217〜219
左肺静脈　219,303
左肺動脈　211,217〜219,301,327
左腕頭静脈　327

ふ

副耳下腺　361
副膵管　369
副鼻腔後部蜂巣　37
腹側陥凹　279
腹大動脈　313,317
腹部食道　247〜249
腹筋　223
腹腔動脈　305
噴門　247〜249
分界線　149

へ

閉鎖孔　61,67〜71,146,149〜153,157
閉鎖動脈　317
辺縁動脈　289

ほ

母指指節間関節　186,205
傍脊椎線　209
傍大動脈リンパ節　355
傍中心動脈　282
膀胱　61,221〜223,265

ま

末節骨　128,145,186〜205

み

右胃大網動脈　305
右胃動脈　305
右下肺静脈　217
右下肺動脈　217
右下葉気管支　233
右肝動脈　305
右気管傍線　209
右結腸静脈　311
右結腸動脈　309
右主気管支　209,219,233
右上肺静脈　303
右上葉気管支　212,233
右腎　223,265
右腎静脈　315,329
右腎動脈　313
右肺　217〜219
右肺静脈　219
右肺動脈　211,219,233〜235,301,327
右腕頭静脈　211,327

む

無名線　3,11〜13
盲腸　255〜259
門脈　307,311
　右枝　311
　左枝　311

ゆ

有鈎骨　129〜143
　鈎　133〜137
有頭骨　129〜143
幽門　249〜251
幽門洞　249〜253

よ

葉間耳下腺管　361〜363
葉間静脈　315
葉間動脈　313
葉間肺動脈　211
葉気管支　357〜359
腰動脈　317
腰リンパ節　351〜353
腰リンパ本幹　351〜353
翼口蓋窩　22,29
翼状突起　22
翼突窩　29
翼突筋静脈叢　287

ら

ラムダ縫合　3〜7
卵円孔　9,29
卵管　365
卵管采　365
卵管子宮開口部　365

り

梨状陥凹　229〜231,241〜245
立方骨　181〜191,197〜203
鱗部蜂巣　33

る

ルシュカ関節　45

れ

裂孔リンパ節　353〜355

ろ

漏斗部　217
肋横突関節　83,91
肋椎関節　83
肋骨　49〜53,59,83,99〜101
　頸　51,83
　頭　51〜53,83
肋骨横隔膜角　209,221
肋骨切痕　85

わ

腕尺関節　117〜119,123〜124
腕頭動脈　297,299
腕橈関節　117〜119,123〜124

欧文

A2部　281〜283
A3部　281
Chopart関節　186,203
Citelli角　33
CM関節　133,143
Cooper靱帯　225〜227,367
DIP関節　128〜131,145,186,201〜205
Galen大静脈　285〜287,295
Hilgenreiner線　63
Houston弁　261
IP関節　186,205
Köhlerの涙痕　149
Labbe静脈　287
Lisfranc関節　186,203
M1部　281
M2部　281〜283
MP関節　128〜131,143〜145,186,189,201〜205
Perkin線　63
PIP関節　128〜131,145,186,201〜205
Roland静脈　285
Rosenthal脳底静脈　285〜287,295
Shenton線　63
Stensen管　361〜363
S状結腸　259
S状静脈洞　37,285〜287,293〜295
S状洞溝　33
Trolard静脈　285〜287
Vater乳頭　251,369
WibergのCE角　63
Wirsung管　369

欧文索引

A

abdominal aorta 313,317
accessory bones 187
accessory pancreatic duct 369
accessory parotid gland 361
acetabulum
 convexity 61～63,149
 floor 69～71,149～151,155
 promontory 61～63,149
 rim 61
  anterior 69～71,149～157
  posterior 69～71,149～153,157
  superior 151～153
 roof 63,69～73,149,153～155
 teardrop 61
Achilles tendon 181,191
acromioclavicular joint 89～111,115
acromion 83,89～115,273～275
adrenal artery, inferior 313
air cells 7,29～33,37
alveolar recess (maxillary sinus) 9,23
ampulla of Vater 249～253
anal canal 263
anastomotic vein
 inferior 287
 superior 285～287
anatomical neck (humerus) 103,113
angiography
 ankle 324～325
 aorta, pelvic 317
 aortic arch 298～299
 celiac trunk 304～307
 cervical vessels 296～297
 foot 324～325
 knee 320～321
 leg, lower 322～323
 thigh 318～319
angle of Citelli 33
angle of acetablar inclination 63
angle of mandible 3,17～23
angular gyrus 281～282
ankle 147,178～185,189

ankle (続き)
 angiogram 324～325
 arthrogram 278～279
 recesses
  anterior/posterior 279
  supracalcaneal 279
  tendon 279
ankle joint space 183～185,195,279
anorectal junction 261
anterior arch (atlas) 47～49
anterior cerebral artery 281～283
anterior choroidal artery 281～283
anterior column (pubis) 69～71,149～153
anterior cranial fossa 39
anterior tibial artery 321～325
aorta
 abdominal 313
 ascending 213,217～219,299
 descending 209,213,217～219,233,299
aortic arch 211～213,217～219,233,245,289
aortic bulb 299
aortic valve 211～213
aortopulmonary window 213
appendix 255,259
arcuate arteries 313
arcuate eminence 7,31,35
arcuate line 73
arcuate vein 315
arm
 deep veins 333
 upper 112～115
 →elbow；forearm；shoulder；wristも参照
arthrography
 ankle 278～279
 knee 276～277
 shoulder 272～275
 wrist 268～271
articular facet 47
articular pillar 47
articular processes
 cervical 45～49
 lumbar 55～59
 sacral 75,237
 thoracic 51～53

articular tubercle　33
arytenoid cartilages　229
ascending aorta　213,217〜219,299
ascending colon　257〜259
atlantoaxial joint　11,45
atlas　7,45〜49
　anterior arch　47〜49
　posterior arch　7,47
atrium
　left　211〜213,303
　right　211,217〜219,301〜303,327
auditory canal
　external　5,33,37
　internal　3,7,11,29〜35
auditory vestibule　31,35
axillary recess　273〜275
axillary vein　333
axis　3,29,43〜49,231,243
　body　47〜49
　dens　3,29,43〜45,231
azygoesophageal stripe　209
azygos vein　211,233,327

B

basal vein
　common/inferior　303
　of Rosenthal　285〜287,295
basilar artery　289〜291
basilic vein　335
biceps muscle (tendon sheath of long head)　273〜275
biceps tendon　275
bicipital groove　93〜95,103,107〜113
bipedal lymphangiogram　350〜355
brachial veins　333〜335
brachiocephalic trunk　297〜299
brachiocephalic vein　211,327
breast　209,225〜227,367
bronchogram　356〜359
bronchus　209,213,217〜219,233〜235,357〜359
　intermediate　209,233〜235
　lower lobe　213,233〜235
　main　209,219,233,357〜359
　middle lobe　233〜235
　upper lobe　213,233〜235

C

calcaneocuboid joint　189,201
calcaneus　181〜199,279
　arthrogram　279

calcaneus (続き)
　peroneal trochlea　193
　posterior tuberosity　181,189〜193
　sustentaculum tali　191〜193
callosomarginal artery　281〜283
canine teeth　21〜23
capitate　129〜143
capitellum (humerus)　115〜117,121〜125
capsular recesses, inferior/superior　277
cardia　247
carpal bones　125〜127
　proximal row　125〜127
carpal tunnel　136〜137
carpometacarpal joint　133,143
cauda equina　343〜349
cavernous sinus　287,295
cecum　255〜259
celiac trunk　305
cephalic vein　327,333〜335
cerebellar artery　289〜291
cerebellar veins　293〜295
cerebral artery
　anterior　281〜283
　corpus callosal branch　291
　middle　281〜283
　posterior　289〜291
cerebral veins
　great - of Galen　285〜287,295
　internal　285〜287,295
　superior　293
cerebrum, communicating artery
　anterior　281
　posterior　283,291
cervical artery, ascending　297
cervical canal　365
cervical spine　44〜49,89,243
　intervertebral disk space　45〜47
　intervertebral facet joint　47
　intervertebral foramen　49
cervical vertebrae
　anterior arch (C1)　47〜49
　atlas (C1)　7,45〜49
　　anterior arch　47〜49
　　lateral mass　45
　　posterior arch　7,47
　axis (C2)　3,29,43〜49,231,243
　　body　47〜49
　　dens (=odontoid process)　3,29,43〜49,231
　C1 (atlas)　7,45〜49
　C2 (axis)　3,29,43〜49,231,243
　C7　43,231

cervical vertebrae（続き）
　dens（＝odontoid process）　3,29,43〜49,231
　pedicle　45,49
　posterior arch（C1）　7,47
　spinous process　45〜49
　transverse process　45〜49
　uncinate process　45
cervical vessels　296〜297
cholangiopancreatography, endoscopic retrograde
　（ERCP）　368〜369
cholecystochlolangiography　266〜267
Chopart's joint　187,203
choroidal arteries　281〜283,291
Citelli, angle of　33
circumflex fibular artery　323
clavicle　51,83〜115,209,273〜275
　acromioclavicular joint　93〜95
　conoid tubercle　91,95
Clementschitsch view　21
clinoid processes, anterior/posterior　5,39
clivus　39
coccyx　61,65〜67,75〜81,261
　cornu　75,79
cochlea　29〜31,35
colic arteries, middle/right　309
colic vein, right　311
colon　221,253,257〜259
　haustra　257〜259
　hepatic flexure　259
　splenic flexure　221,259
common bile duct　267,369
common carotid artery　297〜299
communicating artery of cerebrum
　anterior　281
　posterior　283,291
condylar process（mandible）　3
confluence of sinuses　287,293〜295
conoid tubercle　91,95
Cooper's ligaments　225〜227
coracoid process　83,89〜97,101〜111,115,
　273〜275
coronal suture　5
coronoid fossa　115,119,127
coronoid process（mandible）　5,17〜21,27〜29
coronoid process（ulna）　115〜119,123〜127
corpus callosal branch（cerebral artery）　291
costal arch　83
costal notch　85
costodiaphragmatic recess　209,221
costophrenic angle　209,221
costotransverse joint　83,91
costovertebral articulation　83

cranial fossa
　anterior　39
　middle　29
cribiform plate　5
crista galli　11
cubital tunnel　121
cubital vein, median　335
cuboid　181〜191,197〜203
cuneiform bones
　intermediate　183,187〜189,197〜203
　lateral　183,187〜189,197〜203
　medial　181〜183,187〜189,197〜203
cuneonavicular joint　189,199
cystic artery　305
cystic duct　267,369

D

defecography　262〜263
deltoid tuberosity　113
dens（axis）　3,7,11,29,43〜45,231
dentin　23
descending aorta　209,213,217〜219,233,299
descending colon　259
diaphragm　51〜53,209,217,221
　insertions　209
diploe　5
disk→intervertebral diskを参照
disk space→intervertebral disk spaceを参照
dorsalis pedis artery　325
dorsum sellae　31,39
duodenojejunal flexure　253
duodenum　249〜253
dural sac　341〜349

E

ear
　cochlea　29〜31,35
　external auditory canal　33,37
　internal auditory canal　3,7,11,29〜35
　semicircular canals　7,29〜31,35
　tympanic cavity　31,35〜37
elbow　116〜121
enamel　23
endoscopic retrograde cholangiopancreatography
　（ERCP）　368〜369
epidural fat　345
epiglottis　231,241,245
esophageal hiatus　247
esophagus　231,241〜249
ethmoid sinus　3,5,9〜15,41

ethmoidal groove　25
extensor recess(wrist)　271
external auditory canal　5,33,37
external carotid artery　280〜287,297
external jugular vein　327
extradural space　341

F

facet joints
　cervical spine　47〜49
　lumbar spine　55
　thoracic spine　53
facial artery　297
facial nerve　361〜363
fallopian tube　365
femoral arteries　319〜321
femoral vein　337
femur　61〜75,147〜177,261
　greater trochanter　61,69,147〜157
　head　65〜71,75,147〜157,261
　　fovea　149
　intercondylar fossa　161,167〜173
　lateral condyle　147,159〜177
　lateral epicondyle　159,163,167
　lesser trochanter　61,71,149〜157
　medial condyle　147,159〜177
　medial epicondyle　159,163,167
　neck　61,71,149〜157
　　Shenton's line　63
fibula　147,159〜171,175〜197,279
　head　159〜167,171,175〜177
　lateral malleolus　147,175〜187,191〜197
　neck　165〜167,175
fibular artery, circumflex　323
fimbriae, fallopian tube　365
fingers　128〜129,144〜145
fissure
　orbital, superior　13〜15
　sphenopetrosal　35
flexor recess, wrist　271
foot　186〜205
　accessory bones　187
　angiogram　324〜325
　sesamoid bones　187〜189,201〜205
foramen lacerum　29
foramen magnum　5,7,31,45
foramen ovale　9,29
foramen rotundum　9,13
forearm　124〜127
　venogram　334〜335
forefoot　200〜203

Frik tunnel view　166〜167
frontal artery　282
frontal sinus　3〜5,9〜15,31,41
frontal veins　285,287
frontonasal suture　25
frontozygomatic suture　3

G

galactogram　366〜367
Galen, great cerebral vein　285〜287,295
gallbladder　267,369
gastric artery, left/right　305
gastric bubble　209,213,217〜221
gastric folds, posterior wall　249
gastroduodenal artery　305
gastroepiploic artery, right　305
gastroesophageal angle　247
gastrointestinal system, contrast studies　240〜263
genicular artery　321
glandular tissue, breast　225〜227
glenohumeral joint　107
glenoid fossa　89〜91,95,101〜103,107,111,115
glenoid labrum　103,273〜275
glossoepiglottic fold, lateral　241,245
gluteal artery, inferior/superior　317
gluteus minimus, fat stripe medial to　61,149
gonad shield　43
greater sciatic notch　67,75〜77,81
greater trochanter　61,69,147〜157
great toe　187,204〜205
　distal interphalangeal joint　187
　distal phalanx　187

H

hamate　129〜133,137〜143
　hook　133〜137
hand　128〜131
　sesamoid bones　129〜131,143
hard palate　5,13,23
haustra(colon)　257〜259
heart　210〜211
hemidiaphragm　213,219
hepatic artery　305
hepatic duct　267,369
Hilgrenreiner's line　63
hindfoot, standing patient　194〜195
hip　43,67,75〜77,147〜151,156〜157
　joint space　67,147
humeroradial joint　117〜119,123〜125
humeroulnar joint　117〜119,123〜125

humerus 89,105〜127
　anatomical neck 103,113
　bicipital groove 93〜95,103,107〜113
　capitellum 115〜117,121〜125
　coracoid process 83,89〜97,101〜111,115,
　　273〜275
　coronoid fossa 115,119,127
　deltoid tuberosity 113
　epicondyle lateral 113,117〜125
　　medial epicondyle 113〜125
　head 83,89,97,101〜119,127
　metaphysis 105
　neck
　　anatomical 103,113
　　surgical 103〜105,111〜113
　olecranon fossa 113〜119,123〜127
　shaft 99,101,115
　surgical neck 103〜105,111〜113
　trochlea 113〜117,121〜127
　tubercle
　　greater 89,93〜95,103,107〜113
　　lesser 89,93〜95,103,107〜115
hyoid bone 23,231,243
hypopharynx 240〜243
hysterosalpingogram 364〜365

I

ileal arteries 309
ileal veins 311
ileocecal region, spot images 256〜257
ileocecal valve 257〜259
ileocolic artery 309
ileocolic vein 311
ileum 253〜257
iliac crest 57,61,65〜69,77,81,221〜223
iliac lymph channels 353
iliac lymph nodes
　common 351〜355
　external 351〜355
　internal 353〜355
iliac spine
　anterior inferior 67〜69,149〜153,157
　anterior superior 61,65〜69,149〜155
　posterior inferior 61,65,75,237
　posterior superior 61,65,75,237
iliac vein
　common 329〜331,337
　external 329〜331,337
　internal 329〜331
iliac wing 61,65,69,73〜75,237
ilioischial line 149

iliopectineal line 71
iliopubic line 65
ilium 43,73,153〜155,221〜223,237
　child 63
incisor teeth 21〜23
inferior adrenal artery 313
inferior anastomotic vein 287
inferior angle (scapula) 83,99〜101
inferior petrosal sinus 285〜287,293〜295
inferior sagittal sinus 287
inferior vena cava 211〜213,217〜219,301,
　329〜331,337
infraorbital foramen 9
infundibulum 217,327
inguinal lymph nodes 351〜353
inner ear 31
innominate line 3,11〜13
interarytenoid notch 229
intercavernous sinus 285
intercondylar fossa 161,167〜171
intergluteal fat stripe 149
interlobular arteries 313
interlobular vein 315
intermediate cuneiform 183,187〜189,197〜203
internal auditory canal 3,7,11〜13,29〜35
internal jugular vein 287,327
interosseous membrane 125〜127,167,175
interphalangeal joint
　distal 129〜131,145,187,201〜205
　great toe 205
　proximal 129〜131,145,187,201〜205
intertarsal joint 201〜203
intertrochanteric crest 61,149,153〜155
intertubercular sheath 273〜275
intervertebral disk 341〜349
intervertebral disk space
　cervical spine 45〜47
　lumbar spine 55〜59
　thoracic spine 53
intervertebral facet joints
　cervical spine 47〜49
　lumbar spine 55
　thoracicl spine 53
intervertebral foramen
　cervical spine 49
　lumbar spine 55〜59,347
　thoracic spine 53
intradural space 341
intramedullary region 341
intrapatellar fat pad 165
ischium 61〜71,75〜77,81,147〜157
　body 67

ischium（続き）
    child 63
    posterior column 69〜71,149〜151
    spine 61,65〜69,75〜77,81,149〜155
    tuberosity 61,65〜67,71,147〜153,157

J

jejunal arteries 309
jejunal veins 311
jejunum 253〜255
joint space
    ankle 183〜185,195,279
    hip 67,147
    knee 147,169〜171
joints
jugular foramen 7
jugular bulb 293

K

kidney 223,265
knee 147,163〜171,177,277,321
    angiogram 321
    arthrogram 277
    capsular recess, inferior/superior 277
    joint space 147,169〜171
    meniscus 277
    popliteal bursa 277
Köhler's teardrop figure 149

L

Labbé, vein of 287
lactiferous duct 225〜227,367
lactiferous sinus 367
lacunar lymph nodes 351〜355
lambdoid suture 3〜7
lamina（spine） 47,59
larynx 243
    ventricle 229〜231,243
    vestibule 229〜231
lateral malleolus 147,175〜187,191〜197
lateral condyle（femur） 147,159〜177
lateral cuneiform 183,187〜189,197〜203
lateral epicondyle（femur） 159,163,167
lateral epicondyle（humerus） 113,117〜125
lateral malleolus（fibula） 147,175〜187,
    191〜197
lateral sacral crest 75,79〜81
left atrium 211〜213,303
left ventricle 211〜213, 217〜219

lesser sciatic notch 77
lesser trochanter 61,71,149〜157
leg
    angiograms 318〜325
    lower 146〜147,174〜177
        angiogram 322〜323
        venogram, rotational views 336〜337
        →ankle；hip；knee；thighも参照
Lisfranc's joints 187,203
liver 221〜223,307
lumbar lymph nodes 351〜353
lumbar lymphangiography 350〜355
    channel phase 350〜351
    nodal phase 354〜355
lumbar myelography 344〜349
lumbar spine 43,54〜59,344〜349
    intervertebral disk space 55〜59
    intervertebral foramen 57〜59,347
    myelography 344〜349
lumbar vertebrae
    L1 43
    L3, pedicle 43
    L5 73〜77,237
        body 73
        inferior articular process 75
        pedicle 73
        transverse process 73
    pedicle 43,55,59,73
    spinous process 43
lunate 125〜143
lung 209,214〜219,357〜359
    apex 209
    lower lobe 215,357〜359
    middle lobe 215
    segments 214〜215
    upper lobe 215〜217,357〜359
        lingula segment 357〜359
lymph nodes
    common iliac 351〜355
    external iliac 351〜355
    inguinal 351〜353
    internal iliac 353〜355
    lumbar 351〜353
    para-aortic 355
    promontory 351〜355
lymph tracts 351〜353
lymphangiography 350〜355

M

malleolus 199
    lateral 147,175〜187,191〜197,279

malleolus（続き）
　　medial　147,175〜187,195〜197,279
mammography　224〜227
mandible　3〜9,17〜23,27〜37,47〜49,229〜231,243,363
　　angle　3,17〜23
　　condyle　3,7〜9,19〜21,31〜37
　　coronoid process　5,17〜21,27〜29
　　ramus　17〜21
mandibular canal　3,19〜23
mandibular foramen　19
manubrium（sternum）　85〜87,93
marginal air cells　33
marginal artery　289
mastoid air cells　7,29〜33
mastoid antrum　31〜37
mastoid process　3
maxilla　3,9,16〜17,21〜25
　　alveolar process　9
maxillary sinus　3〜5,9〜17,21〜23,27〜31,41
　　alveolar recess　9,23
　　zygomatic recess　27
medial condyle（femur）　147,159〜177
medial cuneiform　181〜183,187〜189,197〜203
medial epicondyle（femur）　159,163,167
medial epicondyle（humerus）　113,117〜125
median antebrachial vein　335
median sacral crest　75〜81
medial malleolus　147,175〜187,195〜197
mediastinum　214
medullary cone　341〜343
meningeal artery, middle, groove of　5
meniscus
　　knee　277
　　wrist　269〜271
mental foramen　19〜23
mental protuberance　3,19〜21
mesenteric vein　307,311
metacarpal　129〜145
metacarpophalangeal joint　129〜131,143〜145
metatarsal　181〜183,187〜191,195〜205
metatarsophalangeal joint　187〜189,201〜203,205
middle cerebral artery　281〜283
middle cronial fossa　29
middle meningeal artery, groove of　5
mitral valve　211〜213
molar teeth　21〜23
myelography　341〜349
　　lumbar　345〜349
　　thoracic　340〜343

N

nasal bones　3〜5,9,25
nasal cartilage　25
nasal cavities　11,21,31
nasal septum　3,9〜13,17,29〜31,41
nasal sinuses　8〜11
nasal spine, anterior　17,25
nasal turbinates　41
nasomaxillary suture　25
nasopharynx　5,231
navicular　181〜191,197〜203
nerve root, spinal　345
nerve root sheath　341,345,349
nipple　225,227,367
nose　24〜25
　　vestibule　25

O

obturator foramen　61,67〜71,147〜153,157
　　Shenton's line　63
obturator internus muscle　61,223
occipital artery　289,291
occipital bone　7,45
occipital crest　7
　　internal　35
occipital protuberance
　　external　7
　　internal　7,35
occipital sinus　287
occipital veins　287
occiput　3
odontoid process　47〜49
olecranon　113,127
olecranon fossa　113〜119,123〜127
ophthalmic artery　281〜283
optic canal　15
oral cavity　231
orbit　3,9〜17,29〜31,39〜41
　　floor　13,17
　　lateral wall　11〜15
　　medial wall　41
　　roof　3,11〜15,31,39
orbital artery, frontal　281〜283
orbital fissure, superior　13〜15
orbital plate　13,41
oropharynx　243
os frontale　4
os intermetatarseum　187
os occipitale　4

os parietale 4
os peroneum 187
os sphenoidale 4
os supratalare 187
os temporale 4
os tibiale externum 187
os trigonum 191
os vesalianum 187
os zygomaticum 4
osseous hemithorax 82〜83
osseous labyrinth 37
osseous sinus, wall 37
outer ear 33

P

Paccionian granulations 3
pancreatic duct 369
pancreaticoduodenal artery
  inferior 305,309
  superior 305
pantomogram, facial/jaw bones 22〜23
papilla of Vater 251,369
para-aortic lymph nodes 355
paraaortic stripe 209
paracentral artery 282
paraspinal stripe 209
paratracheal stripe (right) 209
paravertebral line 51
parietal artery
  anterior/posterior 281〜282
  internal, inferior/superior 282
parietal bone 5
parietal vein 285〜287
parieto-occipital artery 289〜291
parotid duct 361〜363
parotid gland 361〜363
  accessory 361
patella 147,159〜173
  multipartite 172
  Wilberg's shape classification 172
patellar ligament 165
patellofemoral joint 161,173
pedicle
  cervical spine 45,49
  lumbar spine 43,55,59
  sacral spine 237
  thoracic spine 51
pelvic region 60〜81
pelvis 60〜71
  aortic angiogram 316〜317
  child 62〜63

perforating artery 319
periantral air cells 33,37
pericallosal artery 281〜282
Perkin's line 63
peroneal artery 321〜323
peroneal trochlea 193
peroneal veins 337
peroneus longus tendon, groove for 193
petrosal sinus
  inferior 285〜287,293〜295
  superior 287,293〜295
petrosal vein 293
petrous bone 7,32〜37
petrous pyramid 35
petrous ridge 3,9〜13,31,39
phalanx
  finger
    distal 129,145
    middle 129,145
    proximal 129〜135,143〜145
  toe
    distal 187〜189,201〜205
    middle 187〜189,201〜205
    proximal 187〜189,201〜205
pharynx 241
piriform recess 229〜231,241〜245
pisiform 124〜129,133〜143
pituitary fossa 5,39〜41
plantar aponeurosis 191
plantar artery 325
plexus, pterygoid 287
polar artery
  frontal 281〜282
  temporal 281
popliteal artery 321
popliteal bursa 277
popliteal fossa 161
popliteal vein 337
portal vein 307,311
posterior arch (atlas) 7,47
posterior column (ischium) 69〜71,149〜151
posterior cerebral artery 289〜291
posterior tibial artery 321〜325
prefrontal arteries 281〜283
premolar teeth 21〜23
preperitoneal fat 223
promontory (acetabulum) 61〜63,149
promontory (sacrum) 57,67,77,237
promontory lymph nodes 351〜355
psoas muscle 55,221〜223,265
pterygoid fossa 29
pterygoid plexus 287

pterygoid process 23
pterygopalatine fossa 23,29
pubis 147〜157
   anterior column 69〜71,149〜153
   child 63
pubic ramus
   inferior 61,65〜67,71,151
   superior 61,65〜67,75,79,149〜151
pubic symphysis 61,65〜67,79
puborectalis muscle 263
pulmonary artery
   arteriography 300〜303
   left 211,217〜219,301,327
   lingular branch 301
   main 211〜213,217
   right 211,219〜233,235,301,327
   trunk 301
pulmonary hilum tomogram 232〜233
pulmonary trunk 327
pulmonary valve 211〜213
pulmonary vein 213,217〜219,233,303
pulp cavity 19,23
pyloric antrum 249〜253
pylorus 249〜251

R

radial veins 335
radiocarpal joint 125〜127,133,143
radioulnar joint
   distal 125,129,133
   proximal 117,123〜125
radius 113〜135,139〜143,271,335
   head 113〜127
   neck 117,123〜127
   styloid process 125,129〜135,139,143
   tuberosity 119,123〜125
rectal fold, transverse 261
rectosigmoid junction 261
rectum 81,259〜263
   ampulla 261〜263
renal artery 313〜315
renal veins 315,329〜331
retrocardiac space 213
retrofacial air cells 33
retropharyngeal space 231
retrorectal space 261
retrosinus air cells 37
retrosternal space 87,213
ribs 43,49,59,97,101
   first 45,51
   head 51〜53,83

ribs（続き）
   neck 51,83
   twelfth 265
right atrium 211,217〜303,327
right ventricle 211〜213,219,301,327
rima glottidis 229
root canal 19,23
root of the tooth 23
Rosenthal, basal vein of − 285〜287,295
routine radiography 208〜223

S

sacral ala 65,75,237
sacral canal 77,81
sacral crest
   lateral 75,79〜81
   median 75〜81
sacral foramina 55,73〜75,79,237
sacral hiatus 75,79
sacroiliac joint 43,55,61,69〜73,149〜155,237
sacrum 43,55〜57,61,65〜69,73〜81,149,
   221〜223,237,261,345
   ala 65,75,237
   cornu 75〜79,81
   lateral part 73
   promontory 57,67,77,237
sagittal sinus 285〜287
saphenous veins, great/small 337
scaphoid 124〜143
scapula 53,83,89〜91,95〜107,111〜115,243,
   273〜275
   coracoid process 83,89〜97,101〜111,115,
      273〜275
   glenoid fossa 89〜91,95,101〜103,107,111,
      115
   glenoid labrum 103,273〜275
   glenoid process 89
   inferior angle 83,99,101
   lateral process (neck) 97,107,113
   neck 107
   spine 89〜91,97,101〜105
   superior angle 89〜91,97〜107
sciatic notch
   greater 67,75〜77,81
   lesser 77
secondary cuboid 187
sella turcica 38〜41
sellae, dorsum/tuberculum 39
semicircular canals 7,29〜31,35
sesamoid bones
   foot 187〜189,201〜205

sesamoid bones（続き）
　hand　129〜131,143
Shenton's line　63
shoulder　89,101〜111
　arthrography　273〜275
　axillary recess　273〜275
　glenoid labrum　103,273〜275
sialography　360〜363
sigmoid colon　259
sigmoid sinus　33,37,285〜287,293〜295
sinus tarsi→tarsal sinusを参照
skin, breast　225〜227,367
skull　2〜41
skull base　17,28〜29,47,231
small bowel　221,252〜255
soft palate　5
sphenoid bone　3,5,9〜15,29,39〜41
　greater wing　5,9,13,39
　lesser wing　13〜15
　pituitary fossa　5,39〜41
　pterygoid fossa　29
sphenoid sinus　5,9,15,29,39
sphenoparietal sinus　285
sphenopetrosal fissure　35
sphenosquamous suture　35
spinal cord　341〜343
spinal lamina　47,59
spinal nerve root　345
spine　42〜59
　cervical　44〜49,89,243
　lumbar　43,54〜59
　myelogram
　　lumbar　344〜349
　　thoracic　340〜343
　thoracic　43,50〜53
spinous processes（vertebrae）
　cervical spine　45〜49
　lumbar spine　43,55〜59,75,237
　thoracic spine　51〜53
spleen　221〜223,307
splenic artery　305,313
splenic vein　307,311
squamous air cells　33
Stensen's duct　361〜363
sternal angle　85〜87,213
sternal notch　85
sternoclavicular joint　85,93
sternum　85〜87,93,213,219
　body　85〜87,213
　manubrium　85〜87,93
stomach　246〜253
　angular notch　249

stomach（続き）
　body　249,253
　fundus　249
　greater curvature　249
　lesser curvature　249
　pyloric antrum　249〜253
straight sinus　287,293〜295
subarachnoid space　341〜345
subarcuate fossa　35
subclavian artery　211,297〜299
subclavian vein　327,333
subcutaneous tissue, breast　367
subglottic space　229〜231
subphrenic space　221
subscapula bursa　273〜275
subtalar joint　177,183〜185,191,199
sulcul artery, precentral　281
sulcus of the transverse sinus　7
superior anastomotic vein　285〜287
superior mesenteric artery　305,309
superior mesenteric vein　307,311
superior orbital fissure　13〜15
seperior petrosal sinus　287,293〜295
seperior saggittal sinus　285〜287
seperior vena cava　211,233,301,327,333
supracalcaneal recess　279
supraduodenal artery, superior　305
suprascapular artery　297
suprascapular notch　105
supraspinatus fossa　101
surgical neck（humerus）　103〜105,111〜113
sustentaculum tali　191〜193

T

talocalcaneal joint　183〜185
talocalcaneonavicular joint　189,199〜203
talocrural joint　183〜185,195
talonavicular joint　181
talus　147,175〜177,181〜199,279
　arthrogram　279
　head　181,187,197
　lateral process　181,191
　neck　181
　posterior process　181,189〜191
　trochlea　147,177,181
terminal ileum　257
tarsal joints, transverse　187,203
tarsal sinus　181,191,199
tarsometatarsal joints　187〜189,199,203〜205
teeth　19〜23
temporomandibular joint　7,19〜21

temporomandibular joint fossa 33
temporal artery, posterior 281〜282
temporal bone 5,15,21〜23,27,33〜35
　petrous portion 5,15
　styloid process 23,33
　subarcuate fossa 35
　zygomatic process 27,33
temporal fossa 27
temporo-occipital artery 289〜291
temporozygomatic suture 27
tendon recess(ankle) 279
tendon sheath of long head, biceps muscle 273〜275
terminal line 149
thalamoperforate arteries 289
thalamostriate vein, superior 285〜287
thigh 158〜161,318〜319
thoracic artery, internal 297
thoracic spine 43,50〜53
　intervertebral disk space 53
　intervertebral foramen 53
　myelography 340〜343
thoracic vertebrae 43,214
thyrocervical trunk 297〜299
thyroid artery, inferior/superior 297
thyroid cartilage 229〜231
thyroid vein, inferior 327
tibia 147,159〜171,175〜185,189,195,279
　fibular notch 179
　intercondylar eminence 147,159〜171,175〜177
　　lateral tubercle 159,163,167,175
　　medial tubercle 159,163,167,175
　lateral condyle 147,159,163,169〜171,175〜177
　medial condyle 147,159,163,169〜171,175〜177
　medial melleolus 147,175〜187,195〜197
　plateau 165〜167
　tuberosity 165〜167,175
tibial arteries
　anterior 321〜325
　muscular branch 323
　posterior 321〜325
tibial plateau 165〜167
tibial tuberosity 165〜167,175
tibial veins, anterior/posterior 337
tibiofibular joint 161,169,279
toe, great 204〜205
　distal interphalangeal joint 187
　distal phalanx 187
tongue 9,23,243

tooth→teethを参照
trachea 21,47,51,229〜235,243
　bifurcation 233
　carina 209,219
transverse colon 221,259
transverse processes(vertebrae)
　cervical spine 45〜49
　lumbar spine 55,59,73〜75,79,83,237
　thoracic spine 45,51〜53
transverse sinus 7,285〜287,293〜295
transverse tarsal joints 187,203
trapezium 129〜143
trapezoid 129〜143
triangular fibrocartilage(wrist) 269
tricuspid valve 211〜213
triquetrum 125〜127
triquetrum 129〜143
triradiate cartilage line 63
trochanter
　greater 61,69,147〜157
　lesser 61,71,149〜157
trochlea
　humerus 113〜117,121〜127
　peroneal 193
　talus 147,177,181
Trolard, vein of 285〜287
tuberculum sellae 39
turbinate 13
tympanic cavity 31,35〜37

U

ulna 113〜133,139,271,335
　coronoid process 115〜119,123〜127
　olecranon 113〜127
　styloid process 125〜141,271
ulnar recess(wrist) 269〜271
ulnar veins 335
uncinate process, cervical vertebrae 45
uncovertebral joint 45
upper extremeties 82〜145
　→arm；hand；shoulder；wristも参照
ureter 265
urinary bladder 61,221〜223,265
urography 264〜265
uterine ostium(fallopian tube) 365
uterus 365
uvula 243〜245

V

vagina 365

vallecula 229〜231,241〜243
Vater
　ampulla of − 249〜253
　papilla of − 251,369
vena cava
　inferior 211〜213,217〜219,301,329〜331,337
　superior 211,233,301,327,333
venography 326〜337
　axilla 332〜333
　forearm 334〜335
　inferior vena cava 328〜331
　leg, lower 336〜337
　superior vena cava 326〜327
venous angle 327
venous confluence 211,233
ventricle
　larynx 229,243
　left 211〜213,217〜219
　right 211〜213,219,301,327
vermis, inferior vein of 293
vertebrae
　articular pillar 47
　articular processes
　　cervical 45〜49
　　lumbar 55〜59,75
　　sacral 75,237
　　thoracic 51〜53
　body
　　cervical 49
　　lumbar 55,59,73
　　thoracic 51〜53
　cervical − →cervical vertebraeを参照
　end plate 47,53〜57
　interarticular part 59
　lamina 237
　lumbar − →lumbar vertebraeを参照
　odontoid process 47〜49
　pedicle
　　cervical 45,49
　　lumbar 43,55,59,73
　　sacral 237
　　thoracic 51
　spinous processes 43〜59,75,237
　　cervical 45〜49
　　lumbar 43,55〜59
　　thoracic 51〜53

vertebrae（続き）
　thoracic − 43,214
　transverse process 45〜59,73〜75,79,83,237
　　cervical 45〜49
　　lumbar 55〜59
　　thoracic 45,51〜53
　uncinate process 45
vertebral arch 45
vertebral arteries 289〜291,297〜299
vestibular fold 229
vestibule
　auditory 31,35
　larynx 229〜231
vocal chord
　false 229
　true 229
vocal fold 229

W

Wilberg's center-to-corner angle 63
Wiberg's classification of patellar shapes 172
wrist 125〜135
　arthrography 268〜271
　meniscus 269〜271
　recesses
　　extensor 269〜271
　　flexor 269〜271
　　sacciform 269
　　ulnar 269〜271
　triangular fibrocartilage 269

X

xiphoid process 85,87

Z

zygomatic arch 3,13〜15,26〜27,31
zygomatic bone 5,9〜13,29,37
　frontal process 13
zygomatic process（temporal bone） 5,27,33
zygomatic recess（maxillary sinus） 27

X線画像解剖ポケットアトラス
　　　　　　　　第3版　　定価(本体3,800円＋税)

1995年 4月10日発行　　第1版第1刷
2000年 1月25日発行　　第2版第1刷
2011年 2月25日発行　　第3版第1刷Ⓒ

著　者　トルステン B. メーラー
　　　　エミール レイフ

監訳者　町田　徹
　　　　（まちだ　とおる）

発行者　株式会社 メディカル・サイエンス・インターナショナル
　　　　代表取締役　若松　博
　　　　東京都文京区本郷1-28-36
　　　　郵便番号113-0033　電話(03)5804-6050

　　　　　　　　　　　印刷：三報社印刷/表紙装丁：デザインコンビビア

ISBN 978-4-89592-664-5　　C 3047

JCOPY 〈(社)出版者著作権管理機構　委託出版物〉
本書の無断複写は著作権法上での例外を除き禁じられています．
複写される場合は，そのつど事前に，(社)出版者著作権管理機構
（電話 03-3513-6969，FAX 03-3513-6979，info@jcopy.or.jp）の
許諾を得てください．